MCAT Biology

Content Review

blueprint

2nd Edition Acknowledgments
Reviewers: Elizabeth Flagge and Mackenzie Perkins
Editors: Paul Forn, Michael Leung, Brian McGrew, and Elizabeth Serbia PhD
Copywriters: Aislinn McCormack, Zoe Mikel-Stites, and Emily Soto
Cover Design: Becca Roth and Lona Hill

Special thanks to all of the writers, editors, and reviewers involved in prior editions.

Printed in the United States of America

First Printing, 2022

ISBN 978-1-944935-35-1

Blueprint Education Subsidiary Holdings LLC
6080 Center Drive
Suite 520
Los Angeles, CA 90045

Second Edition

This page left intentionally blank.

Group→ 1 2 3 4 5 6 7 8 9 10 11 12 13 14 15 16 17 18
↓Period

Group→	1	2	3	4	5	6	7	8	9	10	11	12	13	14	15	16	17	18
1	1 H																	2 He
2	3 Li	4 Be											5 B	6 C	7 N	8 O	9 F	10 Ne
3	11 Na	12 Mg											13 Al	14 Si	15 P	16 S	17 Cl	18 Ar
4	19 K	20 Ca	21 Sc	22 Ti	23 V	24 Cr	25 Mn	26 Fe	27 Co	28 Ni	29 Cu	30 Zn	31 Ga	32 Ge	33 As	34 Se	35 Br	36 Kr
5	37 Rb	38 Sr	39 Y	40 Zr	41 Nb	42 Mo	43 Tc	44 Ru	45 Rh	46 Pd	47 Ag	48 Cd	49 In	50 Sn	51 Sb	52 Te	53 I	54 Xe
6	55 Cs	56 Ba	57 La	72 Hf	73 Ta	74 W	75 Re	76 Os	77 Ir	78 Pt	79 Au	80 Hg	81 Tl	82 Pb	83 Bi	84 Po	85 At	86 Rn
7	87 Fr	88 Ra	89 Ac	104 Rf	105 Db	106 Sg	107 Bh	108 Hs	109 Mt	110 Ds	111 Rg	112 Cn	113 Nh	114 Fl	115 Mc	116 Lv	117 Ts	118 Og

*	58 Ce	59 Pr	60 Nd	61 Pm	62 Sm	63 Eu	64 Gd	65 Tb	66 Dy	67 Ho	68 Er	69 Tm	70 Yb	71 Lu
**	90 Th	91 Pa	92 U	93 Np	94 Pu	95 Am	96 Cm	97 Bk	98 Cf	99 Es	100 Fm	101 Md	102 No	103 Lr

STOP! READ ME FIRST!

Welcome and congratulations on taking this important step in your MCAT prep process!

The book you're holding is one of Blueprint's six MCAT review books, and contains concise content review with a specific focus on the science that you need for MCAT success. To get the most out of this book, we'd like to draw your attention to some distinctive aspects of our book set and their role in MCAT prep.

First and foremost, **books are not enough** for MCAT prep. Realistic practice is absolutely essential, and should include both MCAT-targeted practice questions and an ample number of full-length practice exams that simulate the MCAT itself.

Second, **our books reflect our experience**. Our book editing team is made up of a combination of people: they represent people who have been in your shoes and have excelled on the MCAT, people who are truly experts in the field of Biology, and people who are experienced tutors and instructors with a focus on MCAT prep (not to mention a few skilled copywriters and communicators to keep us on our toes!). This makes our books unlike many other MCAT review products, which provide a dry, factual overview of scientific knowledge without MCAT-specific context. Instead, our books recognize that the **MCAT is primarily a test of thinking**—and more specifically, a test that reflects how the American Association of Medical Colleges encourages future physicians to think. The "MCAT Strategy" sidebars throughout the book call out specific points to be aware of as you study, and in general, our approach to presenting science is informed by how science is tested on the MCAT—that is, in a way that draws upon passages, builds connections across subject areas, and prioritizes an understanding of fundamental principles. In a nutshell, it's our hope that by studying with these books, you can benefit from our team's unparalleled MCAT expertise.

Third, after completing a chapter, we urge you to test your knowledge with all of the online practice materials that were included with your Blueprint course: our Learning Modules, Qbank, End of Chapter Quizzes, and of course our Practice Tests.

We wish you the best of luck on your MCAT journey,

The Blueprint MCAT Team

This page left intentionally blank.

TABLE OF CONTENTS

This page left intentionally blank.

Biomolecules: A High-Level Overview

0. Introduction

Molecules are the building blocks of life, and in order to understand the function of biological systems it is crucial to have a high-level understanding of the major types of biomolecules. The goal of this chapter is to focus on how major biomolecules contribute to biological processes and to provide the background information necessary for understanding the topics covered in the rest of this volume. More comprehensive information, with a focus on the underlying chemistry, is provided in the Biochemistry textbook.

1. Polarity and Functional Groups

Polarity is perhaps the single most important chemical concept for the MCAT, because it reappears at conceptual levels ranging from the very small-scale (atomic structure) to the very large-scale (physiology). The MCAT loves to test you on small-scale ways of understanding large-scale systems and on the large-scale implications of small-scale changes.

Polarity describes the **distribution of charge** within a molecule as mediated by electrons. In **nonpolar molecules**, electrons are distributed fairly evenly, although transient and induced dipoles may be present. In **polar molecules**, however, one or more electronegative atoms attract electrons, creating areas of higher electron density (with a partial negative charge, indicated using the symbol δ^-) or lower electron density (with a partial positive charge, indicated as δ^+). Taking polarity to the next level, **charged molecules** have one or more full positive or negative charges. Recall that like charges repel each other and opposite charges attract; this means that molecules with partial or full charges will interact with each other more intensely. As we will see, this simple principle has tremendous ramifications, and can be used as a lens through which to analyze many physiological processes.

The concept of a **functional group** is a useful way to explain the reactivity and chemical/physical properties of classes of molecules. A functional group is a specific group of atoms that contribute in a predictable way to the behavior of a molecule. As shown in Figure 1, you can arrange functional groups on a spectrum of polarity. Here, "polarity"

> **>> CONNECTIONS <<**
>
> Chapter 2 of Chemistry

is used very broadly, encompassing the presence of permanent dipoles, the ability to engage in hydrogen bonding, and the presence of charges.

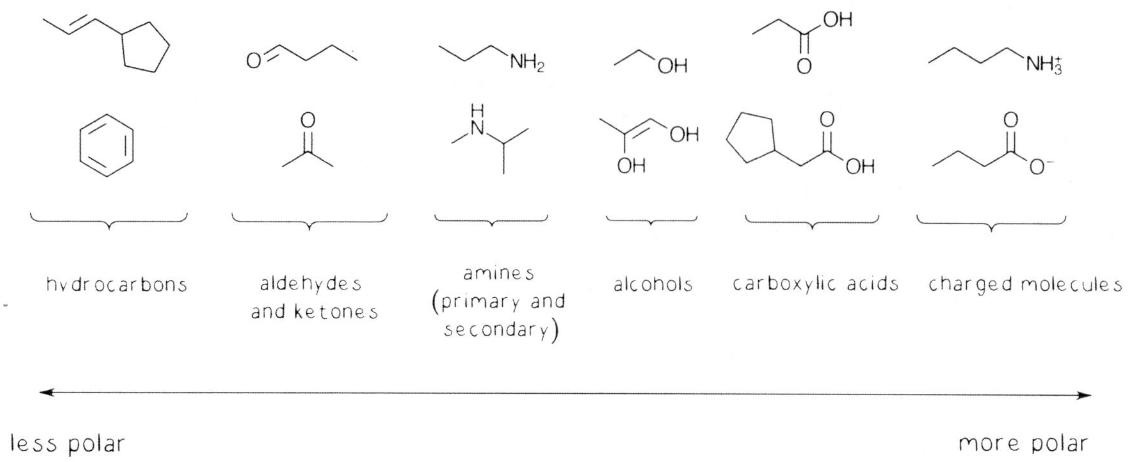

Figure 1. Functional groups and polarity (including charged groups)

What happens if a molecule has more than one functional group? Essentially, you have to make a qualitative assessment of the molecule as a whole. On the MCAT, you will often need to make a snap judgment about whether a molecule is polar or nonpolar, even though polarity is more properly thought of as a spectrum. Essentially, you have to use your judgment. Many "nonpolar" biological molecules do have some degree of polarity, but the polar functional groups are outweighed by much larger nonpolar structures. This is shown below in Figure 2, which illustrates some **steroids**, a large class of nonpolar hormones derived from cholesterol.

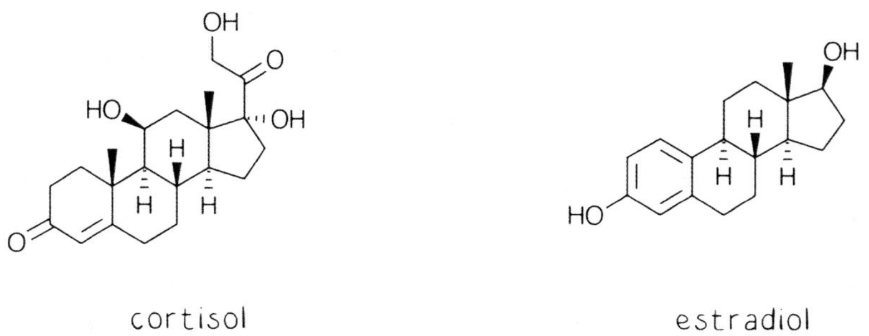

cortisol

estradiol

Figure 2. Nonpolar steroids

Additionally, **amphipathic molecules** exhibit significant polar and nonpolar properties localized to different parts of the molecules. A common example of amphipathic molecules are **fatty acids**, which have a polar head and a nonpolar tail.

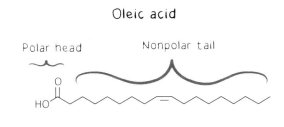

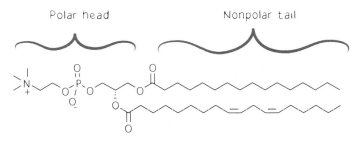

Figure 3. Amphipathic molecules

When determining whether a molecule is polar or nonpolar, be sure to take its **molecular geometry** into account. A molecule can have polar bonds but be nonpolar if those polar bonds are arranged such that the dipoles cancel each other out. Two famous examples of this are carbon tetrachloride (CCl_4) and carbon dioxide (CO_2). Such molecules may occur as trap answers to questions about polarity, so be on the lookout!

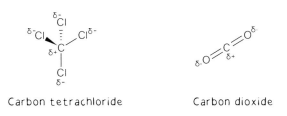

Figure 4. Nonpolar molecules with polar bonds

Polarity is also often discussed in terms of **solubility**. Based on the principle that "like dissolves like," polar molecules are typically soluble in polar solvents (the most well-known of which is water), while nonpolar molecules are soluble in nonpolar solvents. In an organic chemistry lab, nonpolar solvents include compounds like hexane that are toxic physiologically. As such, in a biological context it often makes more sense to think of polar molecules as "liking" aqueous solutions and of nonpolar molecules as "liking" lipid-rich environments, since lipids are one of the most common nonpolar environments that can be found in the body. Thus, polar molecules can be described as **water-soluble**, **hydrophilic**, or **lipophobic** (although "lipophobic" is not commonly encountered). Nonpolar molecules can be described as **non-water-soluble**, **hydrophobic**, or **lipophilic**. For the purposes of the MCAT, these terms are essentially synonyms.

MCAT STRATEGY >>>

Recall that solubility is just a special case of intermolecular interactions. The MCAT could also ask you about which structures are likely to interact with each other in a more specialized environment, such as membrane receptors. The same basic principle applies: like interacts with like, and positive charges interact with negative charges.

Table 1 summarizes the key properties of polar/nonpolar compounds.

Nonpolar ↕ Polar	Examples	Major intermolecular forces	Soluble in water?	Lipophilic?
	Hydrocarbons (alkanes, alkenes, alkynes)	London dispersion forces	N	Y
	Aldehydes and ketones	Dipole-dipole forces	Y	N
	Amines	Dipole-dipole forces, hydrogen bonding (not tertiary amines)	Y	N
	Alcohols	Dipole-dipole forces, hydrogen bonding	Y	N
	Carboxylic acids	Dipole-dipole forces, hydrogen bonding	Y	N
	Charged compounds	Ionic interactions are intramolecular ion-dipole interactions	Y	N

Table 1. Key properties of polar and non-polar compounds

2. Amino Acids and Proteins

Proteins are the building blocks of life, and **amino acids** are the building blocks of proteins. Amino acids are called amino acids because they have an **amine (–NH₂)** functional group and a **carboxylic acid (–COOH)** functional group. Although "amino acid" is a general chemical term that applies to many structures, in the context of the MCAT it refers to the 20 amino acids that are coded for by specific codons and are used in the body to build proteins. Amino acids have a structure characterized by a central carbon to which the following substituents are attached: –NH₂, –COOH, –H, and –R. The –R group is termed the **side chain** of the amino acid, this is where most of the interactions occur; that is, the properties of the side chain are what contributes to the function of the protein or peptide sequence that contain a given amino acid.

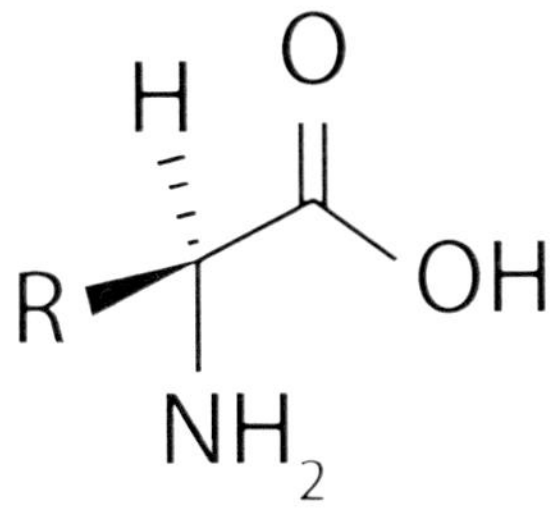

Figure 5. Generic amino acid structure

There are multiple ways that side chains can be classified, and some of them intersect with each other. Probably the simplest classification is into **nonpolar, polar uncharged, negatively charged** (at physiological pH), and **positively charged** (at physiological pH). This classification is illustrated in Table 2, along with the three-letter and one-letter abbreviations for each amino acid, which are essential to memorize for the MCAT. Table 2 also presents subcategories of amino acids, such as **aromatic amino acids, sulfur-containing amino acids,** and **special cases,** and contains information about the pKₐ values and pI values of the amino acids, which are discussed more in Chapter 2 of the Biochemistry textbook.

	Name	Side chain	pK$_a$ values pK$_{a1}$ = COOH pK$_{a2}$ = NH$_2$ pK$_{aR}$ = R	pI
Nonpolar	Glycine (Gly, G)	—H	pK$_{a1}$ = 2.34 pK$_{a2}$ = 9.58	5.97
	Alanine (Ala, A)		pK$_{a1}$ = 2.33 pK$_{a2}$ = 9.71	6.00
	Valine (Val, V)		pK$_{a1}$ = 2.27 pK$_{a2}$ = 9.52	5.96
	Isoleucine (Ile, I)		pK$_{a1}$ = 2.26 pK$_{a2}$ = 9.60	6.02
	Leucine (Leu, L)		pK$_{a1}$ = 2.32 pK$_{a2}$ = 9.58	5.98
	Methionine (Met, M)		pK$_{a1}$ = 2.16 pK$_{a2}$ = 9.08	5.74
	Proline (Pro, P)		pK$_{a1}$ = 1.95 pK$_{a2}$ = 10.47	6.30
	Phenylalanine (Phe, F)		pK$_{a1}$ = 2.18 pK$_{a2}$ = 9.09	5.48
	Tyrosine* (Tyr, Y)		pK$_{a1}$ = 2.24 pK$_{a2}$ = 9.04 pK$_{aR}$ = 10.10	5.66
	Tryptophan (Trp, W)		pK$_{a1}$ = 2.38 pK$_{a2}$ = 9.34	5.89
	Cysteine (Cys, C)		pK$_{a1}$ = 1.91 pK$_{aR}$ = 8.14 pK$_{a2}$ = 10.28	5.07

*Polarity is a spectrum. Tyrosine, while relatively nonpolar, will still show more polar characteristics than an amino acid with no polar elements in its sidechain.

Polar uncharged	Serine (Ser, S)	(structure)	$pK_{a1} = 2.13$ $pK_{a2} = 9.05$	5.68
	Threonine (Thr, T)	(structure)	$pK_{a1} = 2.20$ $pK_{a2} = 8.96$	5.60
	Asparagine (Asn, N)	(structure)	$pK_{a1} = 2.16$ $pK_{a2} = 8.76$	5.41
	Glutamine (Gln, Q)	(structure)	$pK_{a1} = 2.18$ $pK_{a2} = 9.00$	5.65
Positively charged (basic)	Arginine (Arg, R)	(structure)	$pK_{a1} = 2.03$ $pK_{a2} = 9.00$ $pK_{aR} = 12.10$	10.76
	Histidine (His, H)	(structure)	$pK_{a1} = 1.70$ $pK_{aR} = 6.04$ $pK_{a2} = 9.09$	7.59
	Lysine (Lys, K)	(structure)	$pK_{a1} = 2.15$ $pK_{a2} = 9.16$ $pK_{aR} = 10.67$	9.74
Negatively charged (acidic)	Aspartic acid (aspartate) (Asp, D)	(structure)	$pK_{a1} = 1.95$ $pK_{aR} = 3.71$ $pK_{a2} = 9.66$	2.77
	Glutamic acid (glutamate) (Glu, E)	(structure)	$pK_{a1} = 2.16$ $pK_{aR} = 4.15$ $pK_{a2} = 9.58$	3.22

Special cases	
Achiral: Gly	Sulfur-containing: Cys, Met
Aromatic: Phe, Tyr, Trp	Breaks up secondary structure: Pro, Gly

Table 2. Amino acid structures and properties

One complication to be aware of is that amino acids with polar side chains can show hydrophobic behavior. This may seem paradoxical, but recall from Section 1 that hydrophobicity/hydrophilicity is determined on the level of the molecule as a whole, and a molecule that is predominantly nonpolar can still behave in a hydrophobic manner even if it has one or more polar functional groups (see, for example, the steroid molecules in Figure 2).

The side chain of tyrosine has a polar –OH group, and the polar –OH group is attached to a bulky aromatic nonpolar benzyl group. The hydroxyl (-OH) group contributes to the molecule's polarity and is the site for covalent modifications such as phosphorylation.

Interestingly, for cysteine, the S-H bond only has an electronegativity difference of 0.38, but it is considered to be polar for the purposes of amino acid classifications because it can participate in hydrogen bonding.

In addition to this high-level classification, there are some special cases you should be aware of:

>> CONNECTIONS <<

Chapter 2 of Biochemistry

> Glycine is the only **achiral amino acid** because its central carbon is bonded to two hydrogens (one corresponding to the R group of glycine and one that is part of the general structure of amino acids). Because Glycine has the smallest side chain of all the amino acids, it is very flexible and tends to disrupt alpha-helices and beta-sheets, which form the secondary structures of a protein.
> Cysteine and methionine contain sulfur.
> Cysteine residues form disulfide bridges (2 RS–H → RS–SR), resulting in cystine. Disulfide bridges form a crucial part of tertiary structure.
> Tyrosine, phenylalanine, and tryptophan are the **aromatic amino acids**.
> Proline is unique because its side chain binds to the nitrogen of its own amine. This locks it in place and creates so-called **proline kinks** that often disrupt the alpha-helices and beta-sheets, which form the secondary structures of a protein.
> Arginine, lysine, and histidine are **basic amino acids**, while aspartic acid and glutamic acid are **acidic amino acids**. The conjugate bases of aspartic acid and glutamic acid, which are known as aspartate and glutamate, predominate at physiological pH.
> Histidine is often classified as a positively-charged amino acid, although it is not generally positively charged at physiological pH (the pK_a of the side chain NH is 6.04, which means that it *can* serve as a buffer at pH levels slightly more acidic than physiological pH, but the deprotonated, non-charged form is prevalent at physiological pH).

MCAT STRATEGY >>>

Part of why you have to know the above facts inside and out is that the MCAT is likely not just to test you on them directly, but to require you to apply this information in a new context, such as assessing how a mutation might affect the charge and/ or binding properties of an amino acid chain. You can't answer a question like that effectively under time pressure if, for instance, you're struggling to remember how acidity and charge interact and which amino acid beginning with "g" is charged. Think of these facts as crucial additions to your conceptual toolkit, which you can deploy to solve problems.

Amino acids are joined together through **peptide bonds**, in which the –COOH group of one amino acid binds with the –NH$_2$ group of another, releasing water. Peptide bonds have important biochemical properties that are discussed in Chapter 2 of the Biochemistry volume. Sequences of two amino acids are called **dipeptides**, and sequences of three amino acids are called **tripeptides**. The term "**oligopeptide**" is used as a catch-all term to refer to sequences of relatively few amino acid residues (generally

2-20), while **polypeptides** contain more than 20. Peptide chains have an N-terminus (the terminal $-NH_2$ group) and a C-terminus (the terminal $-COOH$ group), and are conventionally written from the N-terminus to the C-terminus, which also corresponds to the order that they are synthesized in.

Proteins are biologically relevant molecules that are made up of one or more long amino acid chain. They have up to four levels of structure, which are essential to know for the MCAT:

>>CONNECTIONS<<

Chapter 2 of Biochemistry

> **Primary structure** is defined as the sequence of amino acids itself.
> **Secondary structure** is formed by hydrogen-bonding interactions between the carboxyl and amine components of the amino acid backbone—that is, *not* the side chains. Two common types of secondary structure are alpha-helices and beta-sheets.
> **Tertiary structure** is defined by side-chain interactions, including:
  - Hydrophobic interactions between side chains.
  - Hydrogen bonding between side chains.
  - Salt bridges formed by interactions between charged side chains.
  - Disulfide bonding between cysteine residues.
> **Quaternary structure** is formed by interactions between polypeptide chains.
  - Typically involves interactions between protein subunits.

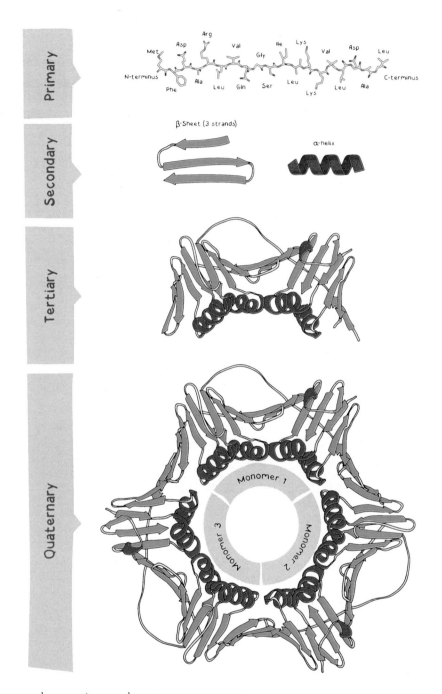

Figure 6. Primary, secondary, tertiary, and quaternary structure

All proteins have primary, secondary, and tertiary structure, but not all proteins have quaternary structure. In general, predicting the secondary and especially the tertiary structures of proteins is computationally challenging. These levels of structure reflect protein folding that maximizes entropy, but it is very difficult to predict exactly what the optimal outcome can be. A tremendous amount of computational resources has been dedicated to protein folding simulations because it is a fundamentally important question for drug design and many other aspects of medical research, and it is an area of ongoing research.

Polarity is the driving force that determines how proteins interact with their surroundings. Nonpolar amino acid residues "like" to interact with other nonpolar substances, while polar and charged amino acid residues "like" to interact with other polar substances. The MCAT can test this principle in many ways, with some common contexts provided below:

> In aqueous solution (which corresponds to the majority of the human body), nonpolar amino acids tend to be part of the **internal core** of a protein's three-dimensional structure, while polar and charged amino acid residues tend to be on the outside.
> **Transmembrane proteins** cross through the lipid bilayer plasma membrane of cells and have three domains: an extracellular domain (facing the outside of the cell), an intracellular domain (facing the cytosol), and a transmembrane domain that spans the plasma membrane. The extracellular and intracellular domains interact with aqueous solution and are therefore largely composed of hydrophilic amino acid residues, while the transmembrane domain is dominated by hydrophobic residues because it crosses through the nonpolar layer of the lipid membrane.
> Proteins interact with other molecules at specialized areas known as **binding sites**. Altering the binding site by replacing one amino acid with another that has similar characteristics in polarity and charge is unlikely to significantly affect the behavior of the protein, whereas replacing one amino acid residue with another one that has different polarity/charge properties is likely to significantly disrupt the behavior.

> **CONNECTIONS** <<

Chapter 3 of Biochemistry

Although proteins are also thought of primarily in terms of structure, they also play a major role in signaling, most notably in peptide hormones and in intracellular signaling pathways. Another crucial role of proteins is that they serve as enzymes, or biological catalysts. The enzymatic function of proteins is essential in regulating the reactions necessary for life.

3. Lipids

Lipids are hydrophobic, and have a diverse range of structural functions in the body, contributing to energy storage, structure, and signaling. For the MCAT, you should be aware of four main classes of lipids: (1) fatty acids and derivatives; (2) cholesterol and its derivatives, such as steroid hormones; (3) eicosanoids, including prostaglandins; and (4) terpenes and terpenoids.

Fatty acids are relatively long-chain carboxylic acids. Short-chain fatty acids are defined as those with five or fewer carbons on the chain, medium-chain fatty acids have six to 12 carbons, long-chain fatty acids have 13 to 21 carbons in their tail, and very long chain fatty acids have even more. Most of the fatty acids you will see for the MCAT are long-chain fatty acids, although it is occasionally useful to note the presence of medium-chain fatty acids as well.

> **CONNECTIONS** <<

Chapter 9 of Biochemistry

Triacylglycerols have three fatty acid chains (R–COOH) attached to a glycerol backbone. The esters formed between the –COOH groups of the fatty acids and the –OH groups of the glycerol can be broken down under basic conditions in a process known as **saponification**.

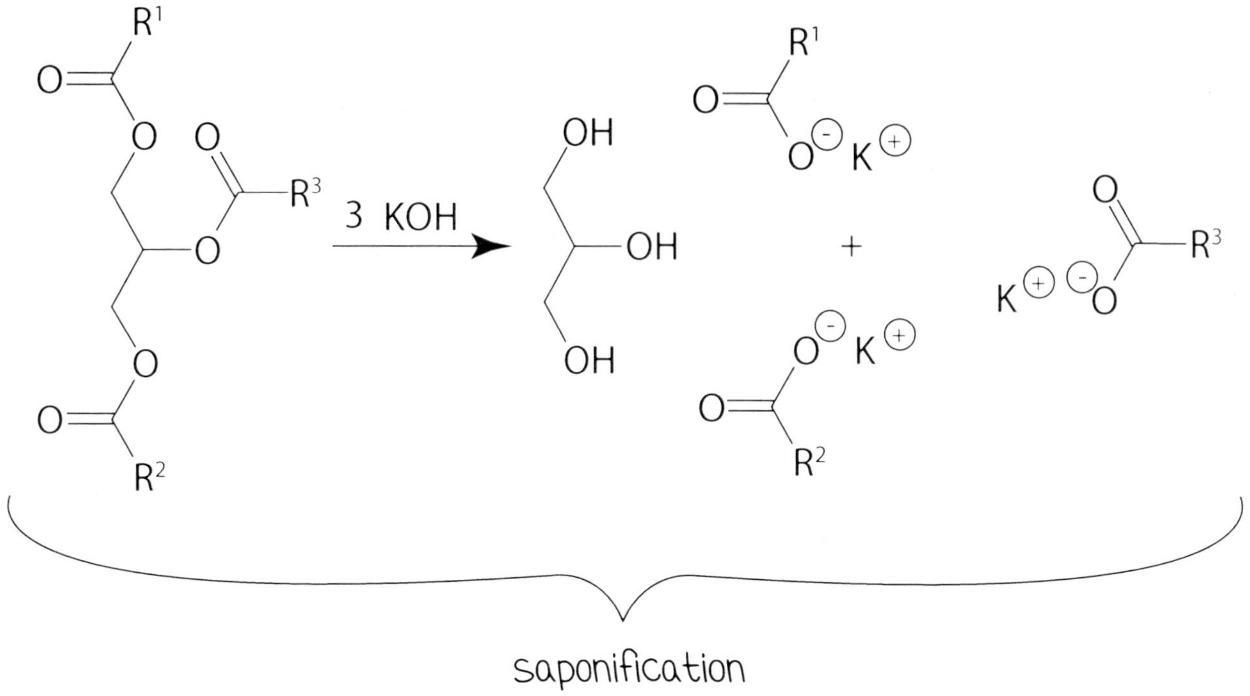

Figure 7. Triacylglycerols and saponification

A diverse range of lipids can be generated by replacing one of the fatty acid chains with something else. In **phospholipids**, this "something else" is a polar phosphate group, which itself can be modified by the addition of other organic substituents. Phospholipids are most well-known for being the major components of the lipid bilayer of the plasma membrane in cells.

MCAT STRATEGY >>>

Recall from our discussion above that fatty acids, one of the components of triacylglycerols, are amphipathic molecules with a polar head and nonpolar tail. How would we expect triacylglycerols to differ from fatty acids? Unlike carboxylic acids or alcohols, the ester functional groups in triacylglycerols cannot participate in hydrogen bonding, so we would expect markedly less polar behavior. To succeed on the MCAT, it is essential to make a habit of engaging in this sort of reasoning that connects structure to function.

Sphingolipids are based on a molecule known as sphingosine, and all have a fatty acid residue bonded to the amine group of sphingosine. The simplest sphingolipids are known as ceramides. However, the terminal –OH group of sphingosine can be additionally modified, resulting in derivatives including glycosphingolipids and sphingomyelins. These molecules are generally found on the outer side of the plasma membrane and play a crucial role in signaling systems.

Additionally, for the MCAT you should be aware of **waxes**, which are complicated, naturally occurring mixtures of lipids that include fatty acid, long-chain alcohols, aromatic compounds, and other functional groups. They are secreted by plants and animals, are solid at room temperature, and have a range of applications.

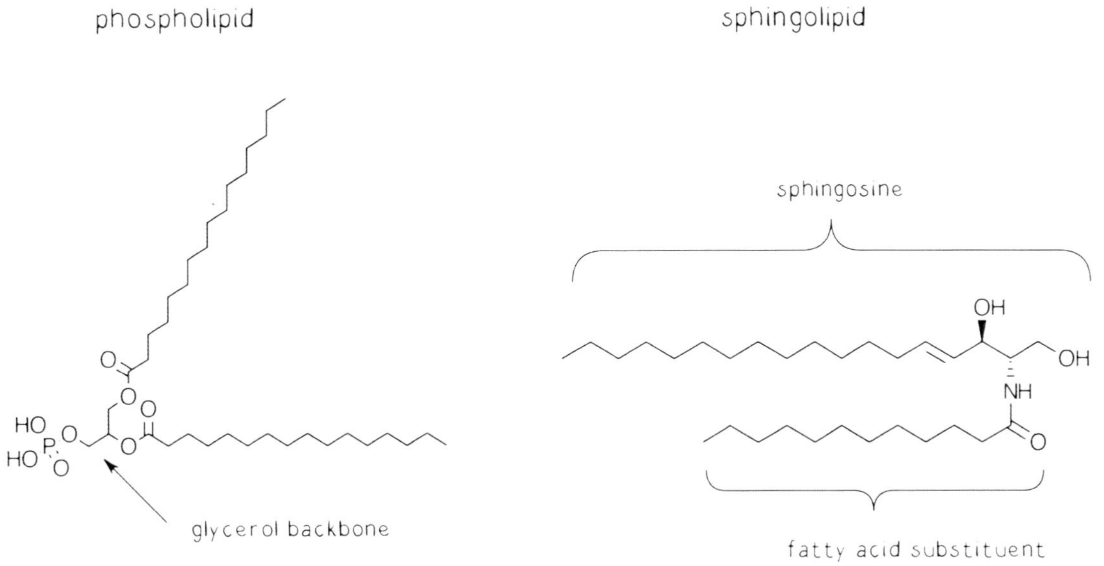

phospholipid

sphingolipid

Figure 8. Phospholipids and sphingolipids

The next major class of lipids includes **cholesterol** and its derivatives, including **steroid hormones** and **vitamin D**. Cholesterol has a characteristic four-ring structure, as do its derivatives. While people often associate cholesterol with heart disease risk, the real story is more complicated. Although cholesterol does play a role in the formation of atherosclerotic plaques, it is also an essential component of life, as it contributes to the fluidity of the plasma membrane and serves as the precursor for steroid hormones and other biologically essential molecules, such as vitamin D.

>>CONNECTIONS <<

Chapter 11 of Biochemistry

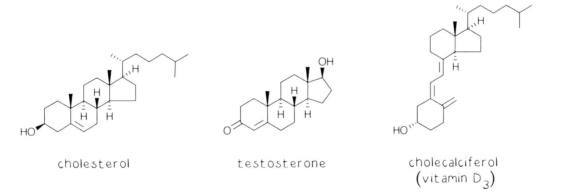

cholesterol

testosterone

cholecalciferol
(vitamin D₃)

Figure 9. Cholesterol and its derivatives

Eicosanoids form a very broad family of signaling molecules, the most important subclass of which is prostaglandins. **Prostaglandins** are synthesized from arachidonic acid, and have 20 carbons and a five-carbon ring, although the other aspects of the structure of prostaglandins may vary widely. Prostaglandins have a wide range of effects. You will have ample opportunity to explore the details in medical school, but one of the most well-known effects of prostaglandins is the regulation of inflammation. Certain prostaglandins contribute to pro-inflammatory environments, while other prostaglandins have anti-inflammatory effects. This is noteworthy because emerging research indicates that inflammation may play a role in the pathophysiology of a surprising number of diseases.

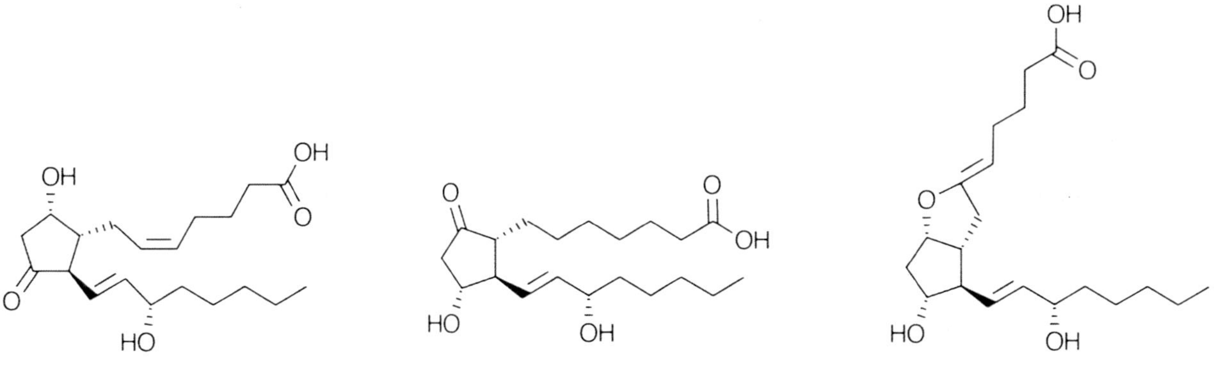

prostaglandin D2   prostaglandin E1   prostacyclin

Figure 10. Prostaglandins

Finally, the MCAT expects you to be aware of **terpenes** and **terpenoids**. Terpenes are hydrocarbons composed of repeating **isoprene units** (C_5H_8), and terpenoids are terpenes that are modified with other organic substituents. Terpenes are produced by many plants and have a variety of applications. However, they are relevant for the MCAT for two major reasons. First, **vitamin A** is a terpene derivative. Second, **squalene**, which is a 30-carbon terpene, is a precursor for the synthesis of cholesterol, steroid hormones, and vitamin D.

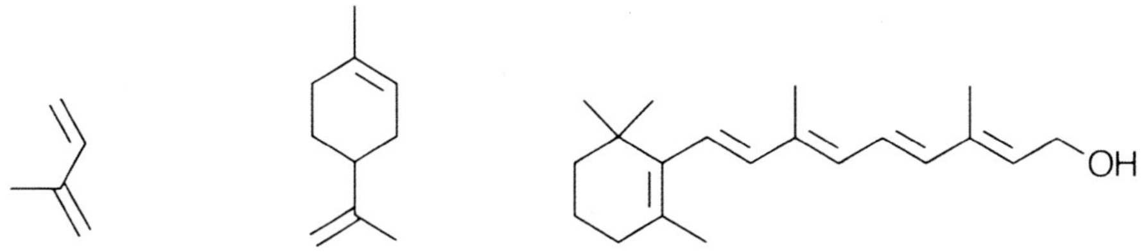

isoprene   limonene   retinol (vitamin A)
                  (a terpene)   (a terpenoid)

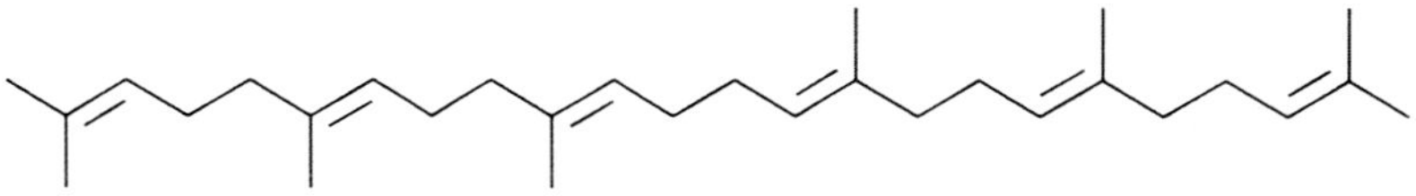

squalene (a triterpene)

Figure 11. Isoprene-containing molecules

We've covered two lipid-soluble vitamins, vitamin A (a terpene derivative) and vitamin D (a cholesterol derivative), but vitamins E and K are lipids as well. Their structures are shown in Figure 12, but they do not belong to any larger classes of lipids that are tested on the MCAT. For more details about the function of vitamins, see Chapter 10 on the digestive system and Chapter 3 of the Biochemistry volume, which deals with enzymes.

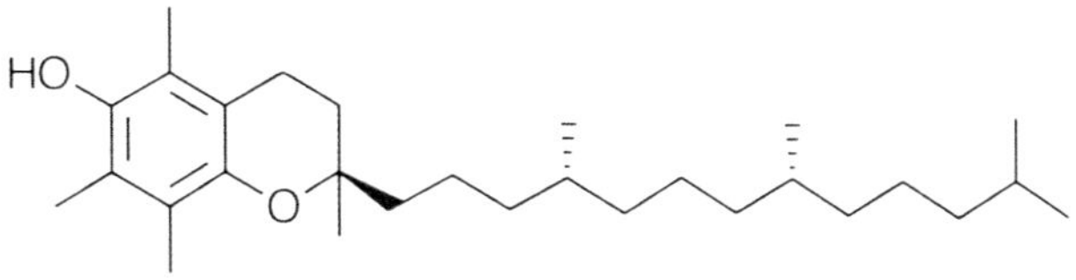

vitamin E

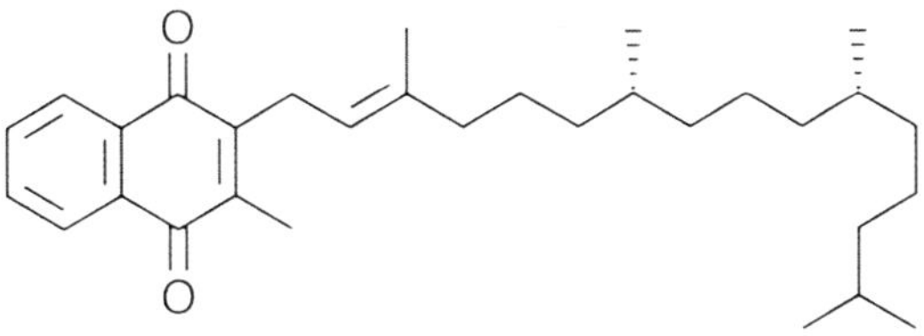

vitamin K

Figure 12. Vitamins E and K

4. Carbohydrates

Carbohydrates are a major source of energy. Their metabolic and biochemical properties are very important topics for the MCAT, and are discussed at length in the Biochemistry textbook. In this section, we will briefly review the classification, structure, and terminology associated with carbohydrates in order to provide a scaffold for understanding how they fit into the cellular and physiological systems explored in other chapters of the present volume.

> **CONNECTIONS** <<

Chapter 10 of Biology

> **CONNECTIONS** <<

Chapters 6, 7, and 8 of Biochemistry

Carbohydrates get their name as many of them have a structural formula that can be written as $C_x(H_2O)_y$—that is, they are composed of carbon and water. They contain a carbon backbone, a carbonyl group (C=O), and at least one hydroxyl group (–OH). If the molecule contains a terminal carbonyl group, it is known as an **aldose** (because it is an aldehyde), while if the carbonyl group is non-terminal, it is known as a **ketose** (because it is a ketone). Depending on the number of carbons, carbohydrates can be referred to as **trioses** (three carbons), **tetroses** (four carbons), **pentoses** (five carbons), or **hexoses** (six carbons).

Carbohydrate chemistry can be challenging in the context of the MCAT for several reasons, the most important of which are outlined below.

> Carbohydrates generally have multiple stereocenters, meaning that their stereochemistry is complex, to the point that a separate nomenclature system has been developed for it. For the purposes of this chapter, it suffices to know that in eukaryotes, carbohydrates occur in their **D-isomers**. This system of nomenclature

(D/L) is based on the orientation of glyceraldehyde and is not equivalent to either *R/S* or dextrorotatory/ levorotatory.

> Carbohydrates exist in linear forms and ring forms, and it is important to be familiar with both.
> Carbohydrates bond with each other to form chains. Isolated carbohydrates are known as **monosaccharides**, groups of two are known as **disaccharides**, and long carbohydrate chains are known as **polysaccharides**. For the MCAT, you must be familiar with biologically relevant monosaccharides and disaccharides, as well as some important polysaccharides.

The stereochemistry of carbohydrates and the interconversion between linear and ring forms is beyond the scope of this chapter, but a familiarity with the nomenclature and structure of the essential carbohydrates will prove helpful in understanding much of the biology content of the MCAT.

MONOSACCHARIDES				
Name	**Type**	**Linear structure**	**Ring form**	**Notes**
Glucose	Aldohexose			Main source of fuel for the organism
Fructose	Ketohexose			Produced by many plants/fruits, commonly used as a sweetener
Galactose	Aldohexose			Found in dairy products and sugar beets; can be rapidly converted to glucose

DISACCHARIDES			
Name	**Composition**	**Ring form**	**Notes**
Sucrose	Glucose + Fructose		Table sugar

| Lactose | Glucose + Galactose | | Found in dairy products. Lactose tolerance depends on continued expression of lactase |
| Maltose | Glucose + Glucose | | Found in beer, cereal, and pasta; produced by breakdown of starch |

POLYSACCHARIDES		
Name	Composition	Notes
Amylose	Linear chains of glucose linked by α(1,4) glycosidic bonds	A major component of starch (20%-30%); less easily digested than amylopectin
Amylopectin	Linear chains of glucose linked by α(1,4) glycosidic bonds + branching due to α(1,6) glycosidic bonds every 24-30 units	Comprises approximately 70%-80% of starch; broken down more easily than amylose
Starch	20%-30% amylose, 70%-80% amylopectin	Major energy store produced by most green plants; most common form of carbohydrate in most diets
Glycogen	Linear chains of glucose linked by α(1,4) glycosidic bonds + branching due to α(1,6) glycosidic bonds every 8-12 units	Similar to amylopectin, but more branched; synthesized in liver and stored primarily in liver cells and muscle cells; how the body stores glucose to be used
Cellulose	Linear chain of glucose units linked by β(1,4) bonds	Produced by many plants; not digestible by humans; often referred to as dietary fiber

Table 3. Structure and properties of important carbohydrates

5. Nucleic Acids

Nucleic acids are involved in the storage and transmission of biological information. The discovery that nucleic acids are part of the mechanism through which genetic information is stored and transmitted is one of the most important and fascinating scientific stories of the 20th century, and you should be aware of some of the important experiments and discoveries along that path (see Chapter 3 on molecular genetics). They are made up of **nucleotides**, which have three components: a nitrogenous base, a

>> CONNECTIONS <<

Chapter 10 of Biochemistry

five-carbon sugar, and a phosphate group. You may sometimes encounter the term **nucleoside**, which refers to a nitrogenous base and a five-carbon sugar.

The **nitrogenous bases** include adenine (A), cytosine (C), guanine (G), thymine (T), and uracil (U). Deoxyribonucleic acid (DNA) uses A, C, G, and T, while ribonucleic acid (RNA) uses A, C, G, and U (that is, T is replaced by U in RNA). A and G have two-ring structures and are classified as purines, while C, T, and U have one-ring structures and are classified as pyrimidines. Strict rules govern which nitrogenous bases pair with each other across strands: C and G pair with each other and A and T pair with each other in DNA, while in RNA, U pairs with A. A consequence of this is known as the **Chargaff rule**, which states that in a double-stranded DNA molecule, the percentage of A equals the percentage of T and the percentage of C equals the percentage of G.

The structures of the nitrogenous bases are presented below in Figure 13. They are less high-yield than amino acid structures but are still worth being familiar with at least on the level of recognition. In particular, note that U is a demethylated version of T.

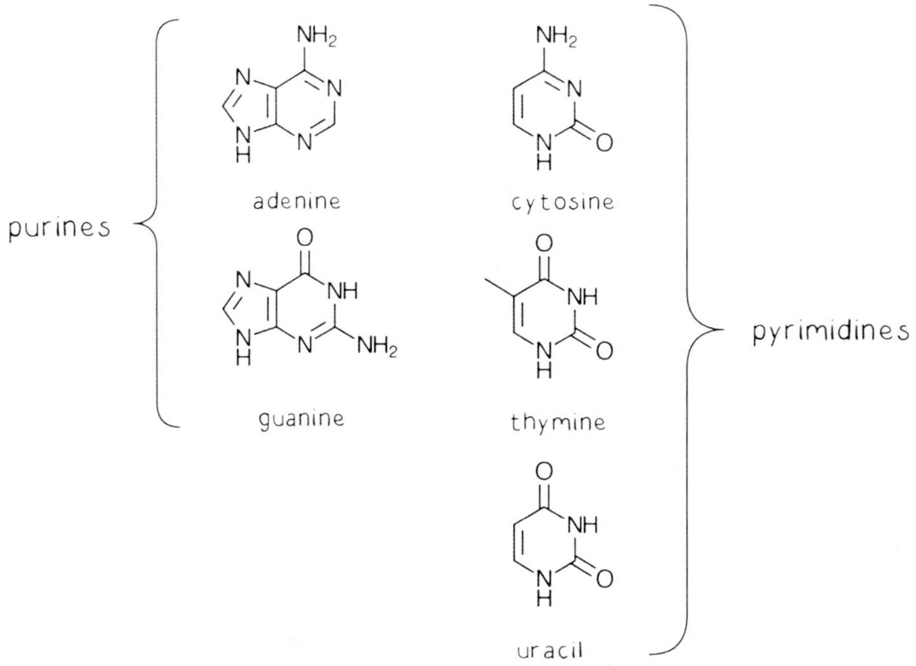

Figure 13. Nitrogenous bases

There are two possibilities for which five-carbon sugar is present in a nucleic acid: **ribose** or **deoxyribose**, in which the 2' hydroxyl group is missing. Ribose is used in **RNA** (*ribo*nucleic acid) and deoxyribose is present in **DNA** (*deoxyribo*nucleic acid).

MCAT STRATEGY >>>

To remember which nucleobases are purines and which are pyrimidines, you can use the following mnemonics. For purines, think *pure as gold*—i.e., that the *pu*rines are *A* and *G*. For pyrimidines, think *cut the pie*—*cut* is for C, U, and T, and *pie* sounds like pyrimidine.

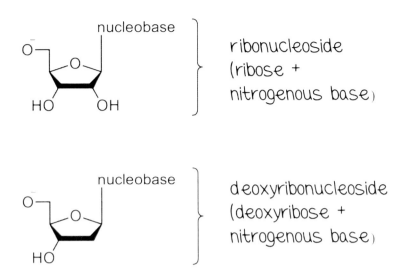

Figure 14. Ribonucleoside vs. deoxyribonucleoside

Nucleic acids are chained together in what is termed a **sugar-phosphate backbone**, connected by **phosphodiester linkages**. In these bonds, a phosphate group forms an ester bond to the 3' carbon of one sugar molecule and the 5' carbon of another. Using this, we can talk about sequences running in the 3' → 5' direction or in the 5' → 3' direction. As we will see, most processes operate in the 5' → 3' direction.

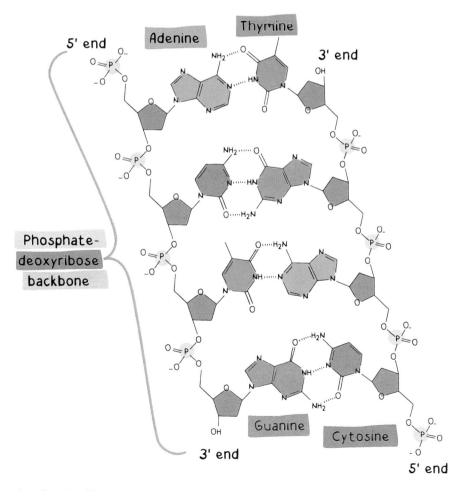

Figure 15. Sugar-phosphate backbone

Nucleic acids can be either **single-stranded** or **double-stranded**. DNA is generally double-stranded, unless the strands are temporarily separated as part of some biological or laboratory process (a process known as denaturing), and RNA is generally single-stranded, although double-stranded RNA does occur as part of some viral genomes and as part of RNA interference in eukaryotes. Additionally, DNA-RNA hybrids can occur, most notably as a temporary step in the transcription of eukaryotic genes. The formation of double-stranded DNA relies on hydrogen-bonding interactions between complementary bases. Two hydrogen bonds are formed between A and T, and three are present between C and G. As a result, sequences in which C and G bases predominate require higher temperatures for the strands to denature (or separate).

Double-stranded DNA has an **antiparallel orientation**: that is, if the 5' → 3' direction of one strand runs "up" the page, the 5' → 3' of the other strand runs "down" the page. Double-stranded DNA is also characterized by a helical shape known as a **double helix**.

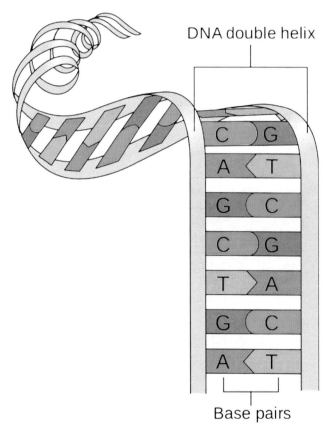

Figure 16. Double helix with antiparallel orientation shown

DNA and RNA play fundamentally different roles in the cell. DNA is used for the long-term storage of genetic information, either in the nucleus (contains the 23 chromosomes of the human genome) or the mitochondria (contain **mitochondrial DNA**, or **mtDNA**, which is inherited maternally). In contrast, RNA is involved in gene expression. The most familiar example of RNA is **messenger RNA (mRNA)**, which is transcribed from DNA and passed to the ribosomes for translation, but you should be aware of some other types of RNA with more diverse functionality as well. **Heterogeneous nuclear RNA (hnRNA)** is the precursor of mRNA, which is generated by several post-transcriptional modifications. **Transfer RNA (tRNA)** serves as the physical link between mRNA sequences and the amino acids that they code for during the translation process in the ribosomes. **Ribosomal RNA (rRNA)** makes up more than 50% of the ribosome by weight and plays an essential role in ensuring that translation successfully happens. **Small interfering RNA (siRNA)** and **microRNA (miRNA)** are RNA sequences that inhibit the expression of specific genes by interfering with the corresponding mRNA. Although these functions of RNA are diverse, a common thread is that they reflect various steps in gene expression-that is, actually *building* the products that genetic sequences code for-instead of long-term storage.

Table 4 summarizes the major structural and functional differences between DNA and RNA.

>>**CONNECTIONS** <<

Chapters 3 and 5 of Biology

PARAMETER	DNA	RNA
Five-carbon sugar	Deoxyribose (no 2' -OH)	Ribose (with 2' -OH)
Nucleobases	A, C, G, T	A, C, G, U
Single- or double-stranded?	Double-stranded	Single-stranded
Basic role	Long-term storage of genetic information	Gene expression
Location in cell	Nucleus, mitochondria	Nucleus, cytoplasm, mitochondria
Subtypes	mtDNA	mRNA, tRNA, rRNA, hnRNA, siRNA, miRNA

Table 4. Major structural and functional differences between DNA and RNA

6. Must-Knows

> Polarity:
  – Polar covalent bonds create permanent dipoles in molecules.
  – Polarity is driving force behind intermolecular forces and physical/chemical compounds of various functional groups.
  – Alkanes = nonpolar, alcohols = polar, carboxylic acids = very polar, charged molecules = extremely polar.
  – Symmetrical polar bonds → overall nonpolar molecule (CCl_4, CO_2).

> Amino acids:
  – Central carbon with $-NH_2$, $-COOH$, $-H$, and $-R$ groups.
  – Nonpolar: glycine (Gly, G), alanine (Ala, A), valine (Val, V), isoleucine (Ile, I), leucine (Leu, L), methionine (Met, M), proline (Pro, P), phenylalanine (Phe, F), tyrosine (Tyr, Y), tryptophan (Trp, W).
  – Polar uncharged: serine (Ser, S), threonine (Thr, T), asparagine (Asn, N), glutamine (Gln, Q), cysteine (Cys, C).
  – Positively charged/basic: arginine (Arg, R), histidine (His, H), lysine (Lys, K).
  – Negatively charged/acidic: aspartic acid (Asp, D), glutamic acid (Glu, E).
  – *Know the structures!*

> Proteins:
  – Building blocks of body, structure and signaling.
  – Primary structure = amino acid sequence, secondary structure = H-bonding between amino acid backbone components, tertiary structure = side-chain interactions, quaternary structure = interactions between polypeptides.

> Lipids: know the structure and functions of the following classes:
  – Signaling, structure, energy storage.
  – Fatty acids and derivatives (triacylglycerols, phospholipids, sphingolipids).
  – Cholesterol and derivatives (steroid hormones and vitamin D).
  – Prostaglandins.
  – Terpenes and terpenoids.

> Carbohydrates:
  – Energy storage; used in metabolism.
  – Important monosaccharides: glucose, fructose, galactose.
  – Sucrose = glucose + fructose, lactose = glucose + galactose, maltose = glucose + glucose.
  – Polysaccharides (starch and glycogen): polymers of glucose used for energy storage in plants and animals, respectively.

> Nucleic acids: differences between RNA and DNA.
  – DNA: deoxyribose base, RNA: ribose base.
  – DNA: A pairs with T, C pairs with G; RNA: A pairs with U, C pairs with G.
  – DNA: long-term storage of genetic information, RNA: gene expression.
  – DNA: double-stranded, RNA: single-stranded.

End of Chapter Practice

The best MCAT practice is **realistic**, with a focus on identifying steps for further improvement. For those reasons, we recommend completing practice questions in an online setting that simulates the real MCAT interface, and taking advantage of advanced analytic features to help you determine how best to move forward in your MCAT study journey.

With that in mind, **online end-of-chapter** questions for Biology, Biochemistry, Chemistry + Organic Chemistry, Physics, and Psychology/Sociology are available through your Blueprint MCAT account.

As a further supplement, given the importance of active learning for effective studying, we also suggest that you consult the Must-Knows at the end of each chapter as a basis for creating a study sheet, in which you list out key terms and test your ability to briefly summarize them.

This page left intentionally blank.

Cellular Biology

0. Introduction

Cellular biology forms much of the basic groundwork for MCAT biology. This subject is important not just because it can be directly tested—although it is very likely that you will encounter at least a few questions on this material—but because it is often a prerequisite for understanding the information presented in passages, especially experimental passages. When studying cellular biology for the MCAT, be sure not to limit yourself to memorizing isolated details. While you do certainly have to have a thorough knowledge of the basic factual material, it is also important for you to be able to integrate the material and understand how cells function in response to various stimuli, how that functionality can be disrupted, and how cells contribute to the larger-scale functionality of the organism.

1. Cell Theory

From 1650 until the mid-19th century, the basic composition of life was a major subject of research, and this process led to the formulation of the following basic tenets of **cell theory** (the first two were proposed in 1839 and the third was proposed in 1855):

1. All living organisms are composed of one or more cells.

2. The cell is the most basic unit of life.

3. All cells arise only from pre-existing cells.

More modern versions of cell theory also incorporate the idea that genetic information encoded by DNA is transmitted from cell to cell. While the statements in cell theory may be easy to take for granted, each of them reflects a remarkable intellectual journey. The MCAT expects you to be familiar with the basics of cell theory and its historical impact on the field of biology, so it is worth reviewing some of the key experimental findings that provided the foundation of cell theory.

The first experiment that identified evidence of cells was conducted by Robert Hooke in 1665, who constructed a simple compound microscope and used it to examine cork, which is composed of dead tissue from the bark of trees. He observed what seemed to be a honeycomb-shaped lattice, and he dubbed the components of that structure "**cells**" because they reminded him of cells (or rooms) within monasteries. In 1674, the self-taught scientist and lens maker Anton van Leeuwenhoek observed so-called "animalcules" ("little animals") under his microscopes; his observations included bacteria and spermatozoa.

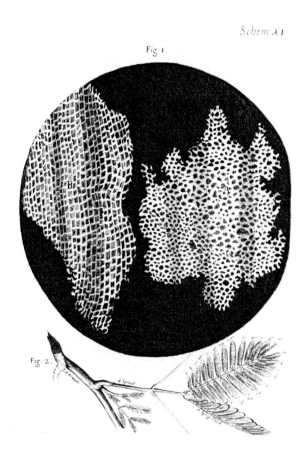

Figure 1. Hooke's observations of the microscopic structure of cork

2. Eukaryotic Cell Structure

Eukaryotes are defined by three major structural/functional features: the presence of a membrane-bound **nucleus**, the presence of **organelles**, and **mitotic division**. In this section, we will discuss the structure of eukaryotic cells.

As mentioned above, eukaryotes are defined by the presence of a membrane-bound **nucleus**, although there are some exceptions to this rule (as is almost always the case in biology). Red blood cells, or erythrocytes, are the most notable exception that you should know for the MCAT: these cells do not contain nuclei. It is also possible for cells to have more than one nucleus, such as what is seen with skeletal muscle fibers.

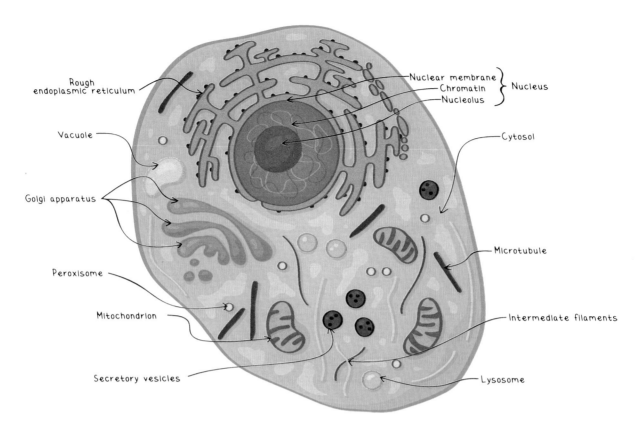

Rough endoplasmic reticulum

Vacuole

Golgi apparatus

Peroxisome

Mitochondrion

Secretory vesicles

Nuclear membrane ⎫
Chromatin   ⎬ Nucleus
Nucleolus   ⎭

Cytosol

Microtubule

Intermediate filaments

Lysosome

Figure 2. Diagram of a eukaryotic cell

The basic function of the nucleus is to compartmentalize and store genetic information, which is encoded in DNA in the form of linear **chromosomes**. The structures that allow the nucleus to carry out this function are the **nuclear membrane** and the **nuclear pores**. The nuclear membrane, also known as the nuclear envelope, is a double membrane composed of two sets of phospholipid bilayers. Nuclear pores are protein complexes that cross the nuclear membrane and allow the selective transport of larger molecules (>40 kDa, most importantly RNA and protein molecules) into and out of the nucleus, while smaller molecules such as ions and fluids can simply diffuse through the membrane. Additionally, the nucleus contains a sub-organelle known as the **nucleolus** ("little nucleus"), which is responsible for ribosome assembly.

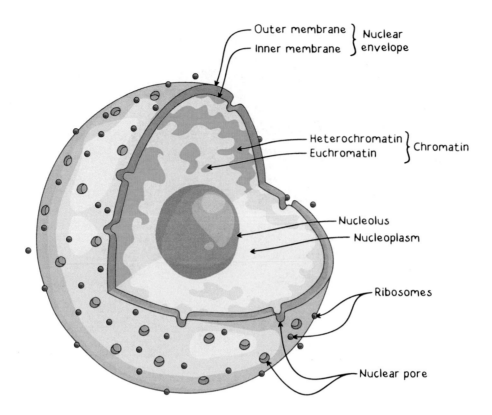

Outer membrane ⎤ **Nuclear**
Inner membrane ⎦ **envelope**

Heterochromatin ⎤ **Chromatin**
Euchromatin ⎦

Nucleolus
Nucleoplasm

Ribosomes

Nuclear pore

Figure 3. Nucleus

The **cytoplasm** is defined as everything else within a living eukaryotic cell (i.e., everything besides the nucleus and the external membrane). It includes all the other organelles and the **cytosol**, which is the dense, gel-like, aqueous solution that comprises the liquid found inside cells. The terms "cytoplasm" and "cytosol" are often used almost interchangeably, but you should be careful to be able to differentiate them if necessary.

The next most basic function of the cell is energy production or metabolism. **Metabolism** is a huge topic, and is covered at length in the Biochemistry textbook. However, when thinking about metabolism generally, you can keep the following points in mind. **Adenosine triphosphate (ATP)** is the source of energy in the cell. ATP is mainly produced by ATP synthase, which is powered by the proton gradient generated by the electron transport chain, which is in turn fed by electron carriers such as NADH and $FADH_2$—meaning that when you see NADH and $FADH_2$, you can essentially think of them as energy precursors. A chain of metabolic processes generates energy. First, **glycolysis** takes place in the cytoplasm and generates a net payoff of two NADH molecules and two ATP molecules per glucose, as well as two molecules of pyruvate. Glycolysis is common in both prokaryotes and eukaryotes, but eukaryotes (and aerobic prokaryotes) exclusively perform the **citric acid cycle** (also known as the Krebs cycle, tricarboxylic acid cycle, or the TCA cycle) and **oxidative phosphorylation** to squeeze every last bit of energy out of the pyruvate generated by glycolysis. In addition, energy can be generated from fatty acids via **beta-oxidation**, and even from amino acids when necessary.

The citric acid cycle, beta-oxidation of fatty acids, and oxidative phosphorylation take place in organelles known as **mitochondria** (singular = mitochondrion), which are the energy powerhouses of the cell. In combination with the products of glycolysis, the citric acid cycle and oxidative phosphorylation allow 30+ molecules of ATP to be obtained from a single molecule of glucose, which is at least a 15-fold increase from what is possible using glycolysis alone. As you can imagine, this was a transformative evolutionary leap in the history of life, and mitochondria are therefore essential to the functioning of all eukaryotic organisms.

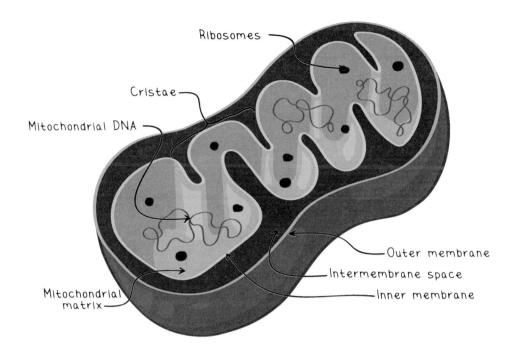

Figure 4. Mitochondrion

Mitochondria are separated from the rest of the cytoplasm by two membranes (an outer membrane and an inner membrane), both of which are composed of a **phospholipid bilayer**. The structure of mitochondria can therefore be subdivided into the outer membrane, the intermembrane space, the inner membrane, and the mitochondrial matrix, which is the innermost part of each mitochondrion. The **mitochondrial matrix** is the site of the citric acid cycle, and oxidative phosphorylation takes place via the action of protein complexes embedded in the **inner membrane** of the mitochondrion. As part of oxidative phosphorylation, the electron transport chain causes a buildup of protons in the intermembrane space, and the resulting proton gradient is used to power the activity of **ATP synthase**.

Mitochondria are also unique in that they are self-replicating organelles. They contain their own DNA (**mitochondrial DNA**, or **mtDNA**), which is circular in structure and inherited maternally, and undergoes binary fission. This remarkable fact has been explained through the **endosymbiotic origin hypothesis**, popularized by the pioneering 20th-century biologist Lynn Margulis. According to this proposal, mitochondria derive from an original prokaryotic cell capable of aerobic metabolism that became engulfed in another cell, resulting in an endosymbiotic lineage. Deleterious mutations in mtDNA can cause mitochondrial disorders, which can vary dramatically in severity, cause wide-ranging symptoms dealing with malfunctioning oxidative metabolism, and are inherited maternally. These disorders are an area of intense ongoing research, and are worth being aware of because they could conceivably be discussed in a passage on the MCAT. Additionally, mtDNA has proven quite useful in research into the genetic history and dispersion of humans, as a result of its maternal inheritance pattern.

Lysosomes can be thought of as the garbage disposal system of the cell. Material from outside the cell enters the lysosomes through **endocytosis**, while material from inside the cells enters through **autophagy**. They are membrane-bound vesicles that contain a diverse range of enzymes that hydrolyze various polymers. These enzymes operate best at acidic pH levels, and the lysosomes are therefore kept at a pH of 4.5-5.0.

The **endoplasmic reticulum** (ER) is a net-like organelle that extends out from the nuclear membrane. It is composed of cisternae, which are flat, round or tube-like structures that are enclosed by membranes. It is divided into the **rough ER** and the **smooth ER**. The rough ER is known as "rough" because it is covered with ribosomes, which are the site of protein synthesis. The smooth ER, which does not have ribosomes, is involved in lipid metabolism (both synthesis and breakdown), the production of steroid hormones, detoxification, and the storage of calcium ions in muscle. Of note, the fact that the smooth ER is involved in lipid production means that it produces the phospholipid components of membranes throughout the cell.

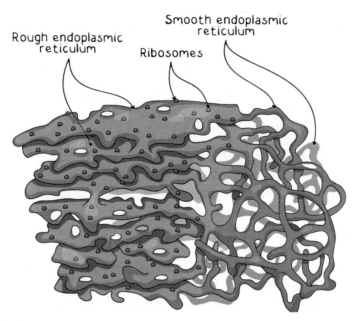

Figure 5. Endoplasmic reticulum

Once proteins are synthesized, the **Golgi apparatus** modifies them and packages them into membrane-bound vesicles that are then sent to the ultimate destination of the proteins. It is composed of stacks of pancake-like chambers known as **cisternae** (similar to those in the ER), and plays a major role in preparing proteins for secretion.

MCAT STRATEGY >>>

The Golgi apparatus is often analogized to a post office. Comparisons like this are sort of silly, but can be helpful to remember the basic functionality of various organelles. As part of your own study process, get creative in thinking about ways to conceptualize how organelles function and what would happen if their function was negatively impacted by some external factor.

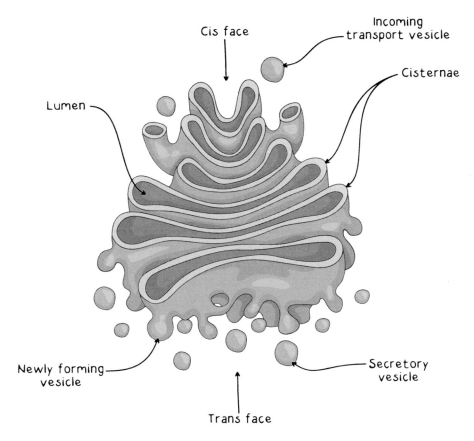

Figure 6. Golgi apparatus

Peroxisomes are the final membrane-bound organelle that you should be aware of for the MCAT. As the name implies, peroxides (such as hydrogen peroxide or H_2O_2) accumulate in the peroxisomes. Functionally, peroxisomes play a major role in the metabolism of very-long-chain lipids by breaking them down to medium-chain lipids that are transported to mitochondria for further processing. Peroxisomes also play a role in detoxification of substances such as ethanol.

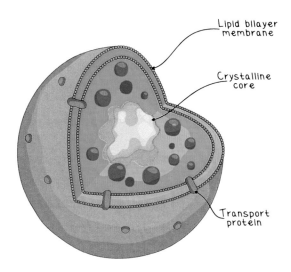

Figure 7. Peroxisomes

The **cytoskeleton** is also a crucial component of the structure of eukaryotic cells. It is sometimes considered an afterthought, but the MCAT considers it to be of comparable importance to the membrane-bound organelles discussed above, so be sure not to skim over it in your study process! Essentially, the cytoskeleton is what provides structural support to a cell and helps it move.

The major components of the cytoskeleton are microfilaments, microtubules, and intermediate filaments. **Microfilaments** are composed of two strands of actin polymers, and play a role in cell motility (or movement), as well as endocytosis and exocytosis. Additionally, microfilaments contribute to the process of cell cleavage during division and to the ability of cells to contract. The actin components of microfilaments also interact with myosin as part of muscle contraction. **Microtubules** are slightly wider than microfilaments and are composed of polymeric dimers of proteins known as alpha-tubulin and beta-tubulin. They help maintain the structure of the cell and make up cilia and flagella. They also help facilitate intracellular transport and make up mitotic spindles, which play a role in chromosome separation during mitosis and meiosis. **Intermediate filaments** constitute a broad category of proteins that provide structural support and are involved in cellular adhesion processes. **Keratin**, which makes up our hair and nails, is a well-known example of an intermediate filament.

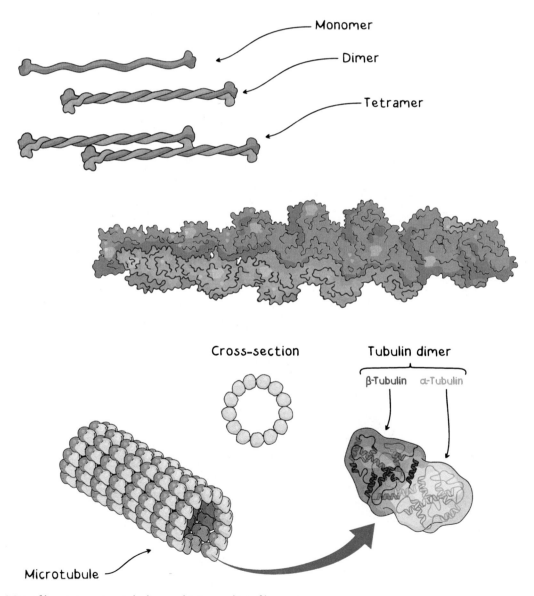

Figure 8. Microfilaments, microtubules, and intermediate filaments

Centrioles are cylindrical structures made up primarily of **tubulin** that help organize the mitotic spindle and are an important constituent of the **centrosome**, which is the major microtubule organizing center within the cell.

Flagella and cilia are two structures involved in cell motility that are formed from microtubules. **Flagella** (singular = flagellum) are tail-like appendages that protrude from a cell and allow it to move, although they also can serve as sensory appendages. Flagella are found in both prokaryotes and eukaryotes, but they are structurally distinct. **Cilia** are relatively small projections that help move substances along the cell surface. A well-known example in the human body is the presence of cilia in the respiratory tract to help move mucus out of the lungs. In eukaryotes, both cilia and flagella are characterized by what is known as a 9+2 structure, in which an outer ring of nine pairs of microtubules surrounds an inner ring of two microtubules. Eukaryotic flagella flap back and forth and their movement is powered by ATP. In contrast, prokaryotic flagella use a rotary motion, are powered by a proton gradient, and are composed of a protein known as flagellin.

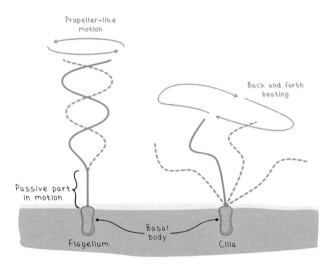

Figure 9A. Prokaryotic flagellum and cilia

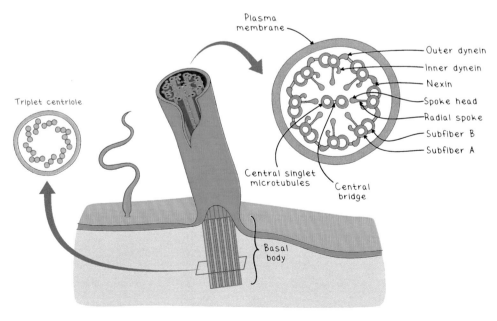

Figure 9B. Structure of a eukaryotic flagellum

A danger when reviewing eukaryotic cell structure for the MCAT is that this material may be quite familiar—perhaps even deceptively familiar, since it is all too easy to allow your eyes to skim over familiar-sounding content without really double-checking it. To combat this tendency, consider making it a point to learn something new about all of the organelles, either from this textbook or from external sources. Even if the new content you learn isn't technically testable content, just the act of learning something new will force you to consolidate your knowledge and identify potential gaps.

3. Transmembrane Transport and Signaling

The **plasma membrane** of a cell separates the cell from the extracellular environment surrounding it, and therefore is critical for maintaining cellular integrity and for mediating the communication of a cell with its surroundings. Biological membranes are discussed in more detail in Chapter 11 of the Biochemistry textbook, but it is worth reviewing some high-level points in the context of eukaryotic cell structure.

The plasma membrane is primarily composed of lipids and proteins. It is defined by the presence of a **lipid bilayer**, created by two layers of phospholipids with hydrophilic heads and hydrophobic tails. The hydrophilic heads face towards the aqueous solutions present in the cytoplasm and the extracellular space, while the hydrophobic tails face inward. **Phospholipids** are a relatively diverse class of molecules that can also be involved in signaling cascades, depending on how the phosphate group is modified (with an example being phosphatidylinositol, a major secondary messenger). **Sphingolipids** are present in the membrane as well, with roles in signaling. **Cholesterol** is another major component of the cell membrane and promotes fluidity at low temperatures by preventing crystal structures from being formed among phospholipid tails and stability at high temperatures by inhibiting the movement of phospholipids in the lipid bilayer. **Waxes** are present in the cell membrane of some types of plants and provide structural support and waterproofing. Carbohydrates are also present in the cell membrane, but only on the outer layer (due to their hydrophilicity), where they modify proteins and lipids in a variety of ways, usually with implications for signaling and/or recognition pathways.

The structure of the plasma membrane is commonly described in terms of the **fluid mosaic model**. The fluid mosaic model states that the plasma membrane can be thought of as a two-dimensional liquid in which the lipid and protein components can shift relatively freely. It is possible for phospholipids to shift from one side of the membrane to another (i.e., from facing the cytoplasm to facing the extracellular space), but this is energetically costly and is catalyzed by enzymes. As a result of these structural aspects of membrane dynamics, very small and nonpolar molecules can diffuse easily through the cell membrane, whereas large and polar molecules must be transported.

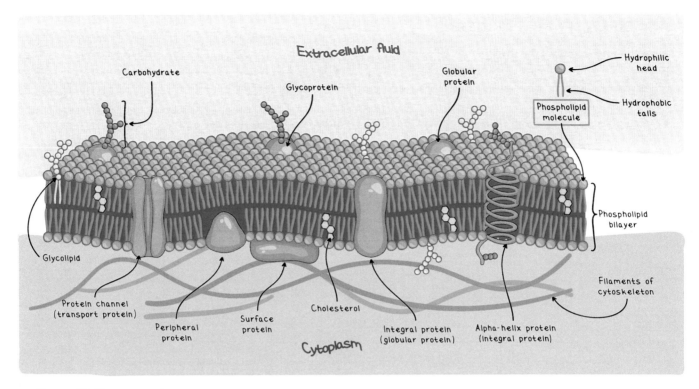

Figure 10. Plasma membrane structure

The plasma membrane contains some notable structures in addition to the phospholipid bilayer. **Lipid rafts** are held together by large amounts of cholesterol and contain relatively high concentrations of sphingomyelins. They can diffuse within the lipid bilayer, and their main functions include contributing to the fluidity of the membrane and helping to regulate signaling processes. The interior and exterior surfaces of the plasma membrane contain **embedded proteins**, and **membrane-associated proteins**, which are held in place by non-covalent interactions with other structures present on the surface of the plasma membrane. The plasma membrane is also traversed by many different types of **transmembrane proteins**, including membrane receptors and transport proteins (channels and pores).

> **>> CONNECTIONS <<**
>
> Chapter 11 of Biochemistry

> **>> CONNECTIONS <<**
>
> Chapter 7 of Biology

The details of transmembrane transport and signaling are discussed in Chapter 11 of the Biochemistry textbook, but for now you should be aware that transmembrane transport is tightly regulated and that the chemical properties of signaling molecules shape how they interact with the cell. Smaller nonpolar molecules, such as steroid hormones, can diffuse directly into the cell, while polar signaling molecules generally exert their effects on cells by interacting with membrane-bound receptors.

4. Cell Cycle and Mitosis

The **cell cycle** describes the rhythm of a cell's life as it goes through phases of division. In this section we will cover the cell cycle and **mitosis**, or asexual reproduction. The cell cycle can be divided into a resting phase, interphase, and cell division.

Resting phase is also known as Gap 0 (G_0). As the name implies, during resting phase nothing in particular happens from the point of view of cell division: essentially, during this period, the cell just goes about its business. However, although we tend to skip over G_0 when covering the cell cycle, it's worth remembering that G_0 is an extremely common state for cells in the body: many fully-differentiated cells remain in G_0 for long periods of time. Because it can last for an essentially indefinite period of time, resting phase is often considered not to be a proper part of the cell cycle itself.

Interphase is when a cell prepares for division, and it can take up approximately 90% of the time of the cell cycle. Two major things happen during interphase: growth and DNA replication. However, interphase is broken into three stages: Gap 1 (G_1), synthesis (S), and Gap 2 (G_2). During G_1 and G_2, the cell grows, and during S, DNA is replicated. Why, then, does S happen in between, meaning that this phase has three stages for two functions? This may seem inefficient, but it has the crucial advantage of allowing checkpoints. The G_1 **checkpoint**, also known as the **restriction point**, is when a cell commits to division. The presence of DNA damage or other external factors can cause a cell to fail this checkpoint and not divide. The G_2 **checkpoint** that takes place before cell division similarly checks for DNA damage after DNA replication, and if damage is detected, serves to "pause" cell division until the damage is repaired. Throughout interphase, chromatin is loosely packaged (euchromatin) to allow transcription and replication.

MCAT STRATEGY >>>

Don't neglect interphase! Many MCAT students focus more intensely on mitosis in introductory biology coursework and carry over that tendency into MCAT prep. However, when studying for the MCAT, you should always keep an eye out for areas of content that have potential implications for disease processes. The fact that two major checkpoints happen in interphase tells you that interphase plays a major role in regulating cell division, with potential implications for cancer.

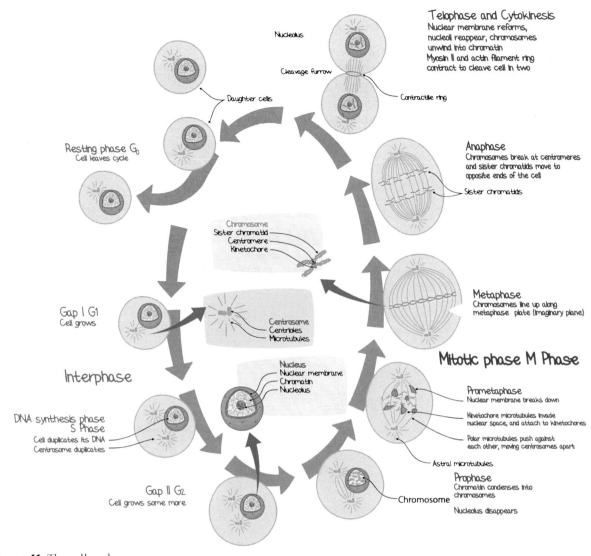

Figure 11. The cell cycle

Cell division, or **mitosis**, takes place in four phases: prophase, metaphase, anaphase, and telophase. For the MCAT, you must be very familiar with these stages, because it is likely that you will have to apply your knowledge of mitosis rapidly in a potentially unfamiliar context. Mitosis (and meiosis, which we will describe in the next section) is a subject that virtually every pre-med student has studied at least twice in various classes, if not more—yet it has a way of remaining a source of confusion.

Essentially, the point of **prophase** is to prepare the cell to go through mitosis. This preparation involves condensing the DNA such that distinct chromosomes become visible, as sister chromatids (or copies of a given chromosome) joined at a region known as the **centromere**. The **kinetochore** assembles on the centromere, and is the site where microtubule fibers that extend from the centrosome and form the mitotic spindle attach to pull the sister chromatids apart in later stages of mitosis. In addition to microtubules that attach to the kinetochore, other microtubules known as **asters** extend from the

MCAT STRATEGY >>>

If you find yourself coming back to study mitosis/meiosis again and again, the best way to solidify your knowledge for the long term is to actively rehearse it. Obtain some pipe cleaner or any other bendy colored structure that you can use to simulate chromosomes and walk through it. Doing so may seem silly, but all measures are on the table for transforming passive knowledge into active knowledge!

centrosome to anchor it to the cell membrane (from the Latin word for "stars"—asters are known for forming star-like patterns around the centrosome). The other major aspect of prophase is preparation of the rest of the structures involved in mitosis. The nuclear envelope and the nucleolus disappear, and the **mitotic spindle** forms.

In **metaphase**, the chromosomes line up at the middle of the cell along an imaginary line that is known as the metaphase plate. This alignment takes place in the center of the cell because the microtubules attached to the kinetochores generally exert the same force. Metaphase is especially important because a final **cell checkpoint** occurs, during which the cell checks to make sure that the kinetochores are attached properly to the microtubules of the mitotic spindle. This serves as a way to prevent improper separation (leading to potential nondisjunction and aneuploidy) in the next phase.

In **anaphase**, the sister chromatids are separated and pulled to opposite sides of the cell by shortening of the microtubules attached to the kinetochores. At this point, each side of the cell should have a complete set of chromosomes.

Telophase can be thought of as the opposite of prophase. A new nuclear envelope appears around each set of chromosomes and a nucleolus reappears within each of those nuclei. The process of mitosis is completed by cytokinesis, which is sometimes considered to be part of telophase and is sometimes presented as an independent process.

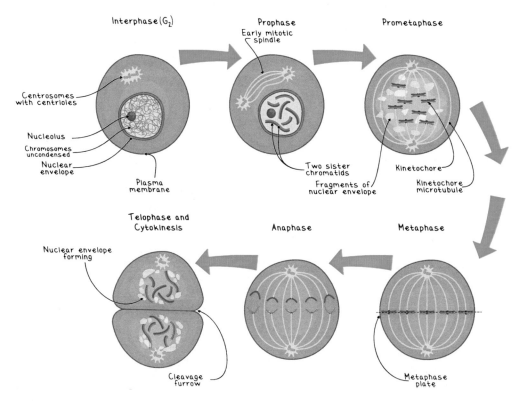

Figure 12. Mitosis

5. Meiosis

Meiosis is a form of cell division that is essential for sexual reproduction. It takes place in germ cells. In humans, gametes are generated by reproductive processes that can be subdivided into **spermatogenesis** (how sperm cells are formed) and **oogenesis** (how eggs are formed). Both involve meiosis, the generation of gametes. For more detail, see Chapter 8, which discusses the human reproductive system.

>>**CONNECTIONS**<<

Chapter 8 of Biology

Meiosis differs from mitosis in that it results in the formation of daughter cells which have only one copy of each chromosome (**haploid**, n). In males, spermatogenesis results in formation of four daughter cells. In females, only one daughter cell and multiple polar bodies are produced. This is in contrast to mitosis, which generates cells with two copies of each chromosome (**diploid**, 2n) that are essentially identical to their parent cell (with the exception of any newly occurring mutations). In meoisis, these daughter cells are known as **gametes**. In sexual reproduction, two haploid cells fuse to create a new diploid cell, known as a **zygote**, which is different from its parents. The variability allowed by sexual reproduction was a tremendously important development in the history of life.

Meiosis and mitosis include the same basic sequence of prophase, metaphase, anaphase, and telophase, but meiosis involves two rounds of cell division and some of the stages are crucially different from their counterparts in mitosis. In the following discussion, we'll focus on the ways in which meiosis and mitosis differ; if not otherwise specified, you can assume that the mechanics involved in the various stages of mitosis transfer over.

Meiosis I is the first round of division, and results in the formation of two haploid daughter cells that contain duplicate sister chromatids. In **prophase I**, **homologous chromosomes** (i.e., the maternal and paternal copies of a given chromosome) pair up with each other in a process known as **synapsis**, forming **tetrads**. While paired up, homologous chromosomes may exchange genetic information in a process known as **crossing over**. The crossing-over points are known as **chiasmata**. This process results in **recombinant DNA** that is another source of variation in sexual reproduction, in addition to the variability inherent to the process.

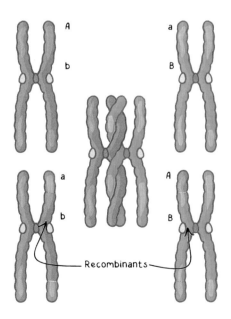

Figure 13. Crossing over

In **metaphase I**, homologous pairs line up at the metaphase plate in the form of tetrads. The orientation of the homologous pairs is random in terms of on which side of the metaphase plate the maternal or paternal copy of a given chromosome in a homologous pair winds up. This is an important point to recognize because it is the mechanical reason for the principle of independent assortment in genetics.

In **anaphase I**, the homologous pairs are separated, and one member of each pair is pulled to each side of the cell. This is when the cell is converted from a diploid cell (maternal and paternal copies of each chromosome) to a haploid cell (only the maternal or paternal copy of each chromosome). Note, however, that each individual member of the homologous pair still has two chromatids.

Meiosis II operates essentially the same way as mitosis. In meiosis II, the sister chromatids are split up into two haploid daughter cells.

Table 1 below summarizes the essential differences between mitosis and meiosis.

MITOSIS	MEIOSIS
Single-stage process	Two-stage process
No pairing of homologous chromosomes	Pairing of homologous chromosomes in synapsis, resulting in tetrads
Results in two diploid cells	Results in one or more haploid cells
Daughter cells are genetically identical to parent cell, except for incidental mutations or malfunctions	Crossing over in prophase I leads to genetic recombination
	Random orientation of homologous pairs in metaphase I leads to principle of independent assortment
Takes place in somatic cells	Only takes place in germ (sex) cells

Table 1. Mitosis versus meiosis

6. Prokaryotic Cells

Prokaryotes are the oldest form of cellular life, and have tremendous effects, both positive and negative, on human health, so a basic knowledge of their structure is fundamental for all physicians.

Prokaryotes are defined by the absence of a nucleus and membrane-bound organelles, and are classified into two domains of life: Bacteria and Archaea. **Archaea** are unicellular organisms that have been traditionally known as extremophiles, capable of inhabiting environments with high salinity or extreme temperatures. Archaea can be thought of as being somewhere between prokaryotic and eukaryotic life; structurally, they resemble bacteria in that they do not have nuclei or membrane-bound organelles, but they resemble eukaryotes in terms of certain genes and enzymes used in metabolic pathways. A notable fact about archaea is that they use a broad range of energy sources, including organic compounds, ammonia, metal ions, and even hydrogen. Additionally, some archaea are photosynthetic. The MCAT places a much heavier emphasis on bacteria than on archaea, so the rest of this section will deal with bacteria and non-living viruses.

Bacteria are ubiquitous: at any given time, it has been estimated that approximately 10^{30} bacteria exist on Earth, with a biomass comparable to that of plants. It is often stated that there are 10 times more bacterial cells than human cells in the body; this has been argued to be an overestimate, but it is still absolutely certain that bacteria, especially in the gastrointestinal tract, are present in huge numbers and play a crucial role in the maintenance of human health. Many bacteria are **commensal**, meaning that the body provides them with nutrients but they have no particular positive or negative effects on the body, except for the marginal effect provided by helping to prevent the overgrowth of harmful bacteria. Some bacteria have a **mutualistic** relationship with the body, which means that they have positive effects on the body. A classic example of this is the fact that vitamins K and B_7 are produced in the gut by bacteria.

Other bacteria, however, are **pathogens**, and can cause infections that negatively impact the organism. The pathogenicity of a bacterium may vary depending on context. For example, methicillin-resistant *Staphylococcus aureus* (MRSA), which is a major problem in hospitals, can asymptomatically colonize the skin of healthy individuals for extended periods of time, but can also cause life-threatening infections, especially in individuals with a weakened immune system. Pathogenic bacteria can damage their human hosts in a variety of mechanisms; while we often think of an infection as simple out-of-control reproduction, there are some bacteria that must reproduce intracellularly (like *Chlamydia*) and others that can reproduce either within host cells or outside of host cells (such as *Yersinia pestis*, the causative agent of plague). Moreover, some bacteria exert a negative effect by producing specific toxins; for example *Clostridium tetani*, which causes tetanus. Treating infections of such pathogens can be tricky, because immediately killing off all of the bacteria could cause a massive release of toxins, which would harm the patient.

Although bacteria do have specific genus and species names, they are commonly described in terms of their shape and their ability to engage in certain types of metabolism. The reason for this is that it can be quite time-consuming and challenging to specifically characterize the type of bacteria observed in a patient or in a culture; although the cost of genomics-based identification techniques has dropped tremendously over the last 20 years, it is still often more feasible to discuss bacteria in terms of macro-level properties such as morphology and metabolism.

Spherical bacteria are known as **cocci**, rod-shaped bacteria are called **bacilli**, and spiral-shaped bacteria are known as **spirilla**. The shape of a bacterium may be reflected in its name, so you should be able to guess that *Staphylococcus aureus* is spherical and *Lactobacillus acidophilus* is rod-shaped (moreover, the *acidophilus* part of that name is a clue that this bacterium likes low-pH environments—and in fact, *Lactobacillus acidophilus* is a major component of the gut and vaginal microbiota, as well as a common ingredient in yogurt).

MCAT STRATEGY >>>

Of course, there is no rule saying that the genus and species name of bacteria have to provide any useful information, but you should cultivate the habit of absorbing all the relevant clues you can.

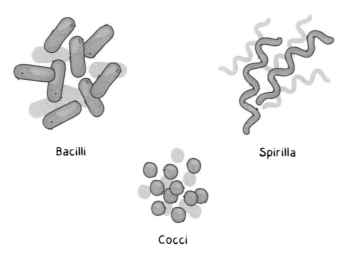

Figure 14. Shapes of bacteria

Bacteria are also classified in terms of how they use oxygen in metabolism. Bacteria that do not require oxygen for metabolism are known as **anaerobes**, and there are several types of anaerobes depending on the details of their relationship with oxygen. For **obligate anaerobes**, oxygen is toxic. (As a historical aside, developing the ability to handle the presence of oxygen in the atmosphere was a major step in the evolution of life. Oxygen, while being vital for a large number species, can also act as a toxin at elevated concentration, because it generates reactive oxygen species that induce major cellular damage. While the MCAT does not expect much familiarity with evolutionary history, you are expected to know about antioxidants, the importance of which derives from this fact.) **Aerotolerant anaerobes** are similar to obligate anaerobes in that they cannot engage in aerobic metabolism, but as their name implies, oxygen is not toxic for them. Other bacteria, known as **facultative anaerobes**, can engage in either aerobic or anaerobic metabolism, depending on the circumstances. Bacteria that require oxygen for metabolism are known as **obligate aerobes**.

Figure 15 shows where you would find different types of bacteria in a culture medium contained in a test tube with a loosely fitting cap. Oxygen would be expected to be present at the top of the tube and absent at the bottom. Therefore, obligate aerobes (number 1 in Figure 15) would only be found at the top, and obligate anaerobes (number 2) only at the bottom. Facultative anaerobes (number 3) would be found throughout the tube, but with a greater distribution at the top due to the increased efficiency of aerobic metabolism. So-called microaerophiles (number 4) are a group of microorganisms that require oxygen for metabolism but at a lower level than found in the atmosphere. Aerotolerant anaerobes (number 5) would be spread evenly throughout the tube.

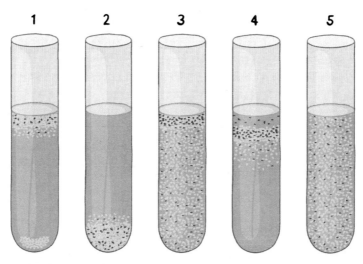

Figure 15. Aerobes and anaerobes in a test tube

Since bacteria by definition do not have membrane-bound organelles, their structure is simpler than that of eukaryotes. Nonetheless, there are some key aspects of the structure of bacteria that help differentiate them from eukaryotes and have clinical implications. In fact, these points are intimately related on a conceptual level. The goal of antibiotics is to kill prokaryotes without negatively affecting eukaryotic (host) cells, so any major structural difference between prokaryotes and eukaryotes can potentially be exploited for that goal.

Unlike eukaryotes, almost all bacteria have a **cell wall** that encloses a **cell membrane**. The cell membrane is similar to that of eukaryotes, but the cell wall is a major structural difference. The basic point of the cell wall is to provide structural support for bacteria in a range of environments. Bacterial cell walls are characterized by the presence of a polysaccharide known as **peptidoglycan**, which gives the cell wall its rigidity.

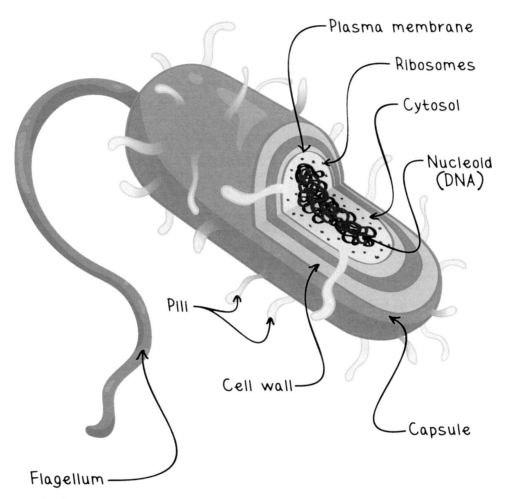

Figure 16. Bacterial cell

There are two main types of bacterial cell walls, containing different quantities of peptidoglycan. They are differentiated in a process known as **Gram staining** (named after the Danish scientist Hans Christian Gram, not after the metric unit of weight). Gram-positive bacteria have cell walls with extensive cross-linked peptidoglycan structures, whereas Gram-negative bacteria have a thin peptidoglycan layer surrounded by a lipopolysaccharide outer membrane. Gram staining depends on a dye that remains trapped within the cross-linked peptidoglycan layers of Gram-positive, while being washed away from the Gram-negative cells.

The steps of Gram staining are as follows:

1. Crystal violet is applied as a primary stain to heat-fixed bacteria.

2. Iodide is added. Iodide binds to the crystal violet stain and traps it within the peptidoglycan layer.

3. An ethanol or acetone wash is applied. This washes away the lipopolysaccharide membrane of Gram-negative bacteria and allows the crystal violet-iodide complexes to be washed away as well.

4. Safranin is applied as a counterstain to visualize Gram-negative cells as pink (otherwise they would just be unstained).

After Gram staining, Gram-positive cells become deep purple in color, while Gram-negative cells become pink. Gram staining is a common first step in the identification of bacteria in clinical settings because, although it has some limitations (not all bacteria yield consistent results), it does correlate to meaningful differences in clinical behavior. Gram-negative bacteria are generally not susceptible to antibiotics such as penicillin that target peptidoglycan cross-linking; however, specific antibiotics exist that target Gram-negative bacteria. The **lipopolysaccharide membrane** of Gram-negative bacteria also has clinical implications because it can induce an innate immune response in humans, causing inflammation and complicating the clinical course of treatment.

Prokaryotes do not have separate mitochondria, but aerobic bacteria carry out **aerobic respiration**, which we usually associate with mitochondria in humans. How can this be? The electron transport chain, which generates a proton pump that powers ATP synthase, requires a membrane. In eukaryotes, the inner membrane of the mitochondria is used for this purpose, but prokaryotes use the **cell membrane** instead.

Prokaryotes do have **ribosomes** (note that these are not *membrane-bound* organelles), but they structurally differ from those in eukaryotes. Prokaryotic ribosomes are made of 30S and 50S subunits, which add up to a 70S ribosome, while eukaryotes have an 80S ribosome composed of a 60S and a 40S component. The unit "S" is a non-metric unit, known as **Svedberg units**, that describes sedimentation rate. It is defined as 10^{-13} seconds, and it refers to how long it takes a particle to sink to the bottom of a test tube under high-intensity centrifugation. The key point here is that Svedberg units are proportional to mass, because larger particles take longer to sediment, but it is not a linear relationship, meaning that Svedberg units are not directly additive. This is why we observe that the 30S and 50S components of the bacterial ribosome add up to 70S. From a clinical point of view this fact about bacteria is important because the structural differences between the subunits of bacterial and eukaryotic ribosomes mean that ribosomes can be a target of antibiotics.

Bacteria also have **flagella** that are used for movement. Unlike in eukaryotes, where the flagellum works by whipping, bacterial flagella work through rotation. They have three components: the **filament**, which extends beyond the cell and is made up of flagellin; the **basal body**, which is embedded in the membrane and is where the rotation takes place; and the **hook**, which connects the basal body with the filament. Movement in response to chemical signals is known as **chemotaxis**.

As mentioned, bacteria lack a nucleus. Their genetic material is contained in a **single circular chromosome** that tends to congregate in a region of the cell known as the **nucleoid region**. Interestingly, prokaryotes can carry out transcription and translation simultaneously. In addition to the main chromosome, prokaryotes often contain small circular pieces of DNA known as **plasmids**.

Plasmids generally code for advantageous but non-essential abilities, and play a major role in antibiotic resistance. Plasmids also often code for **virulence factors**, which refers to anything that allows a bacterial infection to be more virulent, or harmful to the host. For instance, *Vibrio cholerae*, the causative agent of cholera (a disease responsible for millions of deaths in the last two centuries), has virulence factors including motility, adhesion to the intestinal wall, and a toxin. Without these virulence factors, *V. cholerae* would be much less harmful.

Bacteria replicate through a process known as **binary fission**. Remember that although binary fission may be *similar* to mitosis in that it results in two daughter cells that are identical to the parent cell with the exception of any incidental mutations that may take place, it is a *different* process. Mitosis occurs in eukaryotes and binary fission occurs in prokaryotes: do not let any question trick you into answering otherwise! Mitosis involves linear chromosomes lining up on the metaphase plate and being pulled to opposite sides of the cell by elements of the cytoskeleton, while bacteria do not have linear chromosomes. Binary fission involves the following steps: **replication**, in which the chromosome is duplicated while the cell grows; **segregation** and **growth of a new cell wall**, in which the chromosomes are pulled towards different sides of the cell and the cell envelope begins to grow towards the middle of the cell; and then the **separation** of two daughter cells.

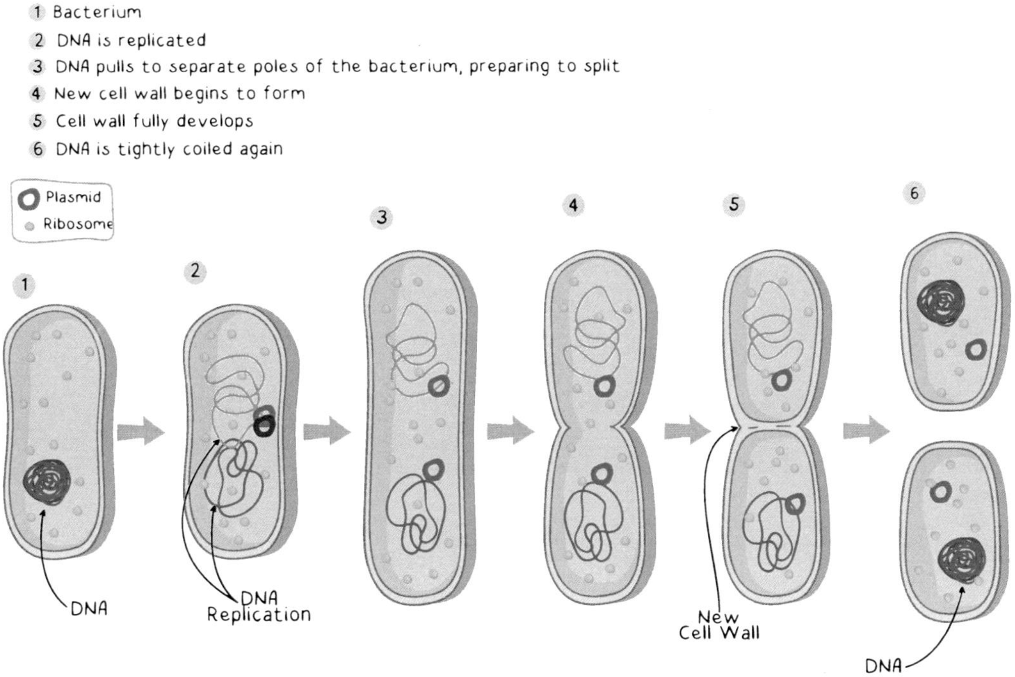

1 Bacterium
2 DNA is replicated
3 DNA pulls to separate poles of the bacterium, preparing to split
4 New cell wall begins to form
5 Cell wall fully develops
6 DNA is tightly coiled again

Figure 17. Binary fission

Binary fission can take place very quickly, and it is easy for bacteria to exhaust the resources available to them in a given setting. The **bacterial growth curve** describes this process. First, when bacteria are introduced to a new environment, they adapt to it during the **lag phase**, which takes place before appreciable growth. They then embark on an exponential growth process, known as the **exponential** or **log phase**. Eventually, the environment can't sustain exponential growth, and growth ceases in the **stationary phase**. Finally, the resources in the environment are exhausted completely and the bacteria die in the **death phase**. This is illustrated in Figure 18. Note that the y-axis of this graph is logarithmic, so the linear increase observed in the log phase actually reflects exponential growth.

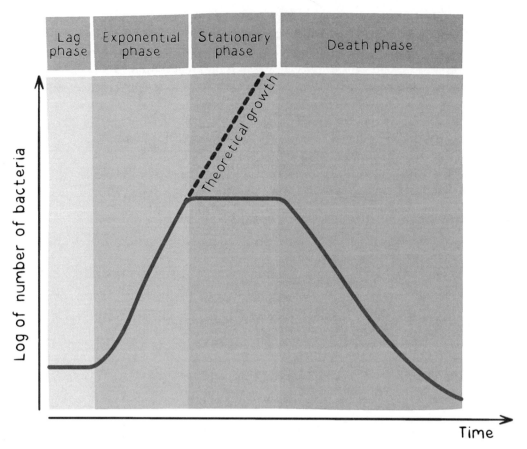

| Lag phase | Exponential phase | Stationary phase | Death phase |

Figure 18. Bacterial growth curve

Bacteria have the remarkable ability to engage in **horizontal gene transfer**. You can think of this as a way of compensating for the fact that binary fission excludes any genetic variability except for what is introduced by chance mutations. There are three mechanisms through which this takes place: transformation, transduction, and conjugation.

Transformation is the simplest of these mechanisms, and refers to the ability of some bacteria to absorb genetic material directly from the environment. Transformation was actually identified before it was securely established that DNA was the material containing genetic information. The first experiment involving transformation was conducted in 1928 by Frederick Griffith, and it was found that harmless strains of *Streptococcus pneumoniae* could be made virulent by exposing it to virulent bacteria that had been lysed with heat. In 1944, the Avery-MacLeod-McCarty experiment did something similar but showed that it was specifically an extract of DNA that led to the transformation of *S. pneumoniae* into a virulent form. This experiment was one of the pieces of evidence suggesting that DNA contains genetic information.

>> **CONNECTIONS** <<

Chapter 5 of Biology

Transduction is virus-mediated gene transfer. The lack of nuclei in bacteria makes it relatively easy for viruses that infect bacteria (bacteriophages) to incorporate part of the bacterial genome during their assembly. Bacteriophages can then infect another bacterial cell, taking the genetic material from a previous cell along for the ride, because it can become integrated into the genome of the new cell after infection. As discussed further in Chapter 5, transduction has been widely applied in biotechnology.

Conjugation can be thought of as the bacterial equivalent similar to sexual reproduction, and involves the transfer of a plasmid through a bridge that is created when a sex pilus on one bacterium (often known as F⁺, which refers to the presence of the fertility factor) attaches to another bacterium (generally known as F⁻). During this process, the fertility factor itself is duplicated and transferred, creating a new F⁺ cell. This is a major mechanism contributing to the spread of antibiotic resistance.

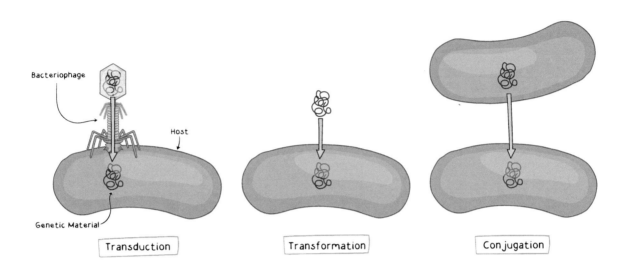

Figure 19. Transduction, transformation, and conjugation

7. Viruses

Viruses are obligate intracellular parasitic particles, which means that they must hijack host cells to replicate. Many do not consider them to be living based on the postulates of cell theory, but they have interacted with prokaryotic and eukaryotic life for billions of years and are a routine part of the clinical practice of medicine.

Viruses exhibit tremendous structural variation, but they all have at least **genetic material** and a protein coat known as a **capsid**. Some viruses also have an **envelope** made up of phospholipids and proteins. Somewhat counterintuitively, lipid envelopes are quite sensitive to the environment; viruses with envelopes can easily be destroyed through light, heat, or desiccation, whereas viruses without envelopes are more resilient. For instance, human immunodeficiency virus (HIV) has an envelope, and cannot survive for long at all in the environment, which explains why it must be transmitted through specific bodily fluids. In contrast, rotavirus, which causes diarrhea in young children, is a non-enveloped virus that is quite persistent in the environment. The term **virion** is used specifically to refer to the fully-assembled, infectious virus; although "virus" and "virion" are sometimes used interchangeably, you should be aware of the difference. Figure 20 presents the structure of the tobacco mosaic virus, a common RNA virus.

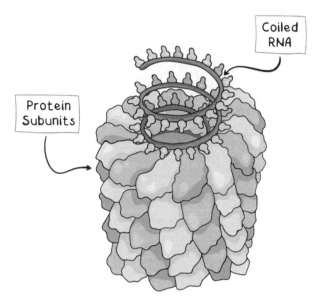

Figure 20. Tobacco mosaic virus structure

Viruses are very small, generally ranging from 20 nm to 400 nm, although some rare exceptionally large viruses have been discovered. Their genomes also vary tremendously in size; for example, the hepatitis B virus encodes only four genes, while a virus known as megavirus encodes approximately 1,100 protein-encoding genes. Viruses can come in a variety of shapes, with some common examples including helical and icosahedral forms.

The genetic material of viruses can be in the form of either **single-stranded** or **double-stranded DNA** or **RNA**. Single-stranded RNA viruses are further subdivided into **positive-sense** and **negative-sense** viruses. Positive-sense RNA viruses can be thought of as simply containing mRNA that can immediately be translated by the cell. In contrast, negative-sense RNA viruses contain RNA that is complementary to mRNA, meaning that mRNA must be synthesized by an enzyme known as **RNA replicase** that is carried in the virion.

Bacteriophages are viruses whose host cells are bacteria. A distinctive fact about them is that instead of entering the cell completely, they inject their genetic material into their host through a syringe-like structure known as a tail sheath. They also contain tail fibers, which are used to attach to the host cell.

MCAT STRATEGY >>>

On one hand, you're not expected to have any specific knowledge about antiviral medications for the MCAT (plenty of time for that in medical school!), but on the other hand, thinking about some of the potential targets for antiviral medications may help you understand the viral life cycle better. Some major approaches include interfering with binding/cell entry, interfering with the process of synthesizing new genetic material, blocking translation, and interfering with the assembly of viral proteins.

Retroviruses are a distinct class of single-stranded RNA viruses with special clinical, evolutionary, and laboratory-related importance. Retroviruses use an enzyme known as **reverse transcriptase** to synthesize DNA from their RNA genome. This DNA is then incorporated into the genome of the host cell, where it replicates along with the host. This makes pathogenic retroviruses very difficult to treat, because they cannot be killed without killing their host cells. Human immunodeficiency virus (HIV), the cause of AIDS, is a retrovirus that is responsible for the deaths of approximately 35 million people worldwide since the HIV pandemic emerged in the late 1970s and early 1980s. The retroviral nature of HIV is one of the reasons why it has been so challenging to develop effective treatments, although combination therapies of antiretroviral drugs now allow persons with HIV to live essentially normal lives. Moreover, it has been proposed that retrotransposons, which account for approximately 40% of the human genome, are fossilized remnants of retroviral infections. On a very practical level, reverse transcriptase is used in the lab to generate complementary DNA (cDNA) sequences from RNA; such applications are discussed more in Chapter 5.

The **life cycle of a virus** within an infected cell depends largely on its genetic material. The basic "goal" of a virus is to replicate by ensuring that its protein-coding genes are expressed. RNA viruses can accomplish this goal in the cytoplasm directly, while DNA viruses are transported to the nucleus for mRNA to be synthesized. The viral genome must also be replicated. Using the machinery of the host cell, new virions are packaged. Virions can be released from a host cell through a process known as **extrusion**, which is similar to exocytosis and does not damage the host cell, or virions can be produced in such quantities that they cause the host cell to lyse and spill out into the environment.

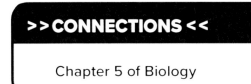

>>CONNECTIONS<<

Chapter 5 of Biology

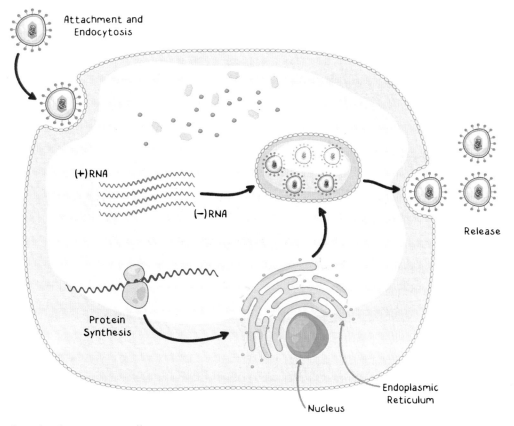

Figure 21. Life cycle of a virus in a cell

Bacteriophages have two distinct life cycles: lytic and lysogenic. During the **lytic cycle**, the bacteriophage essentially works to replicate at full speed, making full use of the host cell's machinery. Eventually, the host cell is filled with virions to the point that it bursts or lyses, and a tremendous number of new virions spill out into the environment. Alternatively, in the **lysogenic cycle**, a bacteriophage can integrate itself into the host genome, at which point it is referred to as a **prophage** or a **provirus**. In response to environmental signals, the prophage can re-emerge from the host genome and resume a lytic cycle.

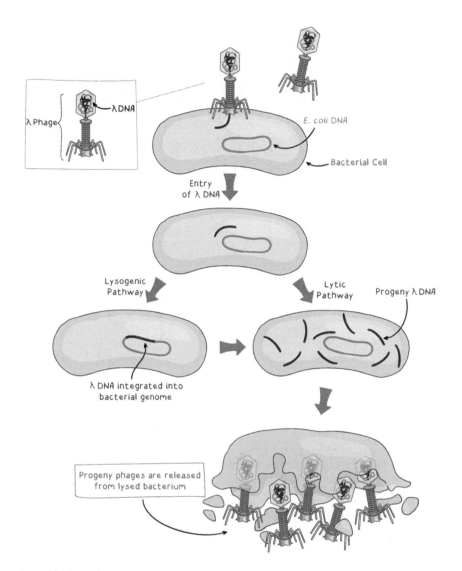

Figure 22. Lysogenic and lytic cycles

The MCAT also expects you to be aware of two types of particles even smaller than viruses: prions and viroids. **Prions** are infectious proteins. This may seem paradoxical, but prions are misfolded proteins that cause other proteins to become misfolded as well, with implications for cellular function. In humans, prions cause Creutzfeldt-Jakob disease (essentially the human form of "mad cow disease"), fatal familial insomnia, as well as a disease known as kuru that was transmitted by cannibalism. **Viroids** are small infectious particles found in plants that can silence gene expression by binding to specific RNA sequences.

8. Must-Knows

> Eukaryotic cell structure:
  - Nucleus: contains DNA and nucleolus; site of DNA replication and transcription.
  - Mitochondria: site of aerobic metabolism; "powerhouses" of the cell; self-replicating and contain mtDNA.
  - Cytoskeleton: made up of microfilaments, microtubules, and intermediate filaments; helps maintain structure of cell and carry out basic functions.
  - Plasma membrane: composed of phospholipid bilayer with lipid rafts and transmembrane proteins; regulates signaling and transport.
> Cell cycle:
  - Resting phase: cell carries out normal activities.
  - Interphase: preparation for division, DNA synthesized and G_1/S and G_2 checkpoints make sure that cell is ready for division.
  - Mitosis: cell division.
> Mitosis:
  - Prophase: nuclear membrane disappears, chromosomes condense, mitotic spindle forms.
  - Metaphase: chromosomes line up along metaphase plate.
  - Anaphase: chromosomes pulled apart.
  - Telophase/cytokinesis: nuclear envelope and nucleolus reappear, cells divide.
> Meiosis:
  - Takes place in sex/germ cells, turns diploid (2n) parent cell into haploid (n) daughter cells; has two stages.
  - Meiosis I → two haploid daughter cells with duplicate sister chromatids.
  - Prophase I: homologous chromosomes pair up in synapsis, exchange genetic information in crossing over.
  - Meiosis itself + homologous chromosomes → major source of genetic variability in sexual reproduction.
> Prokaryotes and viruses:
  - Bacteria: no membrane-bound organelles, no nucleus, circular genome.
  - Bacteria shapes: cocci = spheres, bacilli = rods, spirilla = spirals.
  - Metabolism: obligate aerobes require oxygen, obligate anaerobes require oxygen-free environments, facultative anaerobes can do both.
  - Bacterial cell walls contain peptidoglycan.
  - Gram-positive: turn purple in Gram staining, have thick peptidoglycan cell walls.
  - Gram-negative: turn pink in Gram staining, have thin wall with outer lipopolysaccharide layer.
  - Ribosomes (70S) are structurally different than in eukaryotes (80S).
  - Transformation: DNA from environment, transduction: virus-mediated gene transfer; conjugation: like sexual reproduction for bacteria.
  - Viruses: obligate intracellular parasites, protein capsid coat around genetic material.
  - Lytic cycle: machinery hijacked, host cell killed; lysogenic: virus incorporates itself into host genome and waits. Only in bacteriophages.

End of Chapter Practice

The best MCAT practice is **realistic**, with a focus on identifying steps for further improvement. For those reasons, we recommend completing practice questions in an online setting that simulates the real MCAT interface, and taking advantage of advanced analytic features to help you determine how best to move forward in your MCAT study journey.

With that in mind, **online end-of-chapter** questions for Biology, Biochemistry, Chemistry + Organic Chemistry, Physics, and Psychology/Sociology are available through your Blueprint MCAT account.

As a further supplement, given the importance of active learning for effective studying, we also suggest that you consult the Must-Knows at the end of each chapter as a basis for creating a study sheet, in which you list out key terms and test your ability to briefly summarize them.

This page left intentionally blank.

This page left intentionally blank.

Molecular Genetics

0. Introduction

It is common to distinguish between molecular genetics and genetic inheritance, at least partially for historical reasons: the principles of genetic inheritance were largely worked out in the late 19th to early 20th centuries, before scientists elucidated the actual mechanisms of how genetic information is transmitted. However, we're going to reverse the historical path of research into genetics and cover the mechanisms first. Having a solid understanding of how inheritance works on the molecular level can help you make sense of inheritance patterns and evolution, which are discussed in Chapter 4.

> **>> CONNECTIONS <<**
>
> Chapter 4 of Biology

1. Central Dogma and the Genetic Code

The central dogma of molecular genetics states that information flows **from DNA to RNA to protein**. The term "dogma" may seem somewhat strange in this context because it is frequently encountered when discussing religion or philosophy, but this terminology is a historical relic from a period when scientists were still debating where genetic information was contained. It was only in the 1950s that a series of experiments conclusively showed nucleic acids—specifically DNA—were the medium in which genetic information was stored.

One of the most decisive experiments that concluded DNA contains genetic information was the 1952 **Hershey-Chase experiment**. The researchers used radiolabeled sulfur and phosphorus as a way of distinguishing between proteins (which contain sulfur atoms present in cysteine and methionine residues, but no phosphate groups) and nucleic acids (which contain phosphate groups, but no sulfur). It was known at this point that bacteriophages (viruses that infect bacteria) inject genetic material into bacterial cells. Radiolabeled bacteriophages were added to cell cultures of bacteria, and it was determined that the bacterial cells post-transduction contained radiolabeled phosphate, not sulfur. These results indicated that the genetic material is DNA.

The idea that information flows from DNA to RNA to protein is familiar to anyone who has taken a college-level biology course, but it's still important to review. First of all, because it is a good problem-solving tool to apply to difficult passages and secondly, because some noteworthy exceptions/complications have been discovered. The simplest version of this framework states that genetic information is stored over the long term in **DNA**, and is then transcribed into **messenger RNA (mRNA)**, which are then translated into **proteins**. This correctly describes the basic chain of events in most cells, but it is not the whole story. Most remarkably, **reverse transcriptase** (present in retroviruses; see Chapter 2) allows DNA to be transcribed from RNA, reversing the normal flow of information. Additionally, several forms of non-coding RNA exist, including **transfer RNA (tRNA)**, which assists in translation, and other forms of RNA that affect gene expression (discussed in more depth in Chapter 5). Figure 1 presents the central dogma: the basic logic of the principle is shown on the left side of the image, while the right side of the image contains details that we will discuss in this chapter. It may be worth revisiting Figure 1 after studying this chapter to see how the details align with the big-picture principles.

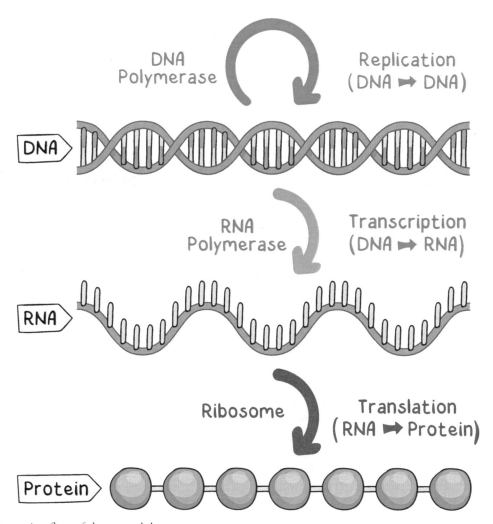

Figure 1. Information flow of the central dogma

The central dogma is also limited in that it is only referring to the flow of *genetic* information. Signaling pathways also transfer information throughout the organism using a wide range of mechanisms: proteins can influence other proteins in secondary messenger systems, steroid hormones can upregulate gene expression, and so on. However, in the context of an MCAT passage, you can apply the central dogma to predict some of the ways a cell might react to a stimulus. For instance, a steroid hormone can bind to a nuclear receptor, increasing the rate at which a specific gene (DNA) is transcribed into RNA, which then is translated into the protein of interest.

In order to understand how information contained in the form of nucleic acids can be translated into proteins, it is useful to think of DNA/RNA as containing a **genetic code**. DNA and RNA each contain four bases (A, C, G, and T for DNA and A, C, G, and U for RNA). Combinations of these letters code for 20 amino acids. A system in which each base corresponds to an amino acid would clearly be too simple, as would a system in which combinations of two nucleobases coded for amino acids. Instead, we have a system in which combinations of three nucleobases, known as **codons**, code for amino acids. There are 64 (4^3) combinations of bases, which is much more than enough to code for the 20 amino acids mentioned above. However, this is actually advantageous in that it provides a certain degree of resilience and tolerance for error. This property of the genetic code is known as **degeneracy**. The genetic code also contains three stop codons that cause the translation process to be halted, and a start codon (coding for methionine) that indicates where translation begins.

MCAT STRATEGY >>>

A mnemonic for the stop codons is: U Are Annoying (UAA), U Are Gross (UAG), and U Go Away (UGA).

The genetic code is presented below in Table 1. However, you should not memorize it. On the other hand, it is important to be able to identify the stop and start codons. Also, note that nearly half (8 of the 20) of the amino acids are completely specified by the first two base pairs in the codons, and that almost all of the amino acids are definitively specified by the first two base pairs. This leaves some room for error in the third base pair. As discussed below in the section on mutations, this room for error, which leads to the third base of the codon as sometimes being referred to as the "wobble" position, provides some degree of protection against mutations.

>>CONNECTIONS <<

Chapters 2 and 6 of Biology

Second nucleotide

First nucleotide	U	C	A	G	Third nucleotide
U	UUU, UUC Phenylalanine	UCU, UCC, UCA, UCG Serine	UAU, UAC Tyrosine	UGU, UGC Cysteine	U C A G
	UUA, UUG Leucine		UAA, UAG (STOP)	UGA (STOP) / UGG Tryptophan	
C	CUU, CUC, CUA, CUG Leucine	CCU, CCC, CCA, CCG Proline	CAU, CAC Histidine / CAA, CAG Glutamine	CGU, CGC, CGA, CGG Arginine	U C A G
A	AUU, AUC, AUA Isoleucine / AUG Methionine (START)	ACU, ACC, ACA, ACG Threonine	AAU, AAC Asparagine / AAA, AAG Lysine	AGU, AGC Serine / AGA, AGG Arginine	U C A G
G	GUU, GUC, GUA, GUG Valine	GCU, GCC, GCA, GCG Alanine	GAU, GAC Aspartic acid / GAA, GAG Glutamic acid	GGU, GGC, GGA, GGG Glycine	U C A G

Table 1. Genetic code

2. DNA Structure and Chromosomes

The structure of nucleic acids (DNA and RNA) was presented in Chapter 1 on biomolecules, but the basic points of the **Watson-Crick model of DNA structure** are presented below for review:

> DNA is organized in a **double helix** of **antiparallel strands**, with a **sugar-phosphate backbone** connected by **phosphodiester bonds** on the outside and **nitrogenous bases** on the inside.
> Complementary **base-pairing** dictates that adenine (A) pairs with thymine (T) and cytosine (C) pairs with guanine (G).
> The interior of the structure is stabilized by **hydrogen bonds** between base pairs (two hydrogen bonds for AT pairs and three for CG pairs), as well as **hydrophobic interactions** between stacked nitrogenous bases.

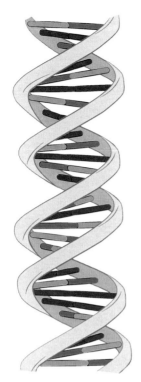

MCAT STRATEGY >>>

A great way to practice applied transcription and translation questions is to create your own MCAT-style question and generate incorrect but tempting answer choices. Regardless of how you do this, work through this carefully and slowly until it becomes reflexive, because this is an instance where investing a relatively small amount of time into really *getting* it is very likely to pay off. When taking the test, remember you can use your whiteboard for these genetic code questions so that you can clearly visualize what's going on.

Figure 2. Double helix structure

The MCAT may ask you to identify the complementary DNA/RNA sequence for a given strand of DNA, either directly or as a step in a more complicated problem. Be very careful about directionality when answering such problems! This is a common source of avoidable missed points on the exam. Standard practice is to list DNA sequences in the 5'→3' order, but remember that the actual complementary sequence must both be complementary *and* antiparallel. Let's work through a sample problem illustrating the correct process and some possible pitfalls:

Example: What is the complementary strand for the DNA sequence AACC?

Solution:

> Step 1: Recognize that the implied directionality in this sequence is 5'-AACC-3'.
> Step 2: Generate a complementary sequence through base pairing: TTGG.
> Step 3: Recognize that this complement must have the directionality of 3'-TTGG-5'.
> Step 4: Be alert to the directionality of the answer choices: the correct answer could *either* be 3'-TTGG-5' (although it is standard to give DNA sequences in 5'→3' order, it is not mandatory) or 5'-GGTT-3'.

Let's consider some potential trap answer choices. Incorrect answer choices might rely on confusion about base pairing. Those are pretty simple to handle: knowing the base pairs is an absolute must, and on the MCAT, it is assumed that most test-takers will have that knowledge. Therefore, we need to look for some more subtle possible missteps. If the answer choices do not specify directionality, then you need to understand that the implied directionality is 5'→3'. A potential trap answer along these lines would be TTGG, because in the absence of explicit marking of directionality, that answer choice would be understood to be 5'-TTGG-3', which would be incorrect. Another possibility would be to include *both* 5'-TTGG-3' (the incorrect answer) and *either* of the two ways of presenting the correct answer (3'-TTGG-5' or 5'-GGTT-3').

In eukaryotes, DNA is organized into **linear chromosomes**, which each contain part of the genome. Human cells normally have 22 distinct chromosomes known as **autosomes**; somatic cells (i.e., non-germline cells) contain two copies of each of these chromosomes, one inherited maternally and the other inherited paternally. Additionally, humans generally have two **sex chromosomes**, with females having two X chromosomes (one inherited maternally and one inherited paternally) and males having an X chromosome and Y chromosome, with the Y chromosome inherited paternally. Therefore, in the standard human cell, there are 46 chromosomes, with two copies of each of 22 autosomes and either two X chromosomes or one X chromosome and one Y chromosome.

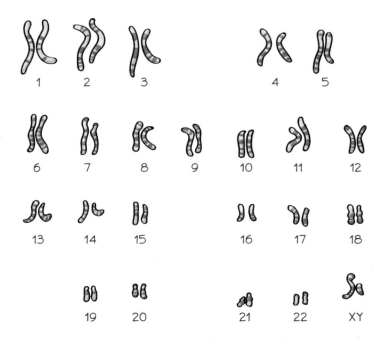

Figure 3. A human karyotype (chromosomes)

The human genome contains approximately 3 billion base pairs, meaning that in diploid somatic cells that contain two copies of each chromosome, there are approximately 6 billion base pairs. One base pair corresponds to approximately 3.4 Å (340 pm or 3.4×10^{-10} m). This means that if stretched out linearly, every body cell would contain approximately 2 meters of DNA. This is obviously incompatible with the size of human nuclei, which are generally about 6 μm (6×10^{-6} m) in size. How do we squeeze so much DNA into the nuclei of our cells? One way is by subdividing the genome into linear chromosomes, but that only accomplishes a relatively small part of the task. The rest of the job is done by histones and chromatin.

Histones are proteins that act as spools for DNA to wind around. They are composed of various subproteins known as H1, H2A, H2B, H3, and H4. The core of a histone contains two dimers of H2A and H2B and a tetramer of H3 and H4, while H1 serves as a linking unit. DNA-histone complexes known as **nucleosomes** contain approximately 200 base pairs each. **Chromatin** is the structure formed by many nucleosomes. This structure is also often referenced by the phrase "beads on a string" because of its appearance under electron microscopy. Two distinct forms of chromatin exist: euchromatin and heterochromatin. **Euchromatin** is a loose configuration that is difficult to see under light microscopy and allows DNA to be readily transcribed. Throughout interphase (i.e., most of the cell cycle), DNA generally exists as euchromatin, which makes sense because this is the form that allows transcription to happen and for cellular activities to be carried out. **Heterochromatin** is the tightly coiled, dense form of chromatin that is visible during cell division and is present to a lesser extent even during interphase.

>> CONNECTIONS <<

Chapter 5 of Biology

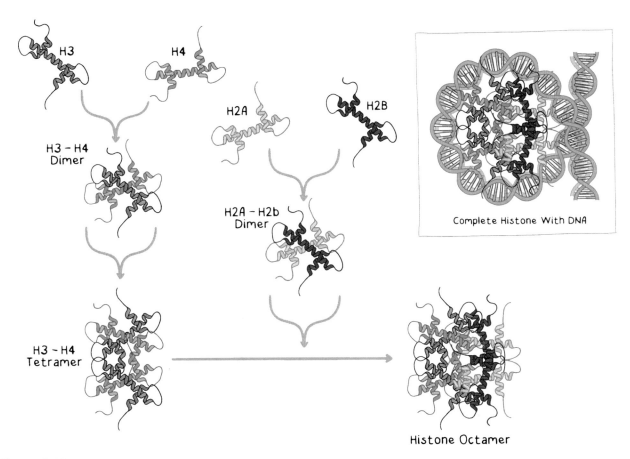

Figure 4. Histones

On a biochemical level, **charge** plays a major role in the interactions between histones and DNA. Histones are highly alkaline and are positively charged at physiological pH, which facilitates their interaction with the highly negatively charged phosphate groups on the backbone of DNA promoting chromatin formation. Modifications like **acetylation** of histones reduce that positive charge, making histones interact with DNA less closely, which in turn facilitates transcriptional activity by downregulating chromatin formation.

3. DNA Replication

DNA replication is the basis for genetic inheritance because it is the process that allows DNA to be passed on to a daughter cell. In replication, a DNA helix unwinds and a new complementary sequence is synthesized from each strand. This process is known as **semiconservative replication**, because each new DNA sequence contains one strand from the original DNA molecule and one newly synthesized complement.

The discovery that DNA replication is semiconservative was determined in 1958 in the **Meselson-Stahl experiment**. This experiment is worth familiarizing yourself with because it provides an elegant example of experimental design related to a specific point of testable content (the semiconservative nature of replication). Given the basic structure of DNA, there are three possibilities for how replication works: (1) the entire DNA molecule could serve as a template for the synthesis of a new DNA molecule, in a process in which the original DNA molecule would denature, replication would take place, the new DNA molecule would be separated, and the original DNA molecule would re-anneal (the conservative hypothesis); (2) each strand of the original DNA molecule could serve as the template for a complementary strand, with the new molecule composed of an old strand and a new strand (the semiconservative hypothesis); and (3) each of the two resulting DNA molecules could contain equally mixed segments of entirely old strands or entirely new strands (the dispersive hypothesis).

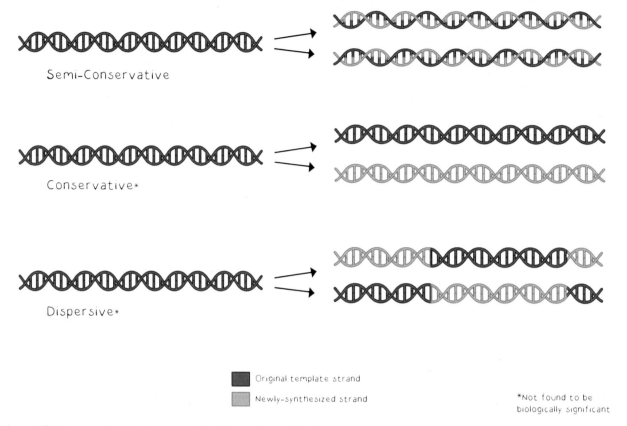

Three postulated methods of DNA replication

Semi-Conservative

Conservative*

Dispersive*

■ Original template strand

■ Newly-synthesized strand

*Not found to be
biologically significant

Figure 5. Conservative/semiconservative/dispersive replication

During the Meselson-Stahl experiment, researchers found a way to distinguish between "old" and "new" DNA. They grew *E. coli* in a medium enriched with ^{15}N (heavier than the normal isotope ^{14}N) until all of the nitrogen atoms in the bacterial DNA were ^{15}N. They then transferred the bacteria to a medium containing ^{14}N. At this point, the "old" DNA would contain ^{15}N and therefore be heavier than the newly-synthesized DNA containing ^{14}N. The researchers carefully used centrifugation to assess the density of DNA samples as a proxy for identifying the mass of the various strands. The three different theories about replication made different predictions for what would happen in these experimental conditions:

> **Conservative replication**: No DNA molecules would have intermediate density. Over progressive rounds of replication, the amount of ^{15}N-containing molecules would remain constant but be overpowered by exponentially-growing quantities of ^{14}N-containing molecules.
> **Semiconservative replication**: After one round of replication, the DNA molecules would have an intermediate weight (something like $^{14.5}N$, although you should note that there is no such isotope in reality). The second round of replication would lead to one set of DNA molecules with only ^{14}N, and one set of molecules with an intermediate weight because the original ^{15}N strands were used as templates.
> **Dispersive replication**: After one round of replication, the DNA molecules would have an intermediate weight (something like $^{14.5}N$). Remember that the fundamental idea behind dispersive replication is that the original DNA would be evenly distributed over new rounds of replication. Therefore, with successive rounds of replication, you would expect to observe uniform intermediate weights converging towards ^{14}N (e.g., first $^{14.5}N$, then $^{14.25}N$, then $^{14.125}N$, etc.), as more and more ^{14}N is incorporated into the molecules.

The results of this experiment clearly confirmed that DNA replication is semiconservative.

Next, let's turn to the actual mechanics of DNA replication. Replication must start somewhere, and that somewhere is known as the **origin of replication**. These are specific sequences that bind with a protein complex known as the pre-replication complex and tend to have high AT content. Bacterial genomes have one origin of replication, from which replication proceeds bidirectionally. Eukaryotic chromosomes have multiple origins of replication.

DNA replication involves several important enzymes:

> **Helicase** unwinds the DNA helix and separates the two strands of DNA.
> **Single-stranded DNA-binding proteins** keep the separated strands from immediately re-annealing.
> **Primase** synthesizes a short RNA primer with a free 3' OH group that is used as the starting point for the synthesis of a new strand.
> **DNA polymerase** reads the DNA template in a 3' to 5' direction and synthesizes the complementary strand in the 5' to 3' direction. This may seem counterintuitive at first, but draw it out: imagine DNA polymerase reading a template from left to right and generating complementary base pairs as it goes, and remember that the new strand is antiparallel to the original strand. This means that the synthesis must proceed from 5' to 3'.
> **DNA gyrase**, also known as DNA topoisomerase II, alleviates the supercoiling that would occur as helicase works its way down the DNA molecule.
> **Ligase** links together **Okazaki fragments**, which are created from the lagging strand of DNA replication.

MCAT STRATEGY >>>

Draw out the function of DNA polymerase as many times as it takes to understand that reading in the 3'-5' direction means synthesizing in the 5'-3' direction. In general, genetics is a subject best approached through understanding rather than just superficial memorization, but this is especially the case for the directionality of DNA.

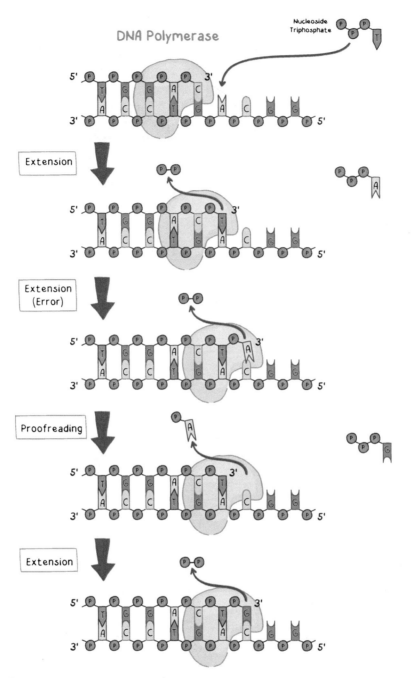

Figure 6. DNA replication

MCAT STRATEGY >>>

The different types of DNA polymerase are relatively low-yield but potentially fair game. They're worth investing a little bit of time into understanding, but don't stay up all night worrying about them at the expense of biochemistry fundamentals (for instance).

While most of these enzymes have relatively straightforward functions, **DNA polymerase** provides some complications that you have to be aware of for the MCAT. First, its directionality has important implications. Recall that DNA polymerase only works in one direction (reading in the 3'→5' direction and synthesizing in the 5'→3' direction). This means that, as helicase works its way in one direction, DNA polymerase can operate straightforwardly on one strand (known as the **leading strand**) but not on the other strand (the **lagging strand**). This problem is solved by having DNA polymerase work piece by piece as the lagging strand is unraveled. The resulting small pieces of DNA are known as Okazaki fragments, and are eventually joined back together by ligase.

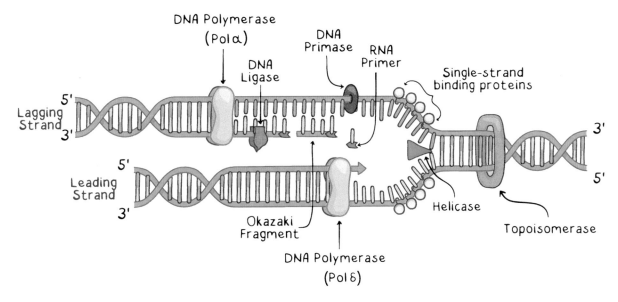

Figure 7. Leading and lagging strands

Additionally, DNA polymerases are more accurately thought of as a family of enzymes, rather than a single enzyme. Roman numerals are used to refer to the different types of DNA polymerases in prokaryotes, and Greek letters are used for the same purpose in eukaryotes. The MCAT does not expect you to be aware of all of the many types of polymerases that exist, but you should be familiar with some of the important examples listed below.

In prokaryotes, **DNA polymerase I** (Pol 1) assists in the joining of adjacent Okazaki fragments and removing the RNA primer through excision repair. **DNA polymerase II** (Pol II) is primarily involved with repair, and **DNA polymerase III** (Pol III) is involved in the main process of DNA synthesis.

In eukaryotes, **DNA polymerase α** initiates synthesis in replication in both the leading and lagging strands, and then **DNA polymerase δ** takes over because it operates more efficiently. Additionally, DNA polymerase δ adds DNA nucleotides when the RNA primer is removed. **DNA polymerase ε** specifically assists in extension of the leading strand, and also assists in DNA repair, as does **DNA polymerase β**. **DNA polymerase γ** replicates mitochondrial DNA.

Some special types of DNA polymerase have their own names. **Reverse transcriptase**, which is discussed in greater depth in Chapter 2 in the context of retroviruses, is a special kind of DNA polymerase that operates with an RNA template. **Telomerase** extends telomeres, which are repetitive sequences at the end of eukaryotic chromosomes that exist because DNA polymerase cannot faithfully replicate the end of the chromosomal sequence. As cells divide, telomeres degrade, and the degradation of telomeres is thought to play a role in the aging process. Telomerase rebuilds telomeres, and is active in stem cells and cancer cells, but not in most somatic cells (with the exception of cell types that need to divide frequently, such as skin cells).

4. Transcription

Recall the central dogma: genetic information flows from DNA to RNA to proteins. The process of going from DNA to RNA—more specifically, messenger RNA (mRNA)—is called transcription. **Transcription** takes place in the nucleus of eukaryotes and in the cytosol of prokaryotes. The end result is the creation of an mRNA copy of a gene that can then be transported to the cytosol for translation into a protein.

The DNA helix must be unzipped for transcription to take place, which means that some of the same machinery that we saw in DNA replication has to be engaged, especially enzymes like **helicase** and **topoisomerase**. **RNA polymerase** is the enzyme responsible for RNA synthesis. In eukaryotes, it doesn't just begin whenever it sees a start codon; instead, it binds to a **promoter region** upstream of the start codon with the assistance of **transcription factors**. The most important promoter in eukaryotes is the TATA box. For more details about promoters, see Chapter 5 on gene expression.

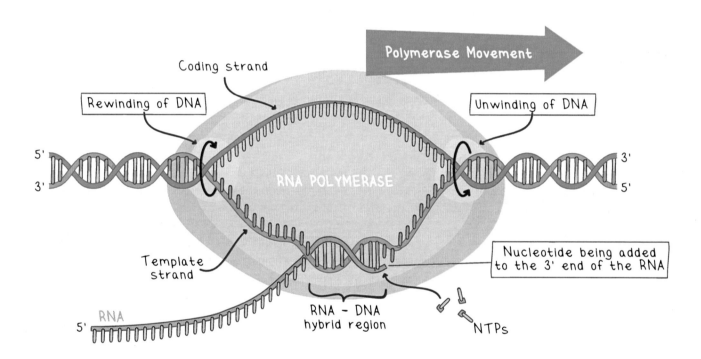

Figure 8. Transcription

It is also important to observe which strand RNA polymerase uses as a template. There is no need for two RNAs to be synthesized at the same time, so there is no equivalent of the leading/lagging strand issues that we saw with DNA replication. Similarly to DNA polymerase, RNA polymerase travels along the template strand in the 3'→5' direction, synthesizing an antiparallel complement in the 5'→3' direction. However, the choice of the **template strand** is far from random. The template strand is known as the **antisense strand**, and the opposite strand is known as the **sense strand**, because it corresponds to the codons on the mRNA that is eventually exported to the cytosol for translation.

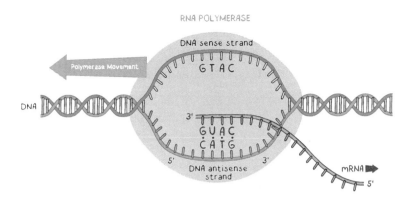

Figure 9. Sense versus antisense strands

Just as DNA polymerase is not a single enzyme, there are also multiple types of RNA polymerase in eukaryotes. Somewhat confusingly, **RNA polymerase II** is the "default" RNA polymerase that synthesizes hnRNA (the precursor to mRNA) and some small nuclear RNA (snRNA). **RNA polymerase I** synthesizes ribosomal RNA (rRNA) in the nucleolus, and **RNA polymerase III** synthesizes transfer RNA (tRNA) and some rRNA.

The immediate product of transcription is not mRNA, but **heterogeneous nuclear RNA (hnRNA)**. This version of RNA must undergo a set of post-transcriptional modifications to become mRNA. There are three post-transcriptional modifications that you must be familiar with for the MCAT: (1) the **3' poly-A tail**, (2) the **5' cap**, and (3) **splicing**. All of these three processes occur only in eukaryotes. In prokaryotes, transcription and translation can occur simultaneously, meaning there is no room for post-transcriptional modifications.

MCAT STRATEGY >>>

Confusion about the sense versus antisense strands is common, and provides the MCAT with an opportunity to test you on specific content about transcription, base pairing, and directionality of DNA within a single question. Be sure to review this carefully and draw it out a few times until it makes sense.

The **3' poly-A tail** is fairly self-explanatory. It is a string of approximately 250 adenine (A) nucleotides added to the 3' end of an hnRNA transcript. It protects the eventual mRNA transcript against rapid degradation in the cytoplasm. The deadenylation of the poly-A tail by a 3' exonuclease is the first step in mRNA degradation, so the speed with which an mRNA molecule is degraded depends largely on how many A residues are left on it. Why does this matter? Essentially, it's important for the cell to make sure that mRNA sticks around for long enough to do its job, but not for too long, because increasing or decreasing the rate of mRNA transcription is an important part of gene regulation. It would interfere with this process to keep mRNA transcripts around indefinitely.

The **5' cap** is also named intuitively. It refers to a 7-methylguanylate triphosphate cap placed on the 5' end of an hnRNA transcript. Similarly to the 3' poly-A tail, it helps prevent the transcript from being degraded too quickly in the cytoplasm, but it also prepares the RNA complex for export from the nucleus.

In **splicing**, noncoding sequences (**introns**) are removed and coding sequences (**exons**) are ligated together. Remember that *ex*ons are *ex*pressed. Genes typically have multiple distinct exons, and they can be ligated in different combinations. That means that if a gene had a set of four introns named A, B, C, and D, possible alternative splicing combinations could include ABCD, ABC, ACD, ABD, BCD, and so on. This dramatically increases the amount of different, but related proteins that can be expressed from a single gene. Splicing explains why there are over 200,000 proteins in the human body, but only approximately 20,000 genes. Splicing is carried out by the **spliceosome**, a combination of small nuclear RNAs (snRNAs) and protein complexes. When combined, they are known as **small nuclear ribonucleoproteins** or **snRNPs**.

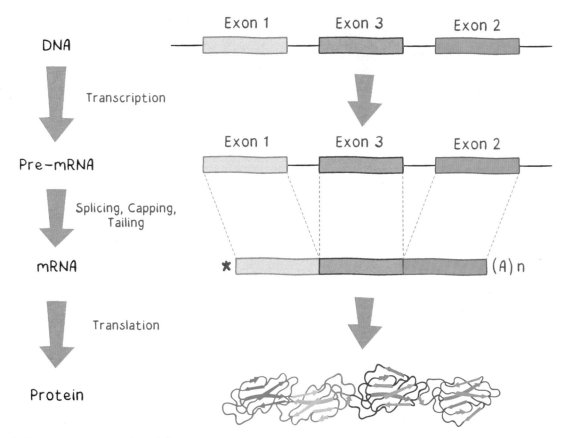

Figure 10. Post-transcriptional modifications

5. Translation

Translation is the process in which an mRNA sequence is translated into a protein, with each codon corresponding to an amino acid. It takes place in the cytoplasm in both prokaryotes and eukaryotes. However, this process occurs a bit differently depending on cell structure. In prokaryotes, translation occurs simultaneously with transcription, but the presence of the nuclear membrane in eukaryotes means that these two processes must be separated.

Transfer RNA, or **tRNA**, is a relatively small RNA molecule characterized by a hairpin structure that is responsible for "translating" between codons and amino acids. At the bottom of the hairpin structure, tRNA molecules contain an **anticodon**, which is specifically complementary to a certain codon of mRNA. Enzymes known as **aminoacyl-tRNA synthetases** do the work of "charging" tRNA molecules with the appropriate amino acids by attaching the C-terminus of the amino acid in question to the 3' end of the tRNA molecule. "Charging" the tRNA molecule requires the investment of two ATP bonds, and this energy is then used to power the formation of a peptide bond during translation. This means that translation (i.e., protein synthesis) is an energy-consuming process. On one hand, this fact may seem obvious, but on the other hand, it has implications for the regulation of gene expression because it implies that it is disadvantageous to synthesize proteins unnecessary for the cell to function.

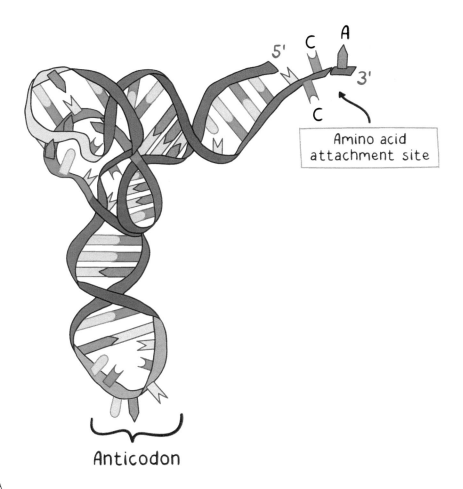

Figure 11. tRNA

Ribosomal RNA (rRNA) is the major part of the structure of **ribosomes**, where translation takes place. Ribosomes contain multiple rRNA strands with associated proteins, and have two major components. These two components are the **large subunit** (50S in prokaryotes and 60S in eukaryotes) and the **small subunit** (30S in prokaryotes, 40S in eukaryotes), with overall sizes of 70S for the prokaryotic ribosome and 80S for the eukaryotic ribosome (recall that Svedberg units describe sedimentation behavior and do not add linearly). The large subunit catalyzes the formation of the polypeptide chain, while the small unit reads the RNA.

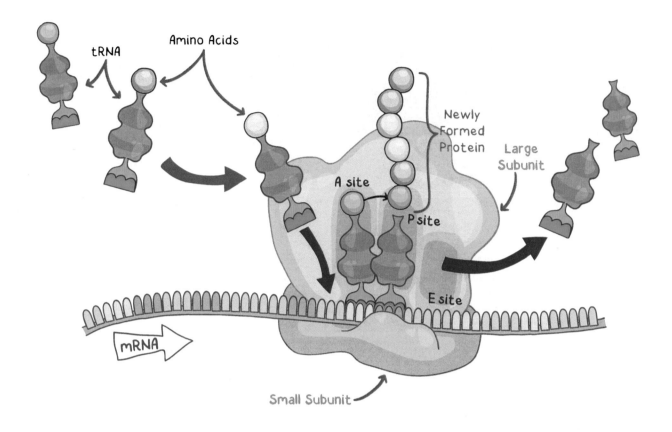

Figure 12. Ribosome structure

Translation occurs in three steps: initiation, elongation, and termination. **Initiation** occurs when the mRNA sequence binds to the small ribosomal subunit. This begins either in the 5' untranslated region known as the Shine-Dalgarno sequence (in prokaryotes) or to the 5' cap in eukaryotes (recall that 5' capping is unique to eukaryotic mRNA). The first tRNA is known as the **initiator tRNA**, and it binds to the start codon (AUG). The initial amino acid is **methionine** in eukaryotes, and **N-formylmethionine** in prokaryotes. Once this happens, initiation factors facilitate the binding of the small ribosomal subunit to the large ribosomal subunit, forming the **initiation complex**.

Elongation is the next step. During elongation, the ribosome reads the mRNA in the 5' to 3' direction and synthesizes a polypeptide from its N terminus to its C terminus. This is one of the reasons why amino acid sequences are traditionally specified in the N-to-C order. Proteins known as **elongation factors** help move this process along. The MCAT expects you to be aware of three binding sites that are involved in elongation. The **A site** contains the next aminoacyl-tRNA complex, and at the **P site** a peptide bond is formed between the growing polypeptide chain and the incoming amino acid. The tRNA, which is now no longer "charged," briefly pauses at the **E site** and detaches from the mRNA. This process continues until **termination,** when a stop codon (UGA, UAA, or UAG) on the mRNA is encountered, at which point a release factor triggers ribosome disassembly and release of the polypeptide.

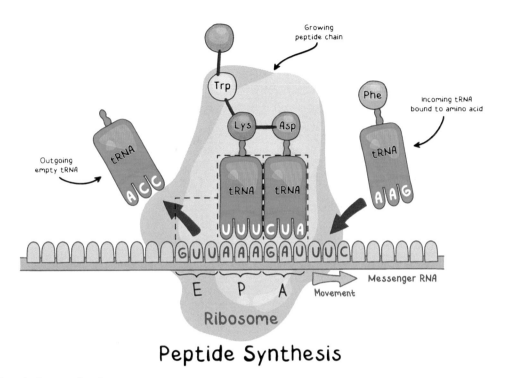

Figure 13. Translation mechanism

Finally, proteins undergo **post-translational modifications**. They may be covalently modified by the addition of various functional groups. These modifications can affect the functionality of a protein or play a role in signaling pathways. **Phosphorylation** is the most common example, and describes the addition of phosphates by enzymes known as kinases, which regulate the activity of enzymes. **Glycosylation** describes the addition of carbohydrates. The effects of glycosylation include improvements in protein stability, regulatory functions, and

>> **CONNECTIONS** <<

Chapter 7 of Biology

structural/functional roles. It is also important to note that glycosylated molecules play a major role in cell adhesion and recognition. For example, the human ABO blood system is based on glycoproteins. These are the two most common types of covalent modifications you will encounter on the MCAT, although many different moieties can be added to proteins. It is possible that you might encounter another type of post-translational covalent modification in a passage, but if so, you can expect that the passage will provide you with the necessary details.

Protein folding is another important modification, because the eventual function of proteins depends greatly on their shape. While protein folding generally follows some large-scale principles regarding polarity (with nonpolar residues more likely to be found towards the inner structure of the core), the details are very challenging to predict. Proteins known as **chaperones** help guide this process.

The formation of **quaternary structure** can also be considered an example of post-translational modification, as can cleavage. **Cleavage** is a frequent occurrence in the synthesis and processing of peptide hormones; the original transcript is a preprohormone, which is then cleaved to a prohormone, which is finally cleaved to the active form of a hormone immediately before release from the cell.

MCAT STRATEGY >>>

Review the types of mutations carefully. If you encounter a question about a type of mutation on your MCAT, that should be a relatively straightforward point. Learn the various types of mutations and how likely each is to have a major effect.

6. Mutations and Repairs

Errors can happen during DNA replication. In this section, we will discuss those errors, their effects, and how the cell combats them.

Let's start by considering **point mutations**, which occur when DNA polymerase incorrectly carries out base-pair matching. This means that the corresponding mRNA codon synthesized from that DNA sequence will be off by one base, such as CAG instead of CGG. The effect of this varies depending on the specific location and outcome of the point mutation, as follows:

> **Silent mutations** occur if the mutated codon codes for the same amino acid as the original codon. Such mutations have no effect on the physiological function of the organism. An example would be GCU [alanine] → GCA [alanine].

> **Conservative point mutations** are examples of **missense mutations** that occur when the mutated codon codes for an amino acid that has similar functional properties (e.g., polarity and size) as the amino acid coded for by the original codon. An example would be GAU [aspartic acid] → GAG [glutamic acid]. Conservative point mutations are expected to have a relatively small effect on the functionality of the protein coded for by the gene, although the word "relatively" is important here; since protein folding is very tricky to predict and biological functionality can be extremely sensitive to small changes, so this is more of a guideline than a rule.

> **Non-conservative point mutations** are **missense mutations** that occur when the mutated codon codes for an amino acid with dissimilar functional properties to the amino acid coded for by the original codon. An example would be GCG [alanine] → GAG [glutamic acid]. All other things being constant, a non-conservative point mutation could be expected to have a significant impact on the functionality of the protein in question.

> **Nonsense mutations** occur when the mutated codon is a stop codon. This truncates the translation process early, and is generally associated with significant malfunctioning in the protein product of the gene, especially if a nonsense mutation occurs relatively early in the gene.

One or more nucleotides can be added to or deleted from the genome, in what are known as **addition** or **deletion mutations**, respectively. If (3 or a multiple of 3) nucleotides are added or deleted, then one or more amino acids are deleted from or added to the protein. These consequences would be difficult to predict; on one hand, it may not be catastrophic, but on the other hand, it could be important, depending on the region of the protein and the specific details of the codon in question. However, if the number of nucleotides added or deleted is *not* a multiple of 3 (i.e., 1, 2, 4, 5, 7...), a **frameshift mutation** occurs, and all of the downstream codons can be expected to code for different amino acids. This is likely to have a massive effect (very likely deleterious) on the functionality of the protein product.

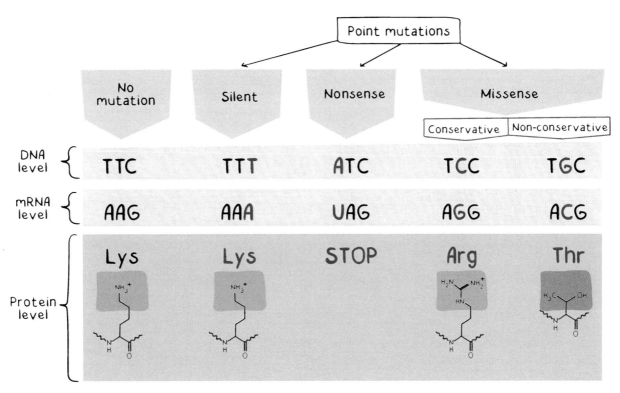

Figure 14. Types of mutations

Additionally, there are larger-scale mutations that can have a more general effect on the structure of a chromosome. Similarly to what we saw with point mutations, there are three large-scale options for what can happen with larger mutations: you can delete a chromosomal region, add extra copies of a chromosomal region, or move chromosomal regions around. Deletion of large chromosomal regions is known simply as **deletion**, while adding extra copies of a region is known as **duplication**. The effect of deletion is straightforward; it removes certain genes from a chromosome, leading either to loss of heterozygosity or a reduction in gene dosage (i.e., the amount that gets transcribed) depending on whether the other copy of the chromosome has a different allele or the same allele. The effect of **amplification** is generally to increase the gene dosage by leading to more transcription of the genes in question. **Inversion** can also occur when a mistake takes place in the directionality of a chromosome, in which a segment is reversed from end to end. All other things being constant, inversions are generally harmless, although they may lead to an increased risk of miscarriage or infertility due to a higher likelihood of problems arising in gametes.

The terms translocation and insertion are used to describe what happens when chromosomal regions are moved around. **Translocation** refers to a scenario in which a sequence of genes switches places from one chromosome to another, while **insertion** describes what happens if a sequence is moved from one chromosome to another. These mutations are slightly different because a reciprocal translocation involves a reciprocal switch and insertion is only a one way change. In balanced translocations, the exchange of genetic material is even, and generally little genetic material is lost or missing, while in unbalanced translocations, the exchange is unequal. Generally speaking, **balanced translocations** are not inherently harmful, although they may increase the likelihood of infertility. However, if the origin point of a balanced translocation lies within the middle of a gene, that can potentially have a negative impact. Translocations should be distinguished from **transposons**, which are generally non-coding genetic elements that can move from chromosome to chromosome. These comprise over 40% of the human genome and are typically not problematic unless they are inserted somewhere that breaks up a coding sequence.

Single chromosome mutations

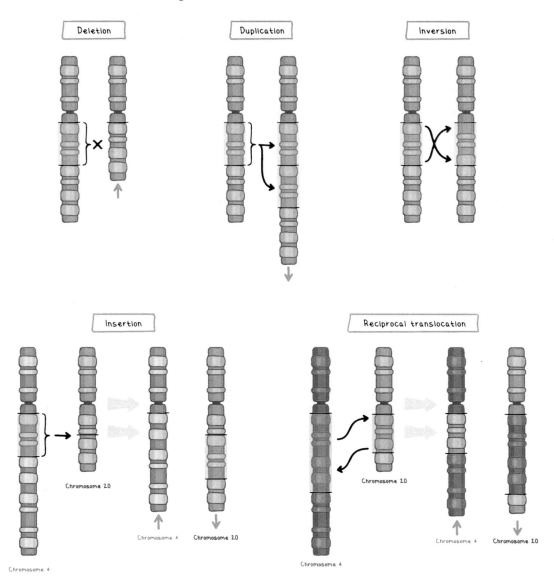

Figure 15. Chromosomal mutations

Another way to generate a chromosomal abnormality is to have too many or too few copies of a given chromosome. This is known as **aneuploidy**, and results from nondisjunction during cell division. Having only one copy of a chromosome is known as **monosomy**, and having three copies is known as **trisomy**. We commonly think of aneuploidy as occurring in meiosis, and indeed, this is the only way for aneuploidy to be inheritable. For this reason, nondisjunction during meiosis is the cause of aneuploidies such as Down syndrome (trisomy 21) or Turner syndrome (monosomy X). However, nondisjunction during mitosis can also occur, with two particularly relevant examples. First, if nondisjunction takes place during mitotic divisions early in embryogenesis, an aneuploidy may affect large proportions of the body, but not all body cells. When applied to Down syndrome, for instance, this leads to a condition known as mosaic Down syndrome, which is generally somewhat less severe. Second, aneuploidies due to nondisjunction during mitosis are extremely common in cancer cells.

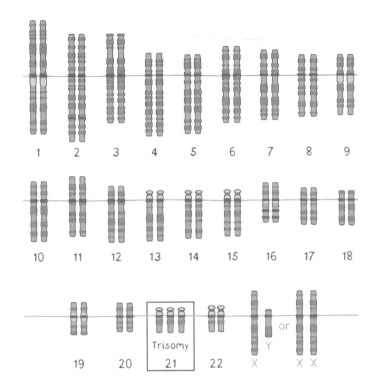

Figure 16. Aneuploidy in Down syndrome

During DNA replication, DNA polymerase occasionally makes errors. The fact that the human genome contains approximately six billion base pairs in diploid cells means that we would still expect to see some errors each time a cell undergoes divisions. This could add up to be a real problem. Fortunately, DNA polymerase also has what is often referred to as a "proofreading" ability. When DNA base pairs are mismatched due to errors in copying, the hydrogen-bonding interactions between the base pairs are relatively unstable, which is detected by DNA polymerase. DNA polymerase can then excise the base pair in question and reinsert the correct base, a functionality that is referred to as 3'→5' exonuclease activity.

DNA damage can also be caused by external sources, such as reactive oxygen species produced by metabolic pathways within the organism, radiation, mutagenic compounds/toxins, and viruses. These substances are known as **mutagens**, and most mutagens are also carcinogens, because mutations ultimately can give rise to cancer. There are several specialized proteins that repair DNA, but you will not be expected to memorize them for the exam.

There are two mechanisms of DNA repair: **base excision repair** and **nucleotide excision repair**. Base excision repair deals with relatively small-scale errors, such as mismatched pairs; oxidized, alkylated, or deaminated bases; and the mistaken inclusion of uracil in DNA. **Mismatch repair** can be thought of as a subset of base excision repair, and has specific proteins dedicated to that functionality during the G_2 stage of the cell cycle. **Nucleotide excision repair** targets larger lesions, such as DNA adducts that include thymine dimers, which result from damage by ultraviolet light.

Additionally, the **mitotic checkpoint** (also known as the spindle checkpoint) takes place in metaphase and is a step that guards against aneuploidy.

7. Must-Knows

> Central dogma: information flows from DNA to RNA to protein.
> Codons: groups of 3 RNA bases that code for amino acids; third position is "wobble"
>   — Stop: UGA, UAA, UAG; start: AUG (methionine)
> Complementary base pairs: A/T, C/G [A/U in RNA], opposite strand is antiparallel.
> DNA coils around histones: euchromatin is loose and transcriptionally active, while heterochromatin is dense and transcriptionally inactive.
> DNA replication is semiconservative. DNA polymerase reads 3'→5' and synthesizes 5'→3'.
> Replication is uninterrupted on leading strand; Okazaki fragments are synthesized from lagging strand and joined together using ligase.
> In transcription, mRNA is synthesized from the antisense/template strand, and is identical (except for containing U instead of T) to sense strand.
> Post-transcriptional modifications of hnRNA → mRNA: 3' poly A tail (anti-degradation in cytoplasm), 5' cap (transport and anti-degradation), splicing (non-coding sequences removed and coding sequences ligated)
> Translation: mRNA → protein in ribosomes through tRNA, which links codon to amino acids.
> Prokaryotic ribosomes: 70S (30S + 50S), eukaryotic ribosomes: 80S (40S + 60S)
> Translation: initiation, elongation, termination; binding sites for elongation are A, P, E.
> Small-scale mutations (point and/or a few nucleotides):
>   — Silent point mutations don't affect amino acids outcome
>   — Point mutations (missense mutations):
>   • Conservative: similar amino acids
>   • Non-conservative: amino acids with different properties
>   — Nonsense mutations: premature stop codon
>   — Insertions/deletions → frameshift mutations, change all downstream amino acids
> Larger-scale mutations:
>   — Translocations: swap of genetic material
>   — Aneuploidy: occurs due to nondisjunction during division.

End of Chapter Practice

The best MCAT practice is **realistic**, with a focus on identifying steps for further improvement. For those reasons, we recommend completing practice questions in an online setting that simulates the real MCAT interface, and taking advantage of advanced analytic features to help you determine how best to move forward in your MCAT study journey.

With that in mind, **online end-of-chapter** questions for Biology, Biochemistry, Chemistry + Organic Chemistry, Physics, and Psychology/Sociology are available through your Blueprint MCAT account.

As a further supplement, given the importance of active learning for effective studying, we also suggest that you consult the Must-Knows at the end of each chapter as a basis for creating a study sheet, in which you list out key terms and test your ability to briefly summarize them.

This page left intentionally blank.

Genetic Inheritance and Evolution

0. Introduction

Now that we've covered the molecular mechanisms of genetics, let's zoom out a little bit to explore how genetic traits are inherited. Historically these were somewhat different branches of scientific inquiry, which is part of why we still tend to consider them separately. After all, livestock and crop breeding, which depends on manipulating the inheritance of genetic traits, is an ancient part of human history, and it is hardly a new observation that children tend to resemble their parents (albeit imperfectly!).

1. Mendelian Genetics

Gregor Mendel, a 19th century Austro-Hungarian monk and scientist of Czech background, is now honored as the founder of genetics, although he had no knowledge of DNA. His findings were largely lost to science for more than three decades before being re-publicized around the turn of the 20th century. Mendel became famous for experiments with breeding pea plants and tracking how various traits were inherited. In doing so, he discovered some classic findings of genetics. For instance, if round and wrinkled peas are crossed, the offspring are all round, but in the next generation, wrinkled peas reappear, with a trait distribution of 25% wrinkled to 75% round. Mendel himself coined the terms "dominant" and "recessive" to describe this behavior of what we now call genes. Several key concepts are associated with the field known as **Mendelian genetics**, and are important for the MCAT. We will outline them below.

First, it is fundamental to distinguish between **phenotypes** and **genotypes**. The term "phenotype" is sometimes understood as "appearance," but is better thought of as the physical manifestation of a genetic trait. In Mendel's experiments, the phenotypes of interest were characteristics visible to the naked eye, such as the color or shape of peas, but in modern genetic research, phenotypes may not be immediately obvious and may take considerable effort to measure. An example might be the efficiency with which cells carry out a certain metabolic pathway. The genotype, in contrast, describes the combination of genes responsible for that phenotype.

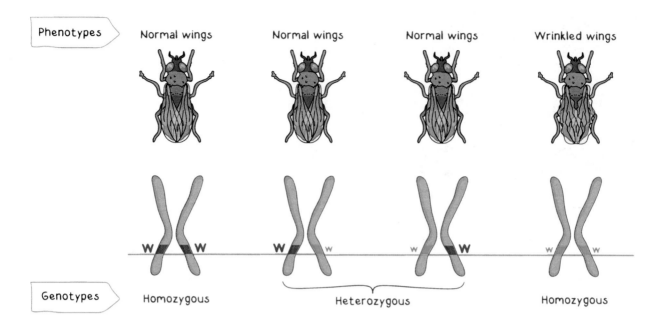

Figure 1. Phenotype versus genotype

The reason why it is important to distinguish between the phenotype and genotype is that the relationship between the two is not one-to-one. That is, a certain phenotype can correspond to multiple genotypes. The converse does not hold, at least within the realm of classical Mendelian genetics, so we will always expect a single genotype to correspond to a single phenotype. This explains Mendel's discovery about the pea plant phenotype distribution across generations: why wrinkled peas "disappear" but "re-emerge" after a generation of only round peas. We must recognize that not all round peas have identical genotypes.

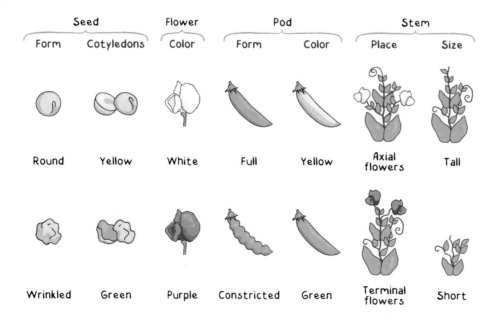

Figure 2. Mendelian experiments with peas

A **gene** is defined as a sequence of DNA that codes for a given trait, and the term **allele** is used to refer to variations of that gene. To continue exploring the example of Mendelian pea shape, the gene for pea shape has a round allele and a wrinkled allele. As discussed in previous chapters, in eukaryotes, DNA is organized into linear chromosomes. Humans have two copies of each autosomal chromosome, one inherited maternally and the other inherited paternally (except sex chromosomes. Recall that females have two X chromosomes and males have an X chromosome and a paternally-inherited Y chromosome). The same basic principle holds true for eukaryotes in general, although plants are known for higher-order ploidies, which may have three, four, or even more copies of each chromosome. Copies of the same chromosome are referred to as **homologues**, because they contain the same set of genes, even if they have different alleles. Moreover, each gene occurs at a specific place on a chromosome, known as a **locus**. This property means that genes can be described in terms of their loci. Combining all of this information, we can conclude that humans inherit two alleles for each gene: one inherited maternally and one inherited paternally (again, with the exception of sex-chromosome genes in males).

Alleles can be described as **dominant** or **recessive**. For dominant alleles, only one copy is necessary for its associated phenotype to be expressed, while for recessive alleles, both alleles must be recessive for expression of the recessive phenotype. Capital letters are used to indicate dominant alleles, while lowercase letters are used for recessive alleles. Mutations can also be classified as **gain-of-function mutations**, in which the mutated protein gains functionality not found in the original protein, or **loss-of-function mutations**, in which the mutated protein loses functionality of the original protein. Loss-of-function mutations tend to be recessive, because the presence of an unmutated allele on the other chromosome compensates for the mutated allele, whereas gain-of-function mutations tend to be dominant. Note that "gain of function" does not necessarily mean advantageous! Some dominant gain-of-function mutations, such as the mutation responsible for Huntingon's disease, can be fatal.

Now we can connect these observations with the Mendelian example of round versus wrinkled pea shape. Let's use a capital R to refer to the round allele, which is dominant, and a lowercase r to refer to the wrinkled allele, which is recessive. In the first round of crosses, Mendel crossed purebred round peas (genotype: *RR*) with purebred wrinkled peas (genotype: *rr*). Let's illustrate this in a **Punnett square**, a common technique for illustrating genetic crosses where the parental genotypes are aligned along the top row and left-hand side of the square, and the genotypic outcomes are obtained by combining one allele from each parent:

	r	*r*
R	*Rr*	*Rr*
R	*Rr*	*Rr*

Figure 3. Punnett square for first generation (F1) cross of round and wrinkled peas

All of the offspring contain one dominant R allele from one parent and one recessive allele from the other parent. This is an excellent time to introduce the important concepts of **homozygosity**, **heterozygosity**, and **hemizygosity**. Homozygous organisms have two copies of the same allele. Therefore, in the cross illustrated in Figure 3, both sets of parents are homozygous (one is homozygous dominant and the other is homozygous recessive). Heterozygous organisms have one copy of two different alleles, as is the case for all of the offspring in Figure 3. Hemizygous is a somewhat less commonly used term that describes a situation in which only one copy of a given allele is present. This can occur due to nondisjunction in an organism with aneuploidy, or more simply, it can occur with regard to genes on the X and Y chromosomes in males.

Referring back to Figure 3, all offspring of the F1 generation are heterozygotes and manifest the dominant (R) phenotype due to the presence of a single dominant allele, R.

Next, let's explore what happens when the F1 generation of all-round peas from Figure 3 is crossed with itself:

	R	r
R	RR	Rr
r	rR	rr

Figure 4. Punnett square for second generation (F2) cross with F1 peas

MCAT STRATEGY >>>

Be prepared to work out probabilities for a variety of genotypes, and also be aware that the MCAT may ask tricky questions in which you have to be careful about wording. Be sure to note whether an inheritance problem is asking about all offspring or just sons or daughters, and to check that any mutation takes place in a germ cell, as mutations in somatic cells are not heritable.

Let's take a close look at the results shown in Figure 4. The genotypes show a 1:2:1 ratio, with 25% of the offspring homozygous dominant (*RR*), 50% heterozygous (*Rr* or *rR*; both of these are functionally the same and are generally noted just as *Rr*), and 25% homozygous recessive. However, the phenotypes show a 3:1 ratio in favor of the dominant phenotype, as only homozygous recessives will actually manifest the recessive phenotype.

What happens if we have a phenotypically dominant individual, but need to know its genotype—that is, whether it is homozygous dominant or heterozygous? In such cases, test crosses can be performed. In a **test cross**, an individual with a dominant phenotype is crossed with an individual with the recessive phenotype. If the phenotypically dominant organism is homozygous, the F1 generation will not have any individuals with the recessive phenotype, whereas if it is heterozygous, approximately 50% of the offspring will express the recessive phenotype. This is shown below in Figure 5:

Test cross of homozygous dominant + homozygous recessive organisms.

	r	r
R	Rr	Rr
R	Rr	Rr

Test cross of heterozygous + homozygous recessive organisms.

	r	r
R	Rr	Rr
r	rr	rr

Figure 5. Test test crosses

Test crossing should be distinguished from backcrossing. Test crossing is a technique used in plant cultivation, animal breeding, and cell culture. Backcrossing is a process in which a hybrid is crossed with a parent or an organism genotypically similar to the parent. The goal of backcrossing is to obtain offspring more similar to the parent.

You should also be aware of the distinction between the terms **wild-type** and **mutated**. Wild-type doesn't apply well to the example of Mendel's peas, because his peas descend from a lineage of plants cultivated by humans. The term wild-type is used to refer to the default phenotype or genotype that is present in most members of a species, in contrast to a mutated genotype. In fruit fly research, this has led to a slightly different pattern of notation than we used above. For example, the wild-type eye color of fruit flies is red, but a mutation exists that results in white eyes. This mutation is known as w, and the wild-type allele is marked with a plus sign, so w corresponds to *having* the mutation, while w^+ means *not having* the mutation. This notation is admittedly confusing, but there's no need to memorize fruit fly genetics for the MCAT–just be aware that interesting genetic notations are sometimes used.

Note that the distinction between the terms wild-type and mutated is *not* the same as the distinction between the terms functional and non-functional. This is a common point of confusion. Wild type refers to the variant of an allele that is most prevalent in a population. It is entirely possible, though, that a new mutation could be advantageous from a functional point of view.

Now that we've covered the basics of Mendelian genetics, let's review some ways in which it can get a little bit more complicated. Not all traits follow Mendelian patterns of inheritance. There is more to inheritance than binary dominant/recessive dichotomies like tall/short, green/yellow, and round/wrinkled. For example, **dominance** is actually considerably more complex than it first appears.

The dominance inheritance pattern we observed in Mendel's experiments, where one copy of the dominant allele is enough to induce the dominant phenotype and there is no phenotypic difference between homozygous dominant and heterozygous individuals, is called **complete dominance**. However, other patterns of dominance exist, including codominance and incomplete dominance.

Codominance takes place when two dominant alleles are phenotypically expressed silmutaneously. The classic example of this is the human ABO blood typing system, which refers to the antigens (known as A and B antigens) expressed on erythrocytes (O refers to the *absence* of either A or B). Individuals can have the following blood types: A, B, AB, or O. An AB phenotype illustrates that these alleles are codominant. Another common example involves the appearance of colored spots in an organism's fur, skin, or outer surface. If B is an allele for black fur and W is an allele for white fur, a pattern of black-and-white spots would reflect a codominant relationship.

Incomplete dominance, in contrast, occurs when a heterozygote displays a blended phenotype. The classic example of this is the snapdragon flower. Homozygous snapdragon flowers are red or white, while heterozygotes express a blended phenotype of pink.

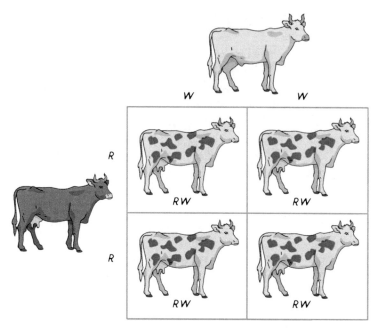

Figure 6A. Codominance

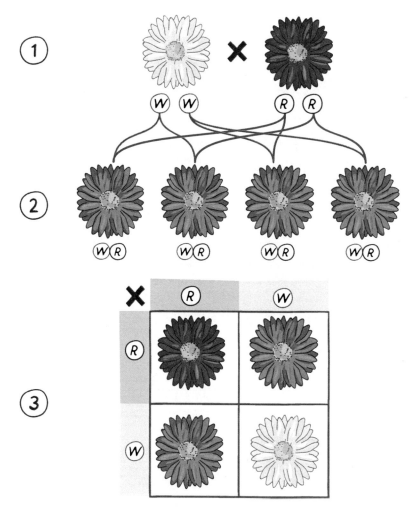

Figure 6B. Incomplete dominance

Other concepts complicate the relationship between a genotype and the associated phenotype. **Penetrance** refers to the likelihood that the carrier of a given genotype (most often associated with a dominant allele) will manifest the corresponding phenotype. An example is the presence of certain mutations in the *BRCA1* gene. A woman with a specific *BRCA1* mutation has an 80% risk of developing breast cancer over the course of her lifetime, meaning that the *BRCA1* mutation has 80% penetrance. The cause of differing penetrances among a population of a certain genotype is mechanistically complicated. In some cases, such as *BRCA1*, environmental factors most likely account for the 20% of women with *BRCA1* mutations who do not develop breast cancer. Other genes may also affect the penetrance of the mutated allele. Additionally, epigenetic modifications can affect gene expression, with potential impacts on penetrance.

Expressivity is a concept that may seem similar to penetrance, but is quite different. While penetrance refers to how often an allele is phenotypically expressed, expressivity refers to the intensity or extent of the phenotype. Another way to conceptualize these concepts is penetrance is a yes/no question (does an organism express a certain phenotype?) while expressivity is a shades-of-gray question (how much of an effect does an allele have on the phenotype?). For mutations associated with human disease, expressivity can be thought of as a condition's severity.

Now that we have these basic concepts in our toolkit, let's move on to take a closer look at specific inheritance patterns, on the level of genes, families, and communities.

2. Inheritance Patterns

A principle underlying Mendelian genetics that is easy to skip over is that alleles are randomly distributed among an organism's offspring. Meaning, there is no relationship between genes in terms of which alleles are inherited. Returning to Mendel's peas, let's imagine what happens if we look at a cross in terms of both pea shape (round vs. wrinkled) and color of the flower (purple vs. white), where *R* and *P* refer to the dominant traits of round shape and purple color, respectively. In this hypothetical experiment, we will cross heterozygotes for both traits. This is known as a **dihybrid cross**.

> **MCAT STRATEGY >>>**
>
> Whenever you're studying a topic that's heavy in terminology, do so with an eye towards how that terminology can be tested. In particular, note key words or phenomena that are associated with certain terms. For example, we could simplify the above outline as follows: codominance → both at once; incomplete dominance → blended; penetrance → do you show it?; expressivity → how much? Shorthand like that would not impress your biology professor, but the good news is that you don't have to. You just have to be able to select the right MCAT answer.

	RP	**Rp**	**rP**	**rp**
RP	RRPP *<round, purple>*	RRPp *<round, purple>*	RrPP *<round, purple>*	RrPp *<round, purple>*
Rp	RRPp *<round, purple>*	RRpp *<round, white>*	RrpP *<round, purple>*	Rrpp *<round, white>*
rP	rRPP *<round, purple>*	rRPp *<round, purple>*	rrPP *<wrinkled, purple>*	rrPp *<wrinkled, purple>*
rp	rRpP *<round, purple>*	rRpp *<round, white>*	rrPp *<wrinkled, purple>*	rrpp *<wrinkled, white>*

Figure 7. Dihybrid cross of pea plants for shape and flower color

This leads to a characteristic trait distribution of a dihybrid cross: 9/16 of the offspring will have the dual dominant phenotype (round, purple), 6/16 of the offspring will have one recessive trait (3/16 will be round and white and 3/16 will be wrinkled and purple), and only 1/16 will show the dual recessive phenotype. The 9:3:3:1 trait distribution for a dihybrid cross of two heterozygotes is important enough to memorize, but don't forget that a dihybrid cross with different genotypes would lead to different results. Therefore, you can always create a Punnett square to calculate the probabilities associated with a specific case.

When calculating the probabilities for the dihybrid cross, it is assumed that there is no link between inheritance of alleles of different genes. In Mendelian genetics, this is known as the **law of independent assortment.**

The law of independent assortment is grounded in molecular genetics. First, alleles of genes on different chromosomes will be inherited independently of each other, due to the random orientation of homologous pairs on the metaphase plate in meiosis. Recall that a eukaryote inherits both a maternal and paternal copy of each autosomal chromosome. Any generated offspring randomly inherit a chromosome copy from each parent. For example, a child may inherit her mother's paternal chromosome 23 and her father's maternal chromosome 23. This process occurs at random. However, independent assortment also applies to genes on the same chromosome due to crossing over, which scrambles the genome within a chromosome during meiosis I. Sometimes it can seem that genetic recombination is anomalous, but that's not actually the case; recombination among homologous chromosomes during prophase I is actually the rule, not the exception.

However, the formation of **chiasmata** (points of crossing over) on the chromosome occur largely at random. However, genes close together on the same chromosome are less likely to undergo recombination than genes that are further away from each other on the same chromosome. If genes are close enough to each other, this tendency can be strong enough to violate the law of independent assortment. This phenomenon is known as **linkage**, and the **recombination frequency (θ)** describes how often a single crossover will occur between two genes during meiosis. If the recombination frequency of two genes is 50%, then the genes obey the law of independent assortment.

The relationship between recombination frequency and distance between genes on a chromosome led to the scientific technique of using recombination frequency to map genes on a given chromosome. The distance associated with a 1% increment in the recombination frequency is known as a **centimorgan (cM)**.

However, we have to account for one more complication. So far, we've discussed a single crossover event between two genes, but **crossover** events are common, and it is possible for more than one to occur in the space between two genes. This event is known as a **double crossover**. The contrast between single and double crossovers is presented in Figure 8.

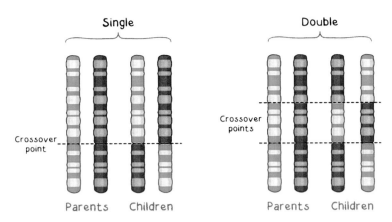

Figure 8. Single and double crossovers

In humans, autosomal dominant and recessive patterns of inheritance exist, as well as sex-linked patterns of inheritance. While you may remember **pedigree analysis** from your coursework in biology or genetics, it is not specifically listed as a required topic for the MCAT. However, pedigrees have appeared in some official AAMC materials, so you should be aware of them. The key principles of pedigrees are that: (1) individuals are arranged in rows that correspond to generations, with older generations at the top and younger generations at the bottom; (2) vertical connections indicate descent by birth, while horizontal connections indicate mating; (3) circles correspond to females and squares to males; and (4) individuals who manifest a certain phenotype have their respective circle or square shaded in. It is also necessary to know the different inheritance patterns and their respective distinctive features.

Autosomal patterns of inheritance are characterized by male and female offspring having an equal likelihood of inheriting a trait. Remember, though, in a family with a small sample size, the even distribution may not be immediately obvious. Just as it wouldn't be *that* remarkable to flip a coin four times and have it come up heads three times instead of two, it wouldn't be particularly unusual for an autosomal trait to manifest in, say, two out of three females and one out of three males. Recessive phenotypes are defined by their ability to skip generations, as we saw with the example of round and wrinkled pea shapes in the classic Mendelian example presented in Figure 2. **Dominant phenotypes** generally do not skip generations.

Recessive phenotypes *can* skip generations, but they do not have to. Imagine a cross between two pea plants with genotypes of *Rr* and *rr*: the recessive allele (*r*) is present in the parental generation, and we can predict that 50% of the offspring will also have the genotype *rr*, thereby expressing the recessive phenotype. However, the pattern of recessive phenotypes skipping generations is typical for genetics as presented on the MCAT, so keep this in mind when answering questions regarding pedigrees and inheritance patterns among families.

Sex-linked inheritance occurs in genes located on the X chromosome. Why not the Y chromosome? Over time, evolution has stripped the Y chromosome of virtually all protein-coding genes other than what is necessary for sex determination. The few genes present on the Y chromosome make Y-linked patterns of inheritance extremely rare. Therefore, for the purposes of the MCAT, **sex-linked is X-linked**.

X-linked inheritance patterns are characterized by males having a higher likelihood of inheriting a trait than females. Let's look at X-linked recessive alleles, because those are much more likely to appear on the MCAT than X-linked dominant alleles. Let's use the notation *X* to refer to a dominant, unaffected allele on the X chromosome and *X'* to refer to a recessive affected allele. Let's review a few possible outcomes of mating: (1) a heterozygote (carrier) female (genotype of *XX'*) with an unaffected male (*XY*), (2) a homozygous dominant (*XX*) female with an affected male (*X'Y*), and (3) a heterozygous female (*XX'*) with an affected male (*X'Y*). The corresponding Punnett squares are shown below in Figure 9, with the affected offspring shown in red and carriers in blue.

XX' female + XY male

	X	Y
X	XX	XY
X'	X'X	X'Y

XX female + X'Y male

	X'	Y
X	XX'	XY
X	XX'	XY

XX' female + X'Y male

	X'	Y
X	XX'	XY
X'	X'X'	X'Y

Figure 9. X-linked recessive inheritance

Females inherit one X chromosome from their mother and one X chromosome from their father, while males inherit their single X chromosome from their mother. As males only have one X chromosome, one recessive mutated allele will result in a recessive phenotype. In the case of X-linked recessive genetic diseases, affected male children can be born to a couple where neither parent has the recessive phenotype. However, it is much rarer for female children to be affected, as this only occurs when both the father is affected and the mother is a carrier. Our take-away here for the MCAT is X-linked recessive mutations are *much* more likely to affect male offspring.

With all of the above in mind, let's look at a flow chart for how to distinguish between autosomal dominant, autosomal recessive, and sex-linked patterns of inheritance.

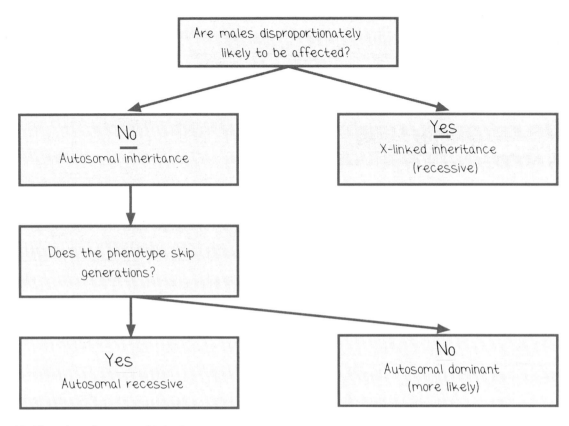

Figure 10. Flow chart for types of inheritance patterns

3. Population Genetics and Evolution

Next, let's zoom out to see how these concepts play out on a population level. To do so, we'll need to look at genetics from the perspective of evolution/natural selection. These concepts were first presented in Darwin's *Origin of Species* in 1859 and currently form the basis for much of modern biology. In the 1973 words of the evolutionary biologist Theodosius Dobzhansky, "nothing in biology makes sense except in the light of evolution."

Many misconceptions exist about **evolution**, and many of those misconceptions make studying evolution much more complex than it needs to be. An **evolutionary system** must have only three structural features: (1) **variations** in phenotypes of individuals of a population, (2) a mechanism for those variations to be passed between generations, and (3) environmental constraints that select for certain variations in traits over others, known as **differential reproduction**. Biological evolution is actually only one example of an evolutionary system. Evolutionary systems have been used in computer modeling and other fields, such as linguistics. In biology, requirement (1) is accounted for by genetic and phenotypic variations within the population. Requirement (2) is accounted for by sexual and asexual reproduction, and requirement (3) is accounted for by natural selection. The key point is that differential reproduction leads to selection for certain traits over time.

Natural selection is the tendency for certain traits to have a higher likelihood of being passed down to offspring or between generations due to environmental pressures. It is not the same thing as evolution. Rather, natural selection is the most common mechanism through which evolution takes place. Natural selection is closely linked to **fitness**, which in the evolutionary context *only* refers to the chance of reproduction associated with a certain phenotype. Fitness *must* be defined in terms of specific environmental constraints. Let's consider two types of bacteria: *Acetobacter aceti*, which grows best in a pH range of 5.4-6.3 and is used industrially to produce vinegar (acetic acid) from the ethanol contained in wine, and *Natronomonas pharaonis*, which likes salty and alkaline conditions (3.5 M

NaCl) of pH 8.5. We ask which bacterium is more fit—but that question does not make sense! The answer depends on the environment, because *A. aceti* grows and reproduces best in acidic conditions and *N. pharaonis* grows and reproduces best in salty, alkaline conditions. Asking which is more "fit" is like asking "which are better, sandals or rain boots?" Rain boots are better for cold rainy days, and sandals are better for a warm day at the beach. Fitness entirely depends on its context within an organism's environment.

MCAT STRATEGY >>>

Evolutionary theory is rarely directly tested on the MCAT, but it's worth investing some time in making sure that you have a clear conceptual foundation. This will help you avoid making mistakes or spending too much time on questions that deal with this topic indirectly. The concepts of evolution and fitness have a way of being relevant in experimental passages that primarily deal with other topics.

The classic Darwinian principles focuses on individual fitness, but many organisms live in groups. While humans form a truly exceptional case of group dynamics, it is common for group dynamics to play a major role in the life cycles of other animals. For example, group selection acts on the level of the group, not the individual. The related concept of **inclusive fitness** expands the rigorous evolutionary definition of fitness (defined in terms of the differential reproduction of traits) to account not just for individuals but their close relatives, who likely share many of the same alleles. This idea helps to explain **altruistic behavior**. From a genetic perspective, it can be advantageous for an individual to engage in altruistic behavior or even self-sacrifice to ensure the survival of similar genotypes in related individuals.

Note how we've switched our perspective from focusing on individual organisms to focusing on genotypes. This is a hallmark of modern genetics. The concept of the **gene pool**, which can be thought of as the combined set of all genotypes in a population, is often used to describe the genetic status of a population. In this framework, evolutionary success can be thought of as an increase in the representation of a certain allele within the gene pool.

Gene Pool

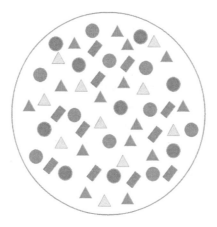

Figure 11. Gene pool

The **Hardy-Weinberg Equilibrium** is a concept used to model stable gene pools. For the Hardy-Weinberg equilibrium to apply to a population it must meet the following criteria:

1. Organisms must be diploid and reproduce sexually.

2. Mating is random.

3. The population size is very large.

4. Alleles are randomly distributed by sex.

5. No mutations occur.

6. There is no migration into or out of the population.

The Hardy-Weinberg equilibirum is hypothetical as no real population meets these criteria. So you may ask why we use this model. The Hardy-Weinberg equilibrium is an example of an analytical simplification that is useful for determining genotype and allele frequencies in a population. Furthermore, the Hardy-Weinberg equations allow us to use allele frequencies to predict the distribution of phenotypes in the population and vice versa. If p and q are the only two alleles of a gene present in the population, then $p + q = 1$. Think of 1 as being like 100% here (how it's used in probability). This equation is just a way of saying that the two alleles p and q account for the whole population. Where things get interesting is if you square the equation: $(p + q)^2 = 1^2 \rightarrow p^2 + 2pq + q^2 = 1$. This second equation allows us to connect genotypes and phenotypes, because the p^2 and q^2 terms correspond to individuals homozygous for p and q, respectively, while the $2pq$ term gives the frequency of heterozygotes. Let's work through an example problem.

Suppose that 9% of a population at Hardy-Weinberg equilibrium has a recessive phenotype. How many people are carriers? We're told that 9% of the population are homozygous recessive; this means that $q^2 = 0.09$, so q is therefore 0.3 (if that math seems tough, remember that 0.09 is 9/100, which makes the square root much easier). We can use the equation $p + q = 1$ to determine p from q. In this case, $p = 0.7$. The frequency of heterozygotes corresponds to $2pq$ or 2(0.7)(0.3), or 0.42. 42% of the population are carriers.

However, as mentioned, Hardy-Weinberg equilibrium often fails to apply perfectly to real-world populations, and exploring some exceptions to the Hardy-Weinberg assumptions can help illuminate some important dynamics in evolutionary biology.

First, selection can operate on the population level. Multiple distinct "types" of selection have been identified to describe the different outcomes associated with different types of selective pressures on phenotypes that vary along a spectrum. That is, some traits show variation along a spectrum, like height or weight. These traits are likely **polygenic**, where multiple genes collectively contribute to the trait. Let's imagine a phenotype such as height with values distributed on a bell curve throughout a population.

Stabilizing selection occurs if both extremes are selected against. For example, if very short and very tall individuals have lower reproductive fitness, the height of the population will be maintained within a tight range. **Directional selection** occurs if only one extreme phenotype is selected against and the other extreme is favored. Returning to our

MCAT STRATEGY >>>

You do need to be aware of all of these details, but don't get bogged down in them. Terms like "directional selection" are really red herrings in a certain sense: there is only one mechanism of selection, natural selection, but it can have different results depending on the external circumstances.

example of height, if for some reason very tall people are selected against, the population would become shorter. **Disruptive selection** occurs when the median phenotype is selected against. Darwin's observations of finches on the Galapagos Islands are a classic example of this. He noted that they had either large or small beaks, but no medium-sized beaks. He proposed that this was due to the size of the seeds they used for food, which were either large or small, such that a medium-sized beak would not be particularly useful. It should be noted that selection acts on phenotypes, NOT genotypes.

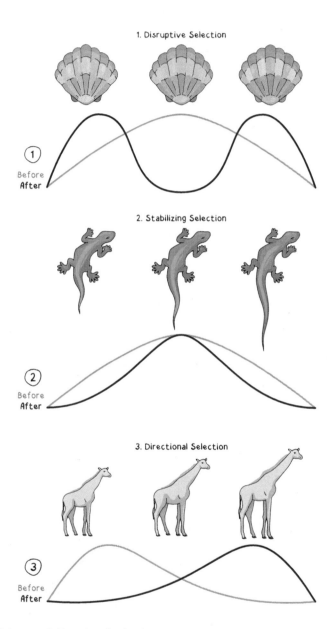

Figure 12. Disruptive, stabilizing, and directional selection

Other mechanisms are associated with changes in the gene pool of a species, such as genetic drift and bottlenecks. **Genetic drift** refers to the role of chance in determining the reproductive fitness of various alleles. In a population no strong pressure may exist for a certain allele, however random chance can cause the allele to increase or decrease in frequency within the population. Genetic drift can have huge effects on a population's evolution. A related, but more specific, concept is **evolutionary bottleneck**. Bottlenecks occur when some external event dramatically reduces the size of a population in a way that is essentially random. For example, a sudden flood wipes out 80% of a population—for the most part, survival will be random. It is possible for a non-representative subset of the gene pool to remain after a bottleneck, with implications for the future evolutionary history of the population. A real-world example is provided by the incidence of Tay-Sachs disease in Ashkenazi Jews (the population of Jews who historically lived in northern Europe). It is thought that Ashkenazi Jews experienced a major bottleneck early in their history, resulting in an unusually high prevalence in that community of Tay-Sachs disease, an autosomal recessive disorder that is fatal in young children.

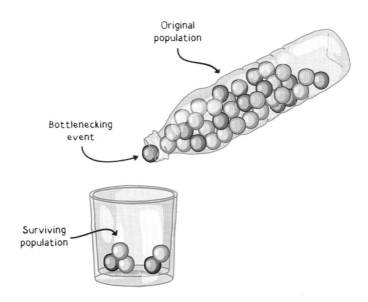

Figure 13. Bottlenecks can drastically affect allele frequencies

Speciation describes how a new species evolves. A species is defined as a group of organisms that can successfully breed to form fertile offspring. The presence of different selective pressures over time can lead to the emergence of new species. However, considerable phenotypic variation can exist within a single species. This is known as **polymorphism**. Examples of polymorphism abound throughout biology, but a helpful example to keep in mind is the ABO blood type in humans discussed earlier in this chapter. Organisms in specific environments may undergo processes of adaptation and specialization, in which certain individuals or subpopulations develop evolutionary strategies specific to certain microenvironments, or niches. These processes do not constitute speciation in and of themselves, but they can help set the stage for speciation. Inbreeding and outbreeding can also occur within populations. **Inbreeding** is breeding between genetically closely related individuals and can lead to the increased manifestation of recessive mutations and other deleterious effects. **Outbreeding**, on the other hand, refers to breeding among genetically distant members of a population.

Since differences between species are defined in terms of reproductive isolation, it is helpful to distinguish between prezygotic and postzygotic barriers to reproduction. **Prezygotic barriers** refer to anything that stops reproduction before the formation of a zygote. This includes occupying different ecological niches, having different patterns of breeding, not engaging in reproductive behavior with members of the other species, incompatible reproductive anatomy, or the inability for fertilization to occur after intercourse.

However, sometimes a zygote is formed, and **postzygotic barriers** describe various forms of reproductive isolation that can occur after a zygote forms. One simple way is for the zygote to simply be unable to develop to term. However, sometimes members of two different species can produce viable offspring. These offspring are known as **hybrids**. Mules are a common example: they are the offspring of a horse and a donkey, and are viable themselves but cannot produce offspring. This is known as **hybrid sterility**. It is also possible for hybrids to be fertile but for fertility to break down in the second generation in a process known as **hybrid breakdown**. On the level of the gene pool, genes can sometimes travel between species, in what is known as **leakage**.

Life has been present on Earth, and subjected to evolution, for a mind-bogglingly long time. The Earth is slightly over 4.6 billion years old, and the first traces of life date to approximately 3 billion years ago, although life may have existed even earlier. All living organisms on Earth, ranging from ourselves to the bacteria that colonize us, are thought to have derived from a single common ancestor due to the presence of many shared biochemical pathways across all forms of life. Eukaryotes are known to have evolved by approximately 2-2.7 billion years ago, and the earliest animal fossils are known from about 890 million years ago. Our species, *Homo sapiens sapiens,* is thought to have evolved approximately 200,000 years ago. You do not have to know these details for the MCAT, but it is useful to have a sense of the depth of evolutionary time and the fact that we are relative newcomers to the scene, so to speak.

Since random errors accumulate on the genome at a relatively fixed rate, the extent to which two genomes differ serves as a proxy for how long ago they had a shared common ancestor. Analytical techniques based on this insight have yielded tremendous results in evolutionary history. This so-called "**molecular clock**" can also be applied to help solve mysteries about emerging disease. Molecular-clock analyses have played a major role, for example, in attempts to determine how the human immunodeficiency virus (HIV; the virus that causes AIDS) originated and spread.

4. Must-Knows

> Phenotype = physical manifestation of a trait; genotype = the specific alleles that an individual carries per gene.

> Allele = specific variant of a given gene, such as round/wrinkled shape of peas.

> Dominant alleles only need one copy present for phenotype to occur. Recessive alleles manifest the corresponding phenotype if no dominant alleles are present.

> Homozygous = both alleles are the same; heterozygous = two different alleles are present.

> Phenotype ≠ genotype. Dominant phenotype can correspond to either homozygous dominant (*RR*) or heterozygous (*Rr*) genotypes.

> Test cross: dominant-phenotype individual crossed with recessive individual to determine phenotype.

> Codominance = two different alleles expressed at the same time (Example: human ABO blood type). Incomplete dominance = blended phenotype in heterozygotes (red × white snapdragon flowers → pink offspring).

> Law of independent assortment: inheritance of various genes not correlated with each other.

> Linkage: exception to independent assortment. Genes physically close to each other on the same chromosome tend to have their alleles inherited together. Recombination frequency can be used to map location of genes on chromosomes.

> Autosomal inheritance: on non-sex chromosomes. Sex-linked inheritance: for genes on X chromosome.

> Recessive inheritance is characterized by skipping generations. Dominant mutations generally do not skip generations.

> X-linked recessive traits affect more males than females because males only have one X chromosome.

> Hardy-Weinberg equilibrium: assumptions include (1) diploid sexual reproduction; (2) random mating; (3) large population; (4) random distribution of alleles by sex; (5) no mutations; (6) no migration. Leads to following equations for allele frequency: $p + q = 1$, $p^2 + 2pq + q^2 = 1$.

> Fitness is defined in terms of reproductive success.

> Speciation: formation of new species, defined by reproductive isolation (inability to produce fertile offspring).

> Stabilizing selection: extremes selected against, phenotype maintained within strict range. Directional selection: one extreme selected against, phenotype moves to the other end. Disruptive selection: middle selected against, population swings to favor both extremes.

> Accumulation of random changes in genome over time → "molecular clock" method of dating divergence from last common ancestor.

End of Chapter Practice

The best MCAT practice is **realistic**, with a focus on identifying steps for further improvement. For those reasons, we recommend completing practice questions in an online setting that simulates the real MCAT interface, and taking advantage of advanced analytic features to help you determine how best to move forward in your MCAT study journey.

With that in mind, **online end-of-chapter** questions for Biology, Biochemistry, Chemistry + Organic Chemistry, Physics, and Psychology/Sociology are available through your Blueprint MCAT account.

As a further supplement, given the importance of active learning for effective studying, we also suggest that you consult the Must-Knows at the end of each chapter as a basis for creating a study sheet, in which you list out key terms and test your ability to briefly summarize them.

This page left intentionally blank.

This page left intentionally blank.

Gene Expression, Biotechnology, and Laboratory Techniques

0. Introduction

In this chapter, we discuss gene expression, biotechnology, and laboratory techniques: three topics that are often treated separately, but actually form a coherent unit within modern biological research.

These topics are important for the MCAT for two main reasons. First, they are a predictable source of questions, usually in the Biological and Biochemical Foundations section. Second, these topics are regularly incorporated into modern biological research, so understanding them will yield major dividends in terms of improving your ability to understand passages about biological research quickly and accurately.

Fundamentally, gene expression refers to all the ways in which cells can regulate the transcription and translation of genes to produce more or less of certain products. It lies at the foundation of how organisms develop, how physiological systems respond to stimuli, and how systemic disorders emerge.

1. Gene Expression and Development

With regard to development, **gene expression** explains why virtually all cells within the human body contain the same genetic code, but have drastically different morphology and functionality. Complex signaling patterns throughout development induce **cell differentiation**, which explains how embryonic stem cells are able to differentiate into the diverse range of specialized cells present in the mature body.

Stem cells—undifferentiated cells that can differentiate into more specialized cells and reproduce through mitosis—are also present in adults. These are known as **somatic stem cells**, and come in a variety of types, with the following notable examples: **hematopoietic stem cells**, which differentiate into various types of blood cells; **intestinal stem cells**, which provide the basis for the constant renewal of the cells lining the surface of the intestines; and **mesenchymal stem cells**, which are capable of differentiating into a wide range of cell types, including adipocytes (fat cells), osteoblasts, and chondrocytes. For the MCAT, you don't need to memorize the different somatic stem cell types, but it is useful to be aware of their existence and general functions.

Stem cells can be classified along a potency scale. **Totipotent cells** are able to differentiate into any any human cell type; in humans, this applies only to the zygote through the stage of the morula. **Pluripotent cells** are able to differentiate into any of the three germ layers (ectoderm, mesoderm, and endoderm), and can be obtained from the internal cell mass of the blastocyst. Adult stem cells are **multipotent**, which refers to the ability to differentiate into several types of cells within a relatively limited functional scope. You may also encounter the term **oligopotent**, which refers to a stem cell that can only derive into a few, closely-related types of cells (Greek oligo- = "few").

Research is currently being conducted into the clinical application of stem cells as treatment for various conditions. Totipotent stem cells have attracted particular interest due to their ability to differentiate into the broadest range of cell types, but ethical dilemmas have arisen from the fact that such stem cells are only found in embryos. For this reason, interest has emerged in the possibility of converting multipotent stem cells found in adults into pluripotent or totipotent cells. Although the clinical applicability of these techniques remains to be established, stem cell research is a fascinating and promising domain of potential future therapeutic strategies.

A final point regarding gene expression and development is the importance of properly regulated apoptosis in development. Although **apoptosis** (programmed cell death) may sound like a negative phenomenon, it plays a fundamental role in proper development as well as maintaining health. In embryonic development, apoptosis plays a major role in defining the boundaries of organs and tissues. A common example of this is in the developing human embryo, where fingers and toes are initially linked by the cells in those structures is what allows fingers and toes to become separate by the time of birth. The pathways regulating apoptosis are complicated, but common causes of apoptosis include failure for a cell to pass the appropriate mitotic checkpoints, cell-internal signaling after mitochondrial dysfunction, and lysosomes bursting (autolysis). Apoptosis also occurs as a response to external signaling pathways that may be misregulated in various disease processes.

MCAT STRATEGY >>>

On one hand, the topic of stem cells is likely to be evaluated by relatively simple questions on their basic definition, degrees of potency, or embryonic versus adult stem cells. On the other hand, though, it's helpful to be aware of the bigger picture regarding stem cells because they could be discussed in a passage, at which point already having a general familiarity with the topic can save you valuable time and mental energy on the exam.

2. Gene Expression in Prokaryotes

For the purposes of the MCAT, gene expression in prokaryotes is synonymous with the concept of the **operon** and the MCAT expects you to be familiar with its workings. If necessary, take some time to review basic facts about prokaryotes (Chapter 2) and the molecular machinery of gene expression (Chapter 3).

Operons are important because they are relatively simple and mechanistic systems that allow a bacterium to respond to changes in its environment by increasing or decreasing the expression of certain genes as appropriate. Operons can be under positive or negative control. In **negative control**, a **repressor** prevents transcription by binding to the operator (a sequence upstream of the first protein-coding region), while in **positive control**, an **activator** stimulates transcription. The classic examples that the MCAT is likely to test you on, the *lac* **operon** and the *trp* **operon**, both involve negative control, but differ in that the *lac* operon is inducible and the *trp* operon is repressible. In a negative inducible operon, the repressor is normally present and the genes are not expressed except under specific conditions. In a negative repressible operon, the genes are usually transcribed, but transcription can be halted by binding of the repressor in appropriate conditions.

The *lac* **operon** was discovered in *Escherichia coli*, but its principles have been subsequently found more broadly in prokaryotes. The basic idea is that *E. coli* has the ability to metabolize glucose, while the *lac* operon gives *E. coli* the ability to metabolize lactose if lactose is present. However, expressing the proteins necessary to metabolize lactose is energetically expensive. Therefore, it is advantageous for *E. coli* to express that cellular machinery only when lactose is present, and even more so, when lactose is present but glucose is absent. The *lac* operon allows *E. coli* to do just that.

>> CONNECTIONS <<

Chapter 2 and Chapter 3 of Biology

The *lac* operon is presented below in Figure 1. The sequences *lacZ, lacY,* and *lacA* are protein-encoding regions necessary for lactose metabolism. The **operator region** is located upstream of those coding sequences and the **promoter region** is located upstream of the operator. The **catabolite activator protein (CAP)** binding sequence is located upstream of the promoter. When no lactose is present, the repressor is bound to the operator and prevents RNA polymerase from transcribing the structural genes.

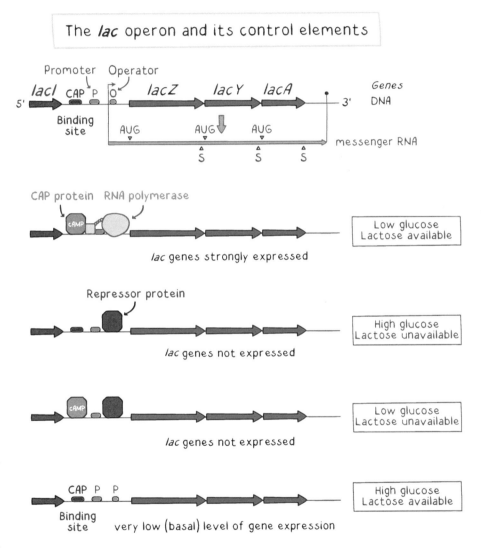

Figure 1. The *lac* operon

When lactose is present, its isomer, allolactose binds with the repressor, dissociating it from the operator. This allows RNA polymerase to transcribe the structural genes. At this point, *E. coli* now has the ability to metabolize lactose. However, in prokaryotic metabolism, just as in life, just because you can doesn't mean that you should! As we mentioned above, there is an energetic cost involved in metabolizing lactose, so it is not advantageous to metabolize lactose if ample glucose is present. This is where CAP comes in. If glucose is low, cellular levels of cyclic adenosine monophosphate (cAMP) are high. cAMP binds to CAP, inducing it to bind to the **CAP binding sequence**. When it does so, CAP promotes elevated transcription of the *lac* structural genes. This is an example of positive control; thus, the *lac* operon is under both negative and positive control.

Table 1 below summarizes the structure and function of the *lac* operon in various environmental conditions.

LACTOSE?	GLUCOSE?	REPRESSOR	CAP	OUTCOME
N	Y	Bound to operator	Absent	No lactose metabolism
Y	Y	Released from operator	Absent	Weak lactose metabolism
Y	N	Released from operator	Binds to CAP binding sequence	Strong lactose metabolism

Table 1: Structure and function of the *lac* operon

The *lac* operon is the most famous example of an operon, but you should also be aware of the **trp operon**, which contains genes for the synthesis of tryptophan. However, it is energetically unfavorable for these genes to be expressed if tryptophan is present. When tryptophan is absent, the repressor does not bind to the operator, and tryptophan synthesis proceeds. However, when tryptophan is present, it binds to the repressor protein and causes it to bind to the operator, thereby inhibiting synthesis. As transcription is not repressed by default (as in the case of the *lac* operon), but can be induced by environmental conditions, the *trp* operon is considered to be an example of an repressible negative operon.

When tryptophan is present, the trp repressor
binds the operator, and RNA synthesis is blocked

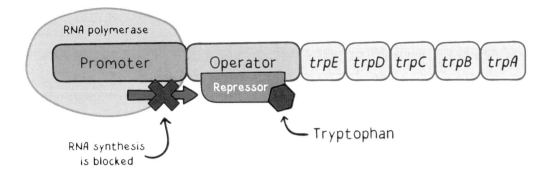

In the absence of tryptophan, the repressor dissociates
from the operator, and RNA synthesis proceeds

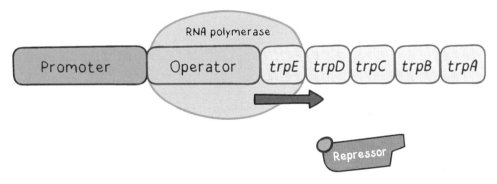

Figure 2. The *trp* operon

3. Gene Expression in Eukaryotes

The regulation of gene expression in eukaryotes is much more complicated than in prokaryotes. For prokaryotes, the MCAT expects you to be able to use the operon model to explain how organisms react to specific stimuli (e.g., the presence or absence of lactose or tryptophan). In contrast, for eukaryotes, it is necessary to be aware of diverse mechanisms that play a role in the regulation of gene expression in response to diverse stimuli and signaling cascades.

First, let's look at regions upstream of the protein-coding elements of a given gene. The main objective is for the transcriptional machinery to identify the right place to start transcription, and to do so in a way that can be regulated. The first step in this process involves sequences of base pairs present in the genome. Upstream regions of DNA where transcription initiates are known as **promoters**. In eukaryotes, many promoters are characterized by specific highly-conserved gene sequences. The TATA box is located approximately 30 base pairs upstream of the coding sequence, while the GC box and CAAT box are located around 60-150 base pairs upstream of the TATA box. These sequences are named for their characteristic base pair sequences (5'-TATAAA-3', 5'-GGGCGG-3', and 5'-GGCCAATCT-3' for the TATA, GC, and CAAT boxes respectively), and their function is to bind to proteins that help recruit RNA polymerase to initiate transcription. For example, the TATA box binds the TATA-binding protein

(TBP), which, in association with some other proteins, comprises a transcription factor that contributes to the binding of RNA polymerase.

In general, **transcription factors** are proteins that regulate expression by binding to a specific DNA sequence through what is termed a DNA-binding domain. Once bound to a sequence of DNA, transcription factors can recruit other regulatory proteins, such as proteins that play a role in acetylation or methylation, discussed below.

In addition to promoters, the eukaryotic genome contains **enhancers**, which increase gene expression of certain genes in response to the particular stimuli. Unlike promoters, enhancers do not have to be located in close proximity to the coding region of the gene. Typically, they may be considerably further upstream than promoters. However, enhancers have been found both upstream and downstream of the coding region, including many base pairs away. Given the tremendous diversity of enhancers, how do they upregulate expression? To answer this question, it is helpful to think three-dimensionally. Enhancers bind transcription factors that twist DNA into a hairpin loop, bringing distant regions into close proximity to each other. These transcription factors may be specific with regard to certain signaling elements. For example, estrogen binds with a nuclear estrogen receptor (ERα or ERβ), which then binds with enhancers (known as estrogen response elements) in the genome to modify transcription.

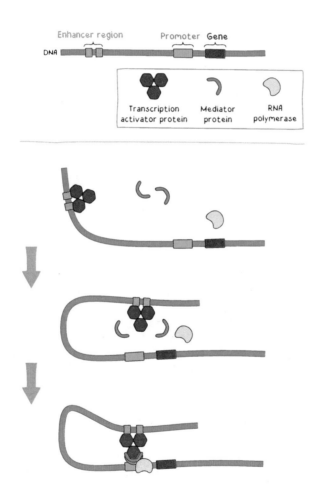

Figure 4. Enhancer region

Silencers are the opposite of enhancers in eukaryotic cells; they are regions of DNA to which transcription factors known as repressors bind. As the name indicates, repressors inhibit the transcription of the gene that they target. However, silencers have been discovered more recently than enhancers, so their function has not been characterized in as much detail.

Another mechanism of increasing the expression of a gene is to duplicate it on the chromosome. Across generations, this can result from sequential mutations, with potential long-term effects on the genome. The duplication of oncogenes is frequently observed in cancer cells, a phenomenon that is linked to the dysregulation of repair mechanisms in cancer cells.

In order for transcription factors to function and for transcription to take place, the relevant molecules must be able to access the DNA. DNA is packaged around **histones**, which are then packaged either densely to form **heterochromatin** or loosely in a "beads on a string" structure to form **euchromatin**. Heterochromatin appears dark under the microscope and is associated with transcriptional inactivity because the DNA is packaged too densely for transcription to take place. In contrast, the less dense structure of euchromatin appears light under the microscope and is associated with transcriptional activity.

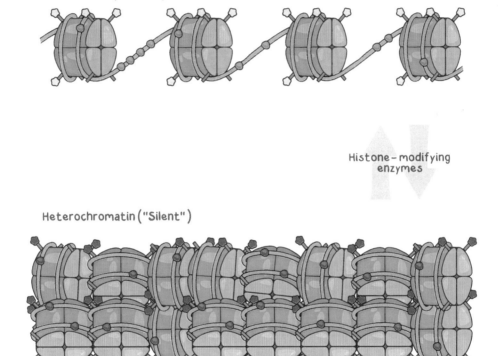

Euchromatin ("Active")

Histone-modifying enzymes

Heterochromatin ("Silent")

Figure 5. Euchromatin and heterochromatin

Certain transcription factors, known as **histone acetyltransferases**, can modify histone structure. As the name implies, histone acetyltransferases transfer acetyl groups from acetyl-CoA to lysine residues on histones. This makes histones less positively charged, weakening their ability to interact with the highly negatively-charged phosphate groups on DNA. This in turn results in a looser wrapping pattern that allows other transcription factors to access the genome more easily. For this reason, acetylation increases transcription. Correspondingly, histone

MCAT STRATEGY >>>

Gene expression in eukaryotes involves a tremendously detailed regulatory apparatus. Focus on the essentials to help you memorize the details. Recall that a cell *must* be able to respond to stimuli by producing more or less of the product of various genes, and then work backwards to figure out the general kinds of functionality (e.g., promoters and enhancers) necessary to do that.

deacetylases remove acetyl groups, which makes the interactions between histones and DNA stronger, reducing transcriptional activity.

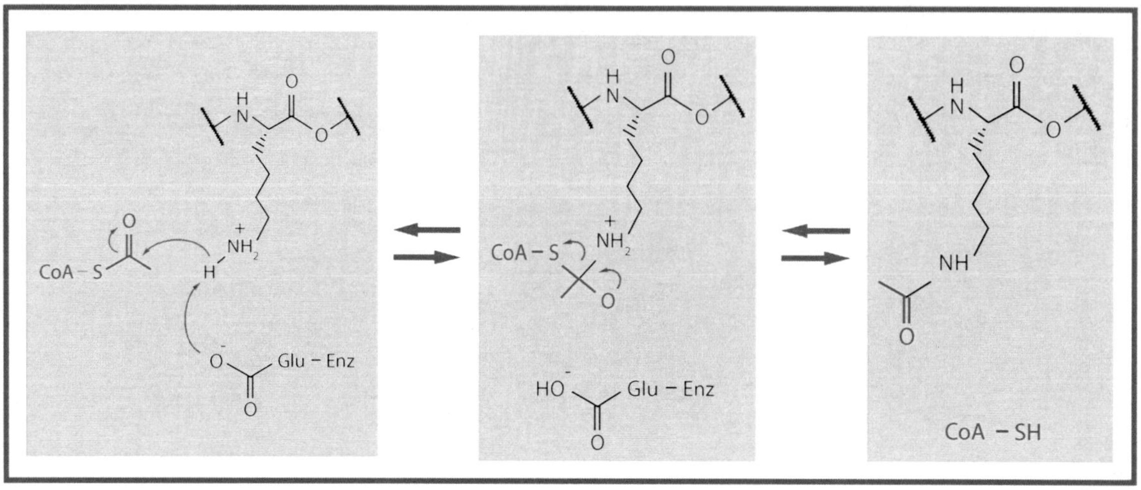

Figure 6. Acetylation of lysine

Figure 6 shows the acetylation of a lysine residue, which is a typical part of histone acetylation. In the context of this chapter, don't worry too much about the mechanism (although it may make sense to revisit this once you have studied organic chemistry mechanisms), but note that the positive charge in lysine is lost.

Gene expression is also affected by **DNA methylation**, in which a methyl group is added to cytosine or adenine nucleotides. Methylation is currently the focus of intense ongoing research because its function is not fully understood. However, it is thought to play a role in processes as diverse as embryonic development, aging, and cancer. For the MCAT, you should be aware that methylation is generally thought to deactivate genes. As shown in Figure 7, methylation can also be the trigger for processes such as the deamination of 5-methylcytosine to result in thymine, which would constitute a point mutation in the DNA code.

MCAT STRATEGY >>>

It's worth taking some time to slowly and carefully walk through why acetylation can increase transcription, because this is an instance where a very low-level property (intermolecular attractions between oppositely-charged molecules) has very high-level effects. Connections like that are MCAT favorites.

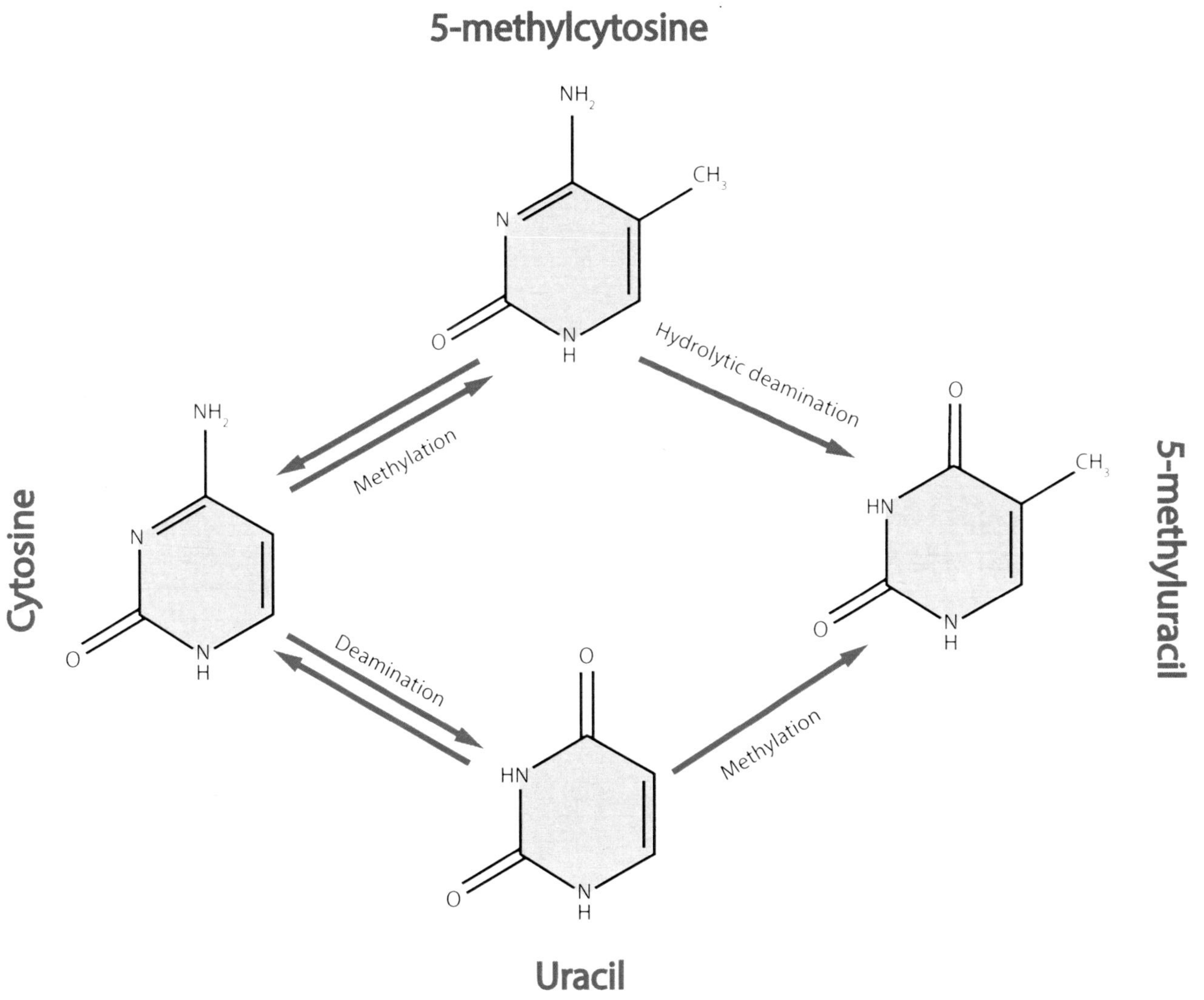

Figure 7. DNA methylation.

Methylation also plays a major role in the phenomenon known as **epigenetics**, which refers to inheritable phenotypic changes involving mechanisms other than the alteration of the genome itself. For example, a 2011 study found altered methylation patterns in the glucocorticoid receptor in adolescents whose mothers experienced intimate partner violence during pregnancy. A 2014 study found that prediabetes in fathers increased the susceptibility of their offspring to diabetes due to methylation changes in gametes. This is an area of ongoing research that the MCAT will not expect you to be responsible for in detail, but it could potentially appear in passages, so a general familiarity with the concept may pay off on Test Day.

In addition to regulatory proteins and the covalent modification of histones and DNA through acetylation and methylation, **non-coding RNA** plays a role in gene expression. The category of non-coding RNA refers to any RNA that is not translated into a protein, with a familiar example being **transfer RNA (tRNA)**. An exciting line of research in the last 20 years has identified a role for non-coding RNA in the suppression of gene expression through the degradation of mRNA sequences before translation. Two categories of such non-coding RNA are **small interfering RNA (siRNA)** and **microRNA (miRNA)**. miRNA and siRNA both silence genes by interrupting expression between transcription and translation.

Although the MCAT in general does not expect you to be aware of the details regarding the pathogenesis of various diseases, there are a few exceptions to this. **Cancer** is one of those diseases. In particular you should be aware of cancer as a disease in which gene expression is abnormal. Let's step back and review the steps involved in oncogenesis, or the development of cancer.

A **tumor** describes any abnormal proliferation of cells; **benign tumors** remain localized, whereas **malignant tumors** can invade other organs and tissues and spread to distant sites in the body in a process called metastasis. The first step in oncogenesis, **tumor initiation**, involves changes that allow a single cell to proliferate abnormally. This means that the cell must develop the ability to bypass regulatory steps of the cell cycle that normally help to restrain mitotic proliferation. **Tumor progression** occurs as a cell develops the ability to proliferate even more aggressively, as its descendants are preferentially selected for and come to predominate the growing tumor. In addition, malignant cells often undergo mutations allowing them to secrete growth factors to stimulate their own growth. These include proteases that digest components of the extracellular matrix and favor **metastasis**, and growth factors that promote the formation of new blood vessels to feed the growing tumor (angiogenesis).

Oncogenesis is associated with mutations that occur by random chance (and elude the normal DNA repair machinery in the cell) or as a result of mutagenic compounds known as **carcinogens**. These mutations alter the functionality of crucial genes in the cell. However, oncogenesis is also associated with dysregulation of gene expression, as abnormally elevated expression of genes involved in growth and proliferation can help contribute to the development of a tumor. Additionally, miRNA activity is abnormal in cancerous cells, further pointing to the importance of gene expression in oncogenesis. Moreover, compounds known as **tumor promoters** help induce the growth of proliferative cells by stimulating the activity of proteins involved in growth and division.

The genes involved in oncogenesis can be divided into **oncogenes** and **tumor suppressor genes**. The basic difference between them is that oncogenes function to promote abnormal growth and proliferation while tumor suppressor genes function to prevent tumorigenic properties.

Oncogenes were first identified based on studies of cancer-causing viruses, known as **tumor viruses**. One example of a tumor virus is the hepatitis B virus, which can cause liver cancer. Many tumor viruses contain retroviral oncogenes, which are reverse-transcribed into the DNA of infected cells. These oncogenes (such as *RAS, RAF,* and *SRC*) often encode proteins that are key components of signaling pathways that stimulate cell proliferation. Tumor viruses, including viruses with DNA genomes (i.e., non-retroviruses), can also induce cancer by hindering the correct function of tumor suppressor genes or promoting the function of oncogenes.

Oncogenes also play a role in driving tumorigenesis in cells that have not been infected with a tumor virus. Genes that function as oncogenes after mutation or inappropriately elevated expression are known as **proto-oncogenes**. Broadly speaking, oncogenes can be classified as genes coding for growth factors, receptor tyrosine kinases (examples include epidermal growth factor receptor [EGFR] and platelet-derived growth factor receptor [PDGFR]), cytoplasmic protein kinases (examples include the Src family and the Raf family), transcription factors (Myc), and regulatory GTPases (the Ras family). Kinases are crucially involved in transducing signals involved in activating cell growth and differentiation, while regulatory GTPases such as the Ras family are likewise involved in signaling in a major growth/differentiation pathway.

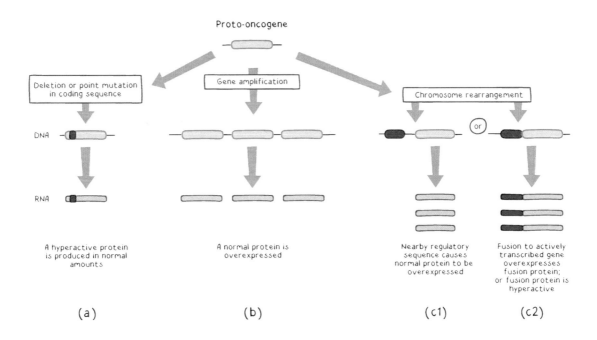

Figure 8. Transition from a proto-oncogene to an oncogene.

As the name suggests, **tumor suppressor genes** inhibit oncogenesis when properly functioning. Mutation-induced dysfunction in these genes means that a cell will not be able to protect itself against oncogenesis as effectively. The major functions of tumor suppressor genes include repressing the expression of genes that are essential for the cell cycle to progress (because uncontrolled cell cycle progression is dangerous), ensuring that the cell responds appropriately to DNA damage detected at cell cycle checkpoints (stopping the cell cycle for repair or inducing apoptosis, as necessary), repairing DNA damage, as well as preventing the changes in adhesion and proliferation involved in metastasis. An important tumor supressor gene to be aware of is the *TP53* gene, which encodes the p53 protein involved in responding appropriately to cell damage, because it is implicated in more than half of all human cancers. Additionally, mutations in the *BRCA* genes, which are responsible for repairing and responding to DNA damage, are associated with dramatically increased risks of breast and ovarian cancer. In many families, these mutations are hereditary, which has led to *BRCA* testing becoming one of the best-known examples of genetic screening.

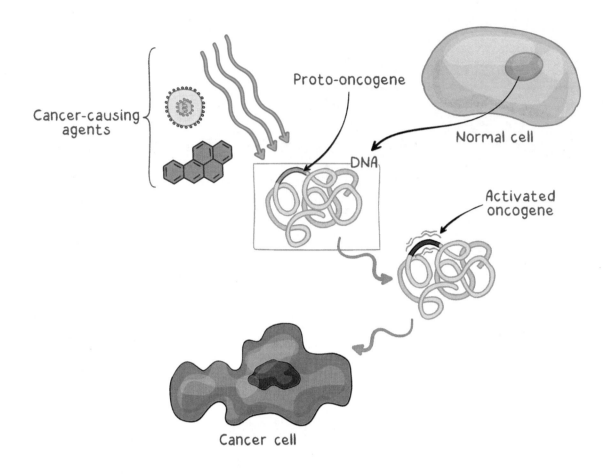

Figure 9. Oncogenesis

The range of mechanisms involved in eukaryotic gene expression is complicated, but for the MCAT, it is really only necessary to be able to associate a given regulatory element with a simple response of "on" (upregulation of target genes through increased expression) or "off" (downregulation of target genes through decreased expression). Table 2 summarizes the components of eukaryotic gene regulation that we have discussed.

ELEMENT	WHAT IS IT?	UPREGULATE OR DOWNREGULATE?
Enhancer	DNA sequence	Upregulate
Silencer	DNA sequence	Downregulate
Transcription factors	Regulatory proteins	Both
Acetylation	Covalent modification of histones	Upregulate
Methylation	Covalent modification of nucleotides	Downregulate
siRNA, miRNA	Non-coding RNA sequences	Downregulate

Table 2. Effects of elements involved in eukaryotic gene expression

4. Recombinant DNA

The creation and application of recombinant DNA is one of the most significant accomplishments in biotechnology over the last 40 years. For the MCAT, you are expected to be aware of the basic mechanisms involved in such research.

The discovery of **restriction enzymes**, also known as **restriction endonucleases**, paved the way for the development of recombinant DNA technologies. In nature, they occur in prokaryotes. These enzymes act as a defense system against invading viruses by cleaving DNA at specific **recognition sites**, which are made up of 4 to 8 base pair sequences. These recognition sites usually involve some degree of symmetry, as reflected by palindromic sequences. These **palindromic sequences** often involve inverted repeats, in which the palindrome is reflected diagonally across the plane of symmetry created by drawing a vertical line through the middle of the recognition site. In other words, the 5'→3' sequences on each strand are the same. When a restriction enzyme cleaves a DNA sequence vertically across the recognition site, the resulting fragments have "blunt" ends, whereas "sticky" ends result from restriction enzymes that cleave a DNA sequence in a zig-zag fashion. Restriction enzymes can cleave DNA either within the recognition site or at some distance from it.

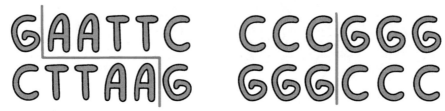

Figure 10. Restriction enzymes and blunt/sticky ends

Restriction enzymes are so important because they generate fragments that can be "tied" back together by DNA ligase without necessarily respecting the original location of the sequences. For example, if you put a sequence of human DNA and a sequence of pig DNA in a Petri dish, digest the sequences with a restriction enzyme, and then treat the fragments with DNA ligase, you will get sequences of human + human DNA, pig + pig DNA, and human + pig DNA. This process is known as **recombination**.

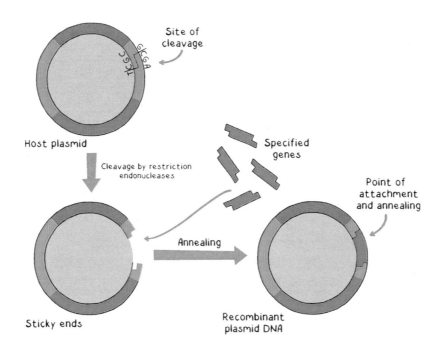

Figure 11. Generation of recombinant DNA using sticky ends

However, for recombinant DNA to be useful, it is essential to be able to recombine novel DNA sequences in significant quantities. To do this, researchers use **vectors**, which are DNA molecules used to carry genetic material into a cell where it can be replicated or expressed. Two main types of vectors are used: plasmids and bacteriophages (viruses that infect bacteria).

Plasmids are short circular DNA molecules that can replicate independently in bacteria. Recombinant plasmids carrying human DNA inserts can be introduced into *E. coli*, where they replicate along with the bacteria to yield millions of copies of plasmid DNA. The DNA of these plasmids can then be isolated, generating large quantities of recombinant molecules containing a single fragment of human DNA. The fragment can then be easily isolated from the rest of the vector DNA by restriction endonuclease digestion and gel electrophoresis, allowing a pure fragment of human DNA to be analyzed and further manipulated. In order to generate recombinant plasmids, human DNA and plasmid DNA are digested with the appropriate restriction enzymes, and then DNA ligase is used for re-sealing. Some human DNA strands re-link together, as do some plasmid DNA strands, but some novel human-plasmid recombinant DNA strands emerge from this process as well.

The next step in the process is to treat *E. coli* cells with the plasmid/DNA mixture. This generates a diverse set of bacteria: some do not take up any plasmids, some take up non-recombinant plasmids, and some take up recombinant plasmids. How do we distinguish between these outcomes? Scientists employ two main techniques. First, plasmids used for genetic engineering generally contain **antibiotic resistance genes**. Treatment with an antibiotic can kill off *E. coli* cells that did not take up any plasmids and therefore only the cells with plasmids remain. The next step is to distinguish between non-recombinant and recombinant plasmids. This can be done through what is known as a **reporter gene**. A reporter gene codes for a product that creates an obvious phenotypic change (such as a change in color) and contains recognition sites for the restriction enzyme that is used in the restriction. This means that *E. coli*

cells with non-recombinant plasmids will express the reporter gene normally, while *E. coli* cells with recombinant plasmids will not, allowing them to be distinguished and sub-cultured. The key features of plasmids used in genetic engineering are presented in Table 3.

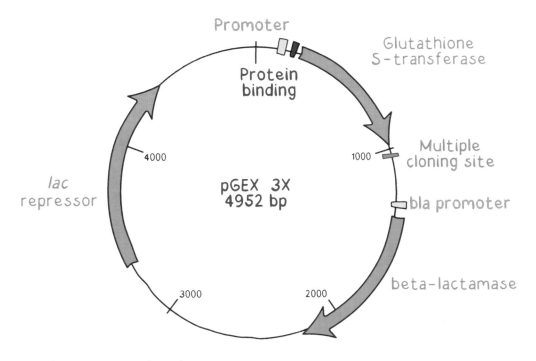

Figure 12. Recombinant DNA in a plasmid vector

FEATURE	FUNCTION
Origin of replication	Interacts with host cell DNA polymerase to initiate replication
Restriction site	Recognition site for a restriction enzyme to cleave DNA
Antibiotic resistance gene	Allows selection of bacteria that have taken up the plasmid
Reporter gene	Distinguishes bacteria with recombinant plasmids from those with non-recombinant plasmids

Table 3. Key elements of plasmids and their functions

Plasmids are not the only vector used for cloning DNA sequences. One limitation of standard *E. coli* plasmids is size, as these plasmids generally contain 2-4 kb of DNA. **Bacteriophage λ** vectors can be used for sequences as large as 15 kb. Additionally, even larger sequences can be transferred using bacteriophage P1 vectors. The principle of bacteriophage vectors is similar to that of plasmid vectors; the major difference is that bacteriophage vectors work by stripping out non-essential genes to carry recombinant sequences.

RNA sequences can also be cloned, through the generation of **complementary DNA (cDNA)**. The first step is to synthesize a DNA copy of the RNA using the enzyme reverse transcriptase. The DNA product is called cDNA because it is complementary to the template RNA. cDNA can then be ligated to vector DNA in the manner previously discussed. Since eukaryotic genes are usually interrupted by noncoding sequences, which are removed from mRNA by splicing, the ability to clone cDNA as well as genomic DNA has been critical for understanding gene structure and function. Additionally, cDNA cloning allows the mRNA corresponding to a single gene to be isolated as a molecular clone. DNA libraries, both of genomic DNA and cDNA, have been developed to allow researchers access to the DNA fragments that interest them in their research.

Plasmid vectors are useful both for amplifying DNA sequences for subsequent analysis and for generating large amounts of the products of the genes of interest. For instance, for approximately the last 30 years, insulin used as a treatment of diabetes has been synthesized using recombinant bacterial plasmids. Incorporating recombinant DNA for insulin into colonies of bacteria allow tremendous amounts of insulin to be generated in a cost-efficient and scalable manner.

Recombinant DNA technology is also widely used in modern research to help elucidate the function of various genes. One common way of doing this is to use **transgenic** or **knockout organisms**. In general, transgenic is a term that refers to any organism whose genome has been modified. This can be done for practical purposes, as in the case of genetically engineered organisms in agriculture, or to elucidate the function of genes. Knockout organisms are those in which one or more genes have been disabled. The goal of such research is to compare the functionality of organisms without a functioning copy of a given gene with that of wild-type organisms in order to obtain more information about the function of a gene. The MCAT will not expect you to be aware of the extended process involved in generating lineages of knockout organisms, but you may be presented with a passage presenting the results of research conducted into knockout organisms. Knockout models of thousands of human diseases have been created, and are a fundamental component of modern biomedical research.

5. Biotechnology: Applications and Ethics

Advances in biotechnology have been applied in several fields, ranging from medicine to pharmacology, forensics, remediation of pollution, and agriculture. The medical applications of DNA technology include the development of relatively widespread and cheap DNA screening techniques which allow individuals to undergo genetic screening to assess their risk of certain disorders. **Gene therapy** is another promising subject of ongoing research and involves splicing a functional allele into the cells of a patient with nonfunctional alleles. This would theoretically allow the effective treatment of currently devastating genetic disorders, but generally has yet to emerge beyond the research stage. DNA technology has also been widely applied in pharmacology. Of particular note, many substances crucial for medical treatment are now produced by recombinant bacteria, such as insulin, tumor necrosis factor, interferons, and components of vaccines. To give a sense of how dramatic a transformation this was, consider that until the 1980s, insulin used to treat diabetics was harvested from pig pancreases!

Biotechnology has also been used in the field of forensics, with DNA analysis used to identify the perpetrators and survivors of various crimes. Additionally, DNA technology revolutionized agriculture, with the development of **genetically engineered strains of crops** that have the ability to be pesticide-resistant, grow in a wider range of conditions, and even contain nutrients that are otherwise unavailable (an example of this is golden rice, which was engineered to contain beta-carotene). However, the use of genetically engineered crops has also been the source of considerable controversy, with concerns being raised about issues including the impact of genetic engineering on food security, the loss of biodiversity, food allergies, consumer safety, and other unintended effects.

Ethical concerns have also been raised regarding **stem cell therapy**, particularly regarding the use of embryonic stem cells, which must be obtained from embryos. In 2001, President George W. Bush implemented a policy restricting federal funding to research on pre-existing human embryonic stem cell lines, although some of those restrictions were removed by President Barack Obama in 2009 via an executive order. Complicated state laws exist regarding stem cells as well. These ethical and legal concerns are part of the reason why so much excitement has accompanied the research into reprogramming adult stem cells to become pluripotent, as discussed in Section 1.

> **MCAT STRATEGY >>>**
>
> Considerations regarding the ethics and applications of DNA technology may seem peripheral, but they have explicitly been identified as testable content by the AAMC, so be sure to have a general sense of the issues.

6. Laboratory Techniques

Along with the spectacular range of applications of biotechnology is a set of important laboratory techniques that you must be aware of for the MCAT. As we saw with recombinant DNA technology, these techniques may be the topic of specific questions, but they are especially likely to occur in passages. Therefore, it is necessary to understand these techniques in order to intepret the data presented in a passage.

Gel electrophoresis is a technique used to separate and analyze nucleic acids (DNA and RNA) by size and charge. The principle of gel electrophoresis is to suspend charged macromolecules in an agarose gel and apply an electric field by applying a positive charge (anode) at one end and a negative charge (cathode) at another end. Note that the anode is positively charged and the cathode is negatively charged in an electrophoresis apparatus because this is an electrolytic cell, not a galvanic cell. Macromolecules will move in response to the charge, but their movement through the gel is affected by size—smaller molecules move more quickly and larger molecules move more slowly. Nucleic acids have such a high degree of negative charge due to the presence of many phosphate groups that they will migrate away from the negatively charged cathode and towards the positively charged anode. Following electrophoresis, the DNA is stained with a fluorescent dye and photographed. Molecular-weight size markers, also known as **ladders**, are fragments with known sizes that can be run parallel to the DNA of interest in an electrophoresis experiment to identify the approximate size of the DNA fragments being analyzed.

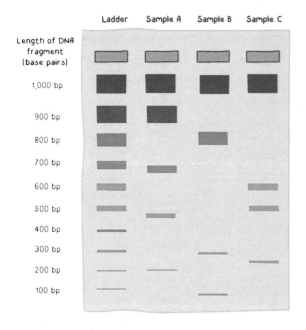

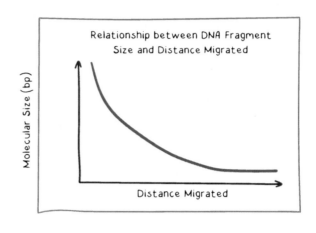

Figure 13. Gel electrophoresis of DNA, with a ladder

>> CONNECTIONS <<

Chapter 5 of Biochemistry

MCAT STRATEGY >>>

If you have ever worked in a lab and performed this technique as part of real-world molecular biology research, you will be aware that the actual processes involved in performing hybridization—or many other of the techniques discussed in this chapter—are more complicated than presented here. However, the MCAT only expects you to be aware of the basic principles of these techniques: what they use, the basic mechanisms involved, and what kind of results they provide.

Another key technique in genetics research is **hybridization**, which refers to the ability of single-strand DNA (or RNA) to join with complementary base pair sequences. The fact that DNA strands can be split ("melted") at elevated temperatures means that single-strand DNA can be generated easily under laboratory conditions, at which point the principle of hybridization can be used in several different ways. As discussed below, hybridization is an important step in **polymerase chain reaction (PCR)**. It can also be used to identify target sequences by using a **hybridization probe**, which is a specific DNA or RNA fragment that can be labeled radioactively. If the fragment is added to a sample of DNA or RNA studied and the sample is heated to generate single-strand DNA or RNA, then the single-stranded radiolabeled probes will anneal with complementary sequences. Analysis of the radiolabeling can then determine the presence of the sequence of interest in the DNA that is tested.

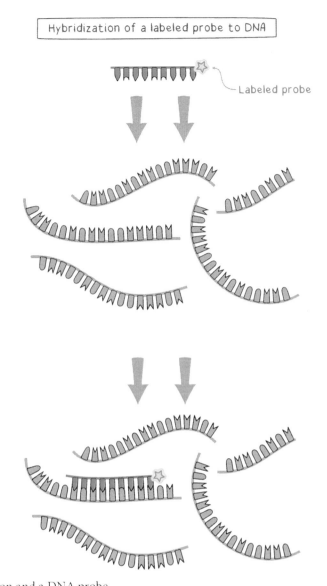

Figure 14. DNA hybridization and a DNA probe

The principles of electrophoresis and hybridization are combined in **blotting techniques**. Several such techniques have been developed, but for the MCAT you should be aware of Southern blotting, northern blotting, and western blotting. **Southern blotting** is a technique used to identify specific DNA sequences, a method discovered by researcher Edwin Southern. The **northern** and **western blots** were named by analogy to the Southern blot (and are therefore often not capitalized), and are used to identify RNA sequences and protein, respectively. In these sequences, the molecules of interest (DNA or RNA fragments, or proteins) undergo gel electrophoresis to separate by size, and then are transferred to a nitrocellulose membrane that can be heated. At this point, probe analysis can be performed (the process is slightly different for western blots, where antibodies are used instead of DNA/RNA probes). This process is outlined below in Figure 15, which shows the details of northern blotting. Nonetheless, the basic principles apply for all types of blotting.

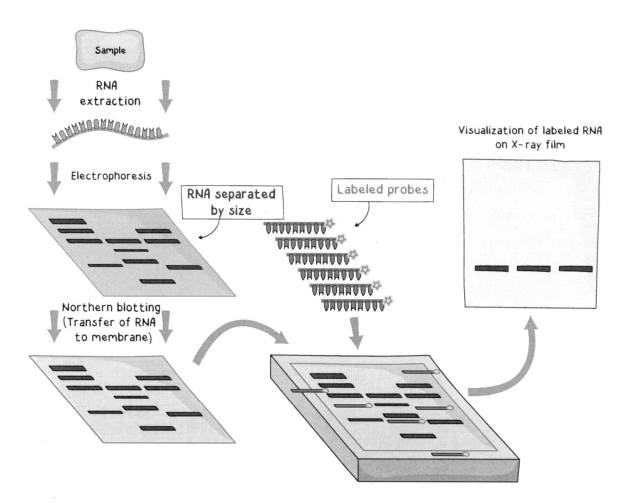

Visualization of labeled RNA
on X-ray film

Figure 15. Northern blotting

DNA microarrays have been developed to leverage hybridization on a larger scale than is possible using Southern blotting, with the possibility of analyzing tens of thousands of genes simultaneously. As the complete sequences of eukaryotic genomes have become available, DNA microarrays operating on the basic principle of hybridization have enabled researchers to undertake global analyses of sequences present in both cellular DNA and RNA samples.

A DNA microarray consists of a glass slide or membrane filter on which oligonucleotides or fragments of cDNA are printed by a robotic system in small spots at high density. Each spot on an array consists of a single oligonucleotide or cDNA. More than 10,000 unique DNA sequences can be printed onto a typical glass microscope slide, making it possible to produce DNA microarrays containing sequences representing all the genes in cellular genomes. One widespread application of DNA microarrays is in the study of gene expression. For example, it can be used to compare the genes expressed by two different cell types. In an experiment of this type, cDNA probes are synthesized from the mRNAs expressed in each of the two cell types (e.g., cancer cells and normal cells). The two cDNA sequences are labeled with different fluorescent dyes (typically red and green) and a mixture of the cDNA is hybridized to a DNA microarray in which 10,000 or more human genes are represented as single spots. It is also possible to synthesize cDNA probes to place on the microarray and have them bind to samples of mRNA as a more direct way of quantifying expression. The array is then analyzed using a high-resolution laser scanner, and the relative extent of transcription of each gene in the cancer cells compared to the normal cells is indicated by the ratio of red to green fluorescence at the a given position on the array.

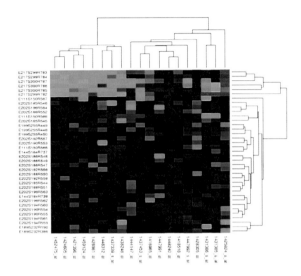

Figure 16. DNA microarray

Various techniques have been used to determine DNA sequences. This is a field that has revolutionized in the last 20-30 years. The human genome was first mapped under the auspices of the Human Genome Project, which started in 1990, took 13 years and cost nearly 3 billion dollars. In 2001, the cost to sequence a human genome was approximately 100 million dollars, which dropped to under 1,000 dollars by 2015.

Novel sequencing techniques have been developed, but the MCAT expects you to be aware of a classic technique, known as the Sanger method or the dideoxy chain termination method. This was the method of choice from the 1980s through the mid-2000s, and was used in the Human Genome Project, before being supplanted by next-generation sequencing methods.

The **Sanger method** of DNA sequencing is based on premature termination of DNA synthesis resulting from the inclusion of chain-terminating dideoxynucleotides, which do not contain the 3' hydroxyl group, in DNA polymerase reactions. DNA synthesis is initiated at a unique site on the cloned DNA from a synthetic primer. The DNA synthesis reaction includes each of four dideoxynucleotides (ddATP, ddCTP, ddGTP, ddTTP), in addition to their normal counterparts. Each of the four dideoxynucleotides is labeled with a different fluorescent dye, so their incorporation into the DNA can be monitored. Incorporation of these dideoxynucleotides stops further DNA synthesis because there is no 3' hydroxyl group available as a site for the addition of the next nucleotide. Thus, a series of labeled DNA molecules is generated, each terminating at the base represented by a specific dideoxynucleotide. Those fragments of DNA are then separated according to size by gel electrophoresis. As the newly synthesized DNA strands are electrophoresed through the gel, they pass through a laser that excites the fluorescent labels. The resulting emitted light is then detected by a photomultiplier, and a computer collects and analyzes the resultant data. The size of each fragment is determined by its terminal dideoxynucleotide, marked by a specific color fluorescence, so the DNA sequence can be read from the order of fluorescent-labeled fragments as they migrate through the gel. High-throughput automated DNA sequencing of this type has enabled large-scale analysis required for determination of the sequences of completed genomes, including that of humans.

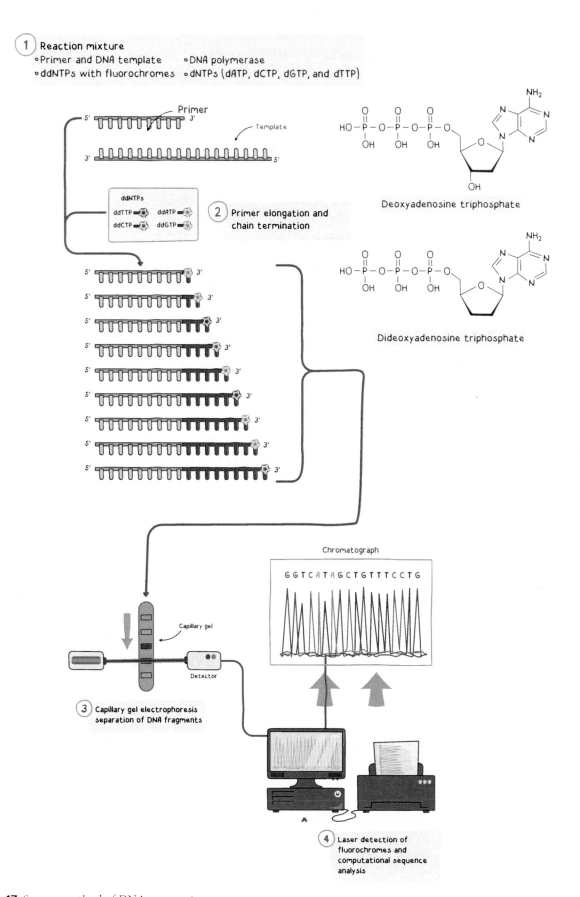

Figure 17. Sanger method of DNA sequencing

DNA sequencing, genetic engineering, and many other applications depend on the ability to produce large quantities of specific DNA sequences. All processes are dependent on a polymerase chain reaction (PCR) to produce the large needed DNA quantity. Essentially, DNA polymerase is used for repeated replications of a defined segment of DNA. Provided that some sequence of the DNA molecule of interest is known, PCR can achieve a striking amplification of DNA via reactions carried out entirely in vitro. The number of DNA molecules increases exponentially, doubling with each round of replication, so a substantial quantity of DNA can be obtained from a relatively small initial sample. For example, a single DNA molecule amplified through 30 cycles of replication would theoretically yield 2^{30}, or more than a billion, progeny molecules. Single DNA molecules can thus be amplified to yield detectable quantities of DNA that can be isolated by molecular cloning or further analyzed directly by restriction endonuclease digestion or nucleotide sequencing. The general procedure for PCR amplification is shown in Figure 18.

Polymerase chain reaction-PCR

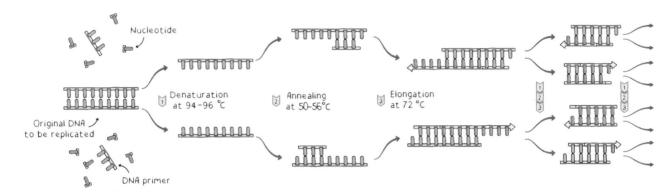

Figure 18. PCR

The starting material in PCR amplification of DNA can be either a cloned fragment or a mixture of DNA molecules; for example, total DNA from human cells. A specific region of DNA can be amplified from such a mixture, provided that the nucleotide sequence surrounding the region is known, so that **primers** can be designed to initiate DNA synthesis at the desired point. Such primers are usually chemically synthesized oligonucleotides containing 15-20 bases of DNA. Two primers are used to initiate DNA synthesis in opposite directions from complementary DNA strands. The reaction is started by heating the template DNA to a high temperature, typically 95°C, to separate the two strands. The temperature is then lowered to allow the primers to pair with their complementary sequences on the template strands. DNA polymerase then uses the primers to synthesize a new strand complementary to each template. Thus, through a single cycle of amplification, two new DNA molecules are synthesized from one template molecule. This process can be repeated multiple times, with a twofold increase in the number of DNA molecules following each round of replication.

The multiple cycles of heating and cooling involved in PCR are performed by programmable heating blocks called thermocyclers. The DNA polymerases used in these reactions are **heat-stable enzymes** from bacteria such as *Thermus aquaticus*, which reside in hot springs where temperatures can exceed 75°C. As these polymerases remain stable even at high temperatures, they are used to replicate the strands of DNA, so PCR amplification can be performed rapidly and automatically. RNA sequences can also be amplified by this method if reverse transcriptase is used to synthesize a cDNA copy prior to PCR amplification.

If the sequence of a target gene is known sufficiently well, a primer for it can be specified. Given this, PCR amplification provides a powerful tool for detecting small amounts of specific DNA or RNA molecules in a complex mixture of other molecules. In such a situation, the only DNA molecules that will be amplified by PCR are those containing sequences complementary to the primers used in the reaction. Therefore, PCR can selectively amplify a specific template from heterogeneous mixtures, such as total cell DNA or RNA. This extraordinary sensitivity has made PCR an important method for a variety of applications, including analysis of gene expression in cells where target DNA is available in only small quantities. The DNA segments amplified by PCR can also be directly sequenced or ligated to vectors and propagated as molecular clones. PCR thus allows the amplification and cloning of any segment of DNA for which primers can be designed. Since the complete genome sequences of many organisms are now known, PCR can be used to amplify and clone a wide array of desired DNA fragments.

7. Must-Knows

> Gene expression: explains how cells with same DNA become different in development.
> Stem cells are capable of differentiation, and can be totipotent (can differentiate into any type of cell), pluripotent (can differentiate into any of the three germ layers), or multipotent (a more limited range). Only embryonic stem cells are totipotent/pluripotent in nature; adult stem cells are multipotent.
> Operons are features of prokaryotes:
>   – Positive vs. negative control: in negative control, a repressor prevents transcription; in positive control, an activator stimulates transcription.
>   – *Lac* operon: negative inducible. In absence of lactose, repressor blocks transcription. When lactose is present, allolactose disengages repressor, allowing transcription. Low glucose levels upregulate transcription through CAP (positive control).
>   – *Trp* operon: negative repressible. Tryptophan is usually synthesized, but when already present, tryptophan causes repressor to bind to operator sequence and block transcription.
> Eukaryotes:
>   – Promoters: upstream DNA sequences that initiate transcription.
>   – Enhancers: DNA sequences that allow increased transcription.
>   – Transcription factors: proteins that regulate expression by binding to a specific DNA sequence.
>   – Heterochromatin: dense, associated with transcriptional inactivity.
>   – Euchromatin: less dense, associated with transcriptional activity.
>   – Histone acetylation: increases transcription.
>   – DNA methylation: decreases transcription.
>   – siRNA and miRNA: decreases protein synthesis.
> Cancer: associated with mutations and altered gene expression patterns leading to uncontrolled proliferation.
>   – Oncogenes: when turned on via mutations, promote division and cancer.
>   – Tumor suppressor genes: normally restrict division; when inactivated, cancer is more likely to develop.
> Recombinant DNA and laboratory techniques:
>   – Restriction enzymes cut DNA at specific points, leading to blunt and sticky ends that can be recombined.
>   – Plasmid and bacteriophage vectors are used to transfer/amplify recombinant DNA.
>   – Electrophoresis separates DNA/RNA molecules by size.
>   – Hybridization: used in Southern, northern, and western blotting to detect specific DNA, RNA, and protein sequences, respectively.
>   – Sanger sequencing method uses dideoxynucleotides to terminate synthesis and electrophoresis to analyze fragment size.
>   – PCR: used to make exponentially large numbers of copies of DNA in a short amount of time; uses primers.

End of Chapter Practice

The best MCAT practice is **realistic**, with a focus on identifying steps for further improvement. For those reasons, we recommend completing practice questions in an online setting that simulates the real MCAT interface, and taking advantage of advanced analytic features to help you determine how best to move forward in your MCAT study journey.

With that in mind, **online end-of-chapter** questions for Biology, Biochemistry, Chemistry + Organic Chemistry, Physics, and Psychology/Sociology are available through your Blueprint MCAT account.

As a further supplement, given the importance of active learning for effective studying, we also suggest that you consult the Must-Knows at the end of each chapter as a basis for creating a study sheet, in which you list out key terms and test your ability to briefly summarize them.

This page left intentionally blank.

This page left intentionally blank.

The Nervous System

0. Introduction

The nervous system is the body's means of taking in information, integrating information, and then controlling and coordinating much of the body's activity through other physiological systems. In this chapter, we will start by discussing general features of the nervous system before moving on to an in-depth discussion of neurons. Neurons are the functional unit in the nervous system. After discussing the mechanisms behind signal transmission, we will discuss some concepts related to electrochemistry and physics, as the MCAT asks cross-disciplinary questions that tie neurons into these other concept areas.

> **>>CONNECTIONS<<**
>
> Chapters 2 and 3 of Psychology

1. Structural Anatomy of the Central Nervous System

Understanding the anatomy of the nervous system requires us to first understand its various divisions and subdivisions. At the highest level are the **central nervous system** (CNS) and the **peripheral nervous system** (PNS). The CNS is at the core of how we interact with the world, and is in charge of processing sensory information and initiating muscle movement. It includes both the **brain** and the **spinal cord**, which are both bathed in **cerebrospinal fluid (CSF)**, encased in tough membranes known as meninges, and protected by skeletal bones—the skull for the brain, and vertebrae for the spinal cord. The PNS contains all other nerves and nervous tissue, including the peripheral neurons that carry information into the CNS, which are known as **afferent fibers**, and those that carry signals from the CNS to the periphery, which are referred to as **efferent fibers**. While the cell bodies of most neurons are found in the central nervous system, there are clusters of cell bodies outside the CNS as well. These clusters are called ganglia and are found along the sides of the spinal cord, in the digestive system, and elsewhere in the body.

During fetal development, the neural tube forms three main regions that give rise to the brain. From anterior to posterior,

> **MCAT STRATEGY >>>**
>
> A helpful mnemonic is the word SAME: sensory afferent, motor efferent.

these regions are the **prosencephalon** (or **forebrain**), **mesencephalon** (or **midbrain**), and **rhombencephalon** (or **hindbrain**). The forebrain is responsible for much of what we associate with behavior and personality, and it itself develops into the diencephalon and the telencephalon. The diencephalon contains three parts: the thalamus, the hypothalamus, and the pineal and posterior pituitary glands. The thalamus relays sensory and motor signals and regulates sleep. The hypothalamus mediates homeostasis and communicates between the nervous and endocrine systems, while the pineal and posterior pituitary glands secrete hormones. The telencephalon contains the **cerebrum**, the largest and among the most important structures of the brain. The cerebrum in turn is divided into a thin, outer layer, known as the cerebral cortex, and subcortical structures such as the hippocampus and basal ganglia. The **limbic system** is not a single structure, but rather a grouping of various structures involved in emotion, memory, and motivation. The limbic system includes the hypothalamus, hippocampus, thalamus, amygdala and a few other structures.

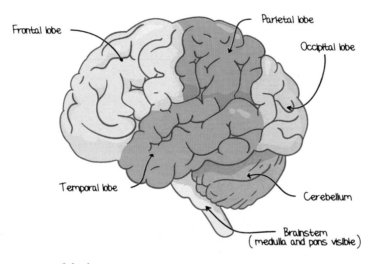

Figure 1. Surface (right) structures of the brain

The cerebral cortex is itself subdivided into lobes: the frontal lobe, parietal lobe, temporal lobe, and occipital lobe. Each of these lobes are responsible for certain higher-order brain functions, including sensation, perception, memory, and cognition. Very broadly, the **frontal lobe** is associated with higher-level cognition and executive functions; while the **parietal lobe** is highly involved in sensory processing. The temporal lobe plays prominent roles in sound and language processing, as well as memory consolidation. The occipital lobe, at the back of the brain, houses the primary visual cortex of the brain. The insula is often categorized as the fifth lobe and is located deep to the lateral sulcus. Parenthetically, some sources indicate there are four lobes of the cerebrum while others indicate there are five. For our purposes and the MCAT, know the names and locations of the lobes and be aware of the insula.

While the forebrain is typically associated with higher-level functions, the **hindbrain** is responsible for more basic functions that have been highly conserved across species throughout the process of evolution. The most prominent structure of the hindbrain is the **cerebellum**, whose name literally means "little cerebrum," as its appearance is similar to the cerebrum, but on a smaller scale. The cerebellum is primarily involved in the coordination of motor control. The hindbrain also consists of the **medulla oblongata**, which controls autonomic functions such as breathing and heart rate, and the **pons**, a relay station through which signals are transmitted between the cerebellum, medulla, and the rest of the brain. The pons also contains clusters of neurons that deal with functions such as sleep, respiration, swallowing, taste, bladder control, and balance.

The **midbrain**, as the name suggests, is located in the central region of the brain, between the forebrain and hindbrain. It contains several structures related to motor control, sleeping, and homeostatic regulation. These structures include the **superior and inferior colliculi**, which modulate sensory pathways, and the **substantia nigra**, which, like the cerebellum, facilitates coordination of voluntary motor control. The midbrain, together with the medulla oblongata and pons, are collectively referred to as the **brainstem**, as they form a stem that connects the brain to the spinal cord.

REGIONS AND PARTS OF THE BRAIN		
Hindbrain	Cerebellum	Coordinated movement.
	Medulla oblongata	Autonomic functions such as breathing, heart rate, blood pressure.
	Pons	Relays signals between the cerebellum, medulla and the rest of the brain. Involved in sleep, respiration, swallowing, taste, bladder control, and balance.
Midbrain	Inferior colliculus	Processes auditory signals and sends them to the medial geniculate nucleus in the thalamus.
	Superior colliculus	Processes visual signals and participates in control of eye movements.
Forebrain	Amygdala	Processes memory, emotions, and decision-making.
	Basal ganglia	Participate in motor control, including eye movements and other voluntary movements as well as procedural and habitual learning.
	Frontal lobe	Involved in voluntary movement, memory processing, planning, motivation, and attention.
	Hippocampus	Consolidation of short-term memory into long-term memory.
	Hypothalamus	Links the nervous system to the endocrine system via the pituitary gland.
	Occipital lobe	Visual processing.
	Parietal lobe	Sensory processing.
	Pineal gland	Modulates sleep through melatonin production.
	Posterior pituitary	Projection through which the hypothalamus secretes oxytocin and ADH (vasopressin).
	Septal nuclei	Part of the reward pathway.
	Temporal lobe	Involved in processing sense information to help form memory and attach meaning to information. Includes Wernicke's area.
	Thalamus	Relays sense and motor signals and regulates sleep and alertness.

Table 1. Gross anatomical divisions and functions of the brain

The **spinal cord** is also considered part of the CNS. It contains bundles of sensory, or afferent, nerve fibers that relay sensory information to the brain, and motor, or efferent, neurons and nerve fibers that relay motor information from the brain to control muscle contractions throughout the body.

The spine (vertebral column) is subdivided into five regions that are categorized based on slight anatomical variations in their vertebrae. Starting from the top, the **cervical spine** corresponds with the neck region and contains seven cervical vertebrae, labeled C1 through C7. The **thoracic spine** corresponds roughly with the curve of the upper back, and contains 12 thoracic vertebrae, T1 through T12. The **lumbar spine** is located in the lower back, and its five lumbar vertebrae are labeled L1 through L5. Then, the sacrum is located at the base of the vertebral column, and the five **sacral vertebrae**, S1 through S5, actually fuse in early adulthood. Finally, the vertebral column ends with the coccyx, or tailbone.

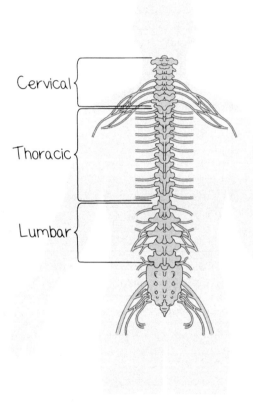

Figure 2. Divisions of the vertebral column

2: Structural Anatomy of the Peripheral Nervous System

The **peripheral nervous system** (PNS) is subdivided into the somatic and autonomic nervous systems. **Somatic nerves** execute voluntary movement, innervating skeletal muscles throughout the body. In contrast, the **autonomic nervous system** controls involuntary responses such as sweating and pupil dilation, and is comprised of two complementary branches: the sympathetic and parasympathetic nervous systems. The sympathetic branch induces the **fight-or-flight response** under conditions of acute stress, whereas the parasympathetic system dampens the acute stress response in order to facilitate relaxation and normal physiological functions like digestion (the **rest-and-digest response**.)

The **sympathetic nervous system** mobilizes body systems to respond to acute environmental stressors, accelerating heart and respiration rates to improve the oxygenation of skeletal muscle tissue, and simultaneously reducing blood flow to organ systems that are less essential in times of acute stress. The sympathetic response also dilates the pupils, allowing more light to enter the eye and heightening visual acuity. The mobilization of these responses is dependent on activation of the sympathetic nervous system and the hormone epinephrine, also referred to as adrenaline, and the closely related norepinephrine, or noradrenaline. Both epinephrine and norepinephrine are produced by the adrenal medulla and norepinephrine is also produced by most sympathetic neurons. By contrast, the **parasympathetic branch** of the autonomic nervous system lowers the heart rate, constricts the pupils, and so on. The parasympathetic response is often referred to as the "rest-and-digest" response, emphasizing its role in physiological processes like digestion.

In both the sympathetic and parasympathetic branches, two neurons act as intermediates propagating the signal from the central nervous system to target organs. The **preganglionic neuron** synapses at a peripheral ganglion on the **postganglionic neuron**, which then synapses and acts on the target organ. In the parasympathetic system, preganglionic neurons are long, synapsing on ganglia near or on the target organ. In the sympathetic system, preganglionic fibers are much shorter. The preganglionic fibers go to the sympathetic trunk. The sympathetic trunk is a chain of ganglia near the spinal cord that extends approximately from the base of the skull to the coccyx. Here, some of the preganglionic neurons will synapse with the postganglionic neurons. The postganglionic sympathetic fibers are longer and extend out to their target organs. While preganglionic and postganglionic fibers of the parasympathetic system, as well as preganglionic fibers of the sympathetic system, primarily use the neurotransmitter acetylcholine, postganglionic sympathetic fibers mostly rely on norepinephrine. Therefore, acetylcholine can be thought of as the default, with the exception that organs targeted by sympathetic activation respond primarily to norepinephrine.

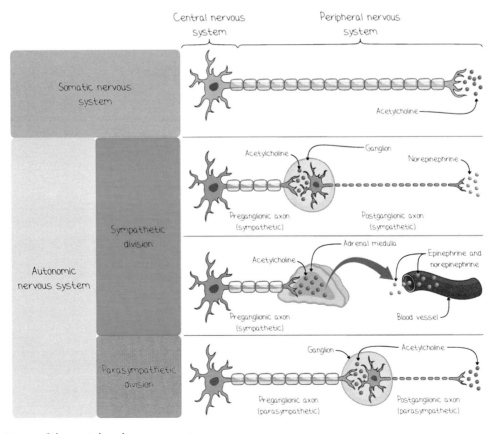

Figure 3. Divisions of the peripheral nervous system

Also underneath the umbrella of autonomic control is the enteric nervous system. This is a highly complex and semi-autonomous branch of the nervous system responsible for regulating and modulating digestive function, so complex that it's sometimes referred to as the body's "second brain."

3. Functional Components of the Nervous System

The primary function of the nervous system is to carry out two parallel and interdependent tasks: processing sensory information from the environment and initiating physiological changes in response to that sensory input. Environmental stimuli are detected by sensory receptors in the body's peripheral nervous system, where they are transduced into electrochemical signals and transmitted via **sensory nerves**, also referred to as **afferent fibers**. These nerves carry sensory information toward the central nervous system, where this information is processed and translated into sensory perceptions.

Distinct regions of the cerebrum specialize in processing certain types of sensory information. Somatosensation, or touch, for example, is processed in the parietal lobe at the primary somatosensory cortex. This is located on a structure called the postcentral gyrus, a fold of brain tissue just posterior to the central sulcus of the brain. Visual processing traverses multiple regions of the brain, beginning in the lateral geniculate body of the thalamus and the superior colliculus, before ultimately being processed in the occipital lobe at the primary visual cortex. The auditory pathway involves several brain structures, including the cochlear nucleus in the medulla oblongata, superior olivary nucleus, inferior colliculus, medial geniculate body of the thalamus, and the temporal lobe. Some nerve fibers from the cochlear nucleus go directly to the inferior colliculus while others go to the superior olivary nucleus prior to being transmitted to the inferior colliculus. The signal is transmitted from the inferior colliculus to the medial geniculate body of the thalamus and ultimately, the primary auditory cortex in the temporal lobe. The gustatory pathway, which is responsible for taste, goes to the thalamus before terminating in the cortex. The olfactory pathway, which is responsible for smell, does not initially go through the thalamus, but rather goes directly to the olfactory cortex.

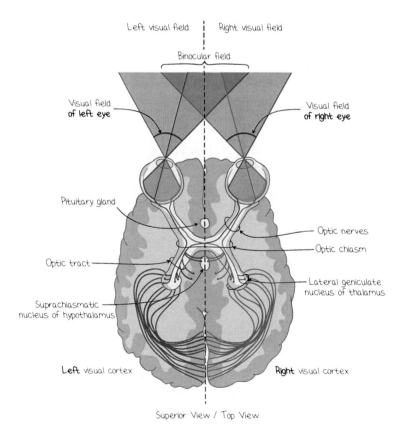

Figure 4A. The visual pathway

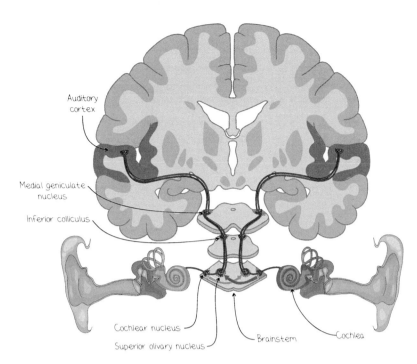

Figure 4B. The auditory pathway

The planning of motor control is initiated in the **premotor cortex**, and executed by the **primary motor cortex**, located in the frontal lobe on a structure called the precentral gyrus. The precentral gyrus is located just anterior to the postcentral gyrus, both of which border the central sulcus separating the frontal and parietal lobes. The electrochemical signals generated in the primary motor cortex will eventually propagate down the spinal cord, but first are modulated by several intermediate structures in the brain. The most prominent of these are the **cerebellum** and the **basal ganglia**, which include the substantia nigra. This modulation helps coordinate the contractions of multiple muscle groups together into unified, directed movement. It is worth keeping in mind that even simple motor actions, such as pointing a finger, require coordination between dozens of different muscles. This coordination is heavily dependent on **dopamine**, a prominent neurotransmitter in the brain, and consequently dopamine dysregulation is implicated in several diseases that involve the deterioration of fine motor control like Parkinson's disease.

Motor impulses are transmitted from the brain along **efferent fibers**, which traverse the spinal cord before exiting the vertebral column at the level of their target muscles. Efferent fibers will eventually terminate at a target muscle, a synaptic connection which we refer to as a neuromuscular junction. At the neuromuscular junction, the presynaptic neuron releases the neurotransmitter acetylcholine upon the muscle cell, stimulating muscle contraction. Even though we often think of motor control in the context of the voluntary control of skeletal muscles, efferent fibers also synapse onto the smooth and cardiac muscles of internal organs, where they transmit commands from brain structures associated with involuntary muscle control.

The two most prevalent neurotransmitters in the entire nervous system are glutamate and GABA. **Glutamate**, an amino acid, is the primary excitatory neurotransmitter in the nervous system, and it is responsible for neuron depolarization and the elicitation of action potentials. **GABA**, in contrast, is the most prominent inhibitory neurotransmitter, by hyperpolarizing neurons, reducing their likelihood of firing.

4. Cells of the Nervous System

All life must respond to its environment. For a microbial organism, the possible responses are limited, as is the distance a signal might need to be sent. As lifeforms become larger, however, it becomes necessary both to integrate complex information from the environment and to send signals across relatively long distances. This must be done quickly, because responding promptly to stimuli can be a life-or-death issue.

The cell type that makes this rapid relay of signals possible is the **neuron**, a non-dividing, highly specialized, and electrically excitable cell type that is the working unit of the nervous system. Like any other piece of highly specialized machinery, neurons require a lot of support and maintenance, which is provided by glial cells. These cells provide nutrients, structure, insulation, and defense from pathogens. They even regulate the growth and pruning of neurons. Glial cells come in many subtypes, each with a specialized function.

Nutrients are transported by astrocytes in the central nervous system. In combination with epithelial cells and pericytes, which surround and support epithelial cells, astrocytes form the **blood-brain barrier**. This structure links the neurons of the central nervous system to the blood supply. The blood-brain barrier is selectively permeable to only a few substances, which helps maintain a stable chemical environment for neurons. One of the most notable functions of astrocytes is the constant, insulin-independent, active transport of glucose from the bloodstream. This process ensures a constant supply of glucose for neurons, which are very demanding in terms of their metabolic requirements. In the peripheral nervous system, satellite cells provide a similar supporting function.

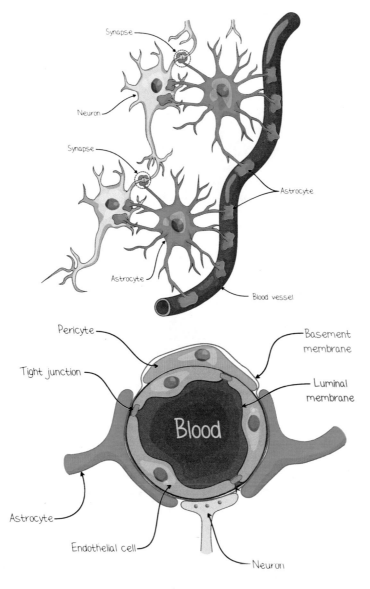

Figure 5. Astrocytes and the blood-brain barrier.

Insulation is provided by **oligodendrocytes** in the central nervous system and **Schwann cells** in the peripheral nervous system. The axons are wrapped in a sheath consisting of a white, fatty substance called myelin. There are also small gaps in this insulation every so often. These gaps are called **nodes of Ranvier**. Even though not all neurons are myelinated, insulating the axons of neurons serves two purposes: preventing cross-talk between axons and massively speeding up signal transmission. The signal, called an **action potential**, then travels from one unmyelinated gap to the next, rapidly "jumping" down the axon in a process known as saltatory conduction.

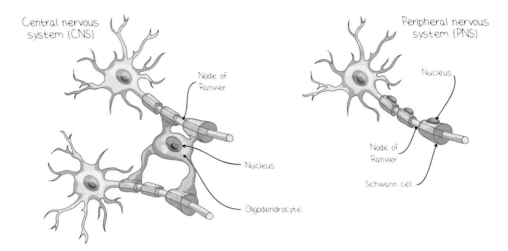

Figure 6. Oligodendrocytes

Infections are very dangerous if they reach the central nervous system, as the CNS is responsible for many functions that are vital to survival. **Microglia** are the first line of defense against invaders in the CNS. They function much like, and are closely related to, macrophages. However, unlike microphages, they also remove waste and damaged cells, prune some neurons, and can even eat away extracellular protein deposits.

GLIAL CELLS	
Oligodendrocytes	Provide myelination in the CNS
Schwann cells	Provide myelination in the PNS
Astrocytes	Provide various support functions to neurons in the CNS
Ependymal cells	Produce cerebrospinal fluid in the CNS
Satellite cells	Control the microenvironment around cell bodies in ganglia in the PNS
Microglia	Macrophages that clean out microbes and debris in the CNS

Table 2. Glial cell types

As mentioned briefly in Section 1, **cerebrospinal fluid (CSF)** bathes and buffers all cells within the CNS. This fluid is secreted by ependymal cells, another type of glial cell. CSF provides a more constant, stable chemical environment and physically cushions the CNS.

Now that we've covered the supporting players, let's look at the neuron itself. In order to understand how a neuron functions, we must first understand its structure. Broadly speaking, neurons have an end that receives input, the **dendrites**, and an end that sends out signals, the **terminal**. Between these two poles, which can be as far as a meter and a half apart in a human, lies its cell body, or **soma**. The soma contains a nucleus and all the normal cellular organelles - that is, all the machinery necessary for a cell to function. Between the soma and the terminal is the **axon**, a long, cable-like structure whose primary function is the rapid relay of signals. Although discussions of nerve transmission often focus on the axon, a thorough understanding of how a neuron transmits information requires grasping how all of its components fit together.

Most dendrites face a **synaptic cleft**, a very small gap between two neurons. This gap lies between the sending end, or terminal, of one and the receiving end, or dendrites, of another. Neurotransmitters released into the synaptic cleft by the previous neuron bind to specialized receptors that allow the influx or efflux of specific ions. This causes a change in the membrane potential called a **graded potential**. The more receptors bind to neurotransmitters, the more graded potentials are created. These graded potentials can travel along the dendrites and the soma, up until a point called the axon hillock, just about adjacent to the axon itself. If enough graded potentials add up in a short enough time to reach a certain threshold, an action potential is generated and travels down the axon. Once the action potential reaches the terminal, it causes voltage-sensitive calcium channels to open. The resulting influx of calcium creates a small signaling cascade that leads to the exocytosis of neurotransmitters, and into the next synaptic cleft. More details are presented in Section 5, but it's worth taking a moment to review and understand the big picture before delving into the details of action potential transmission.

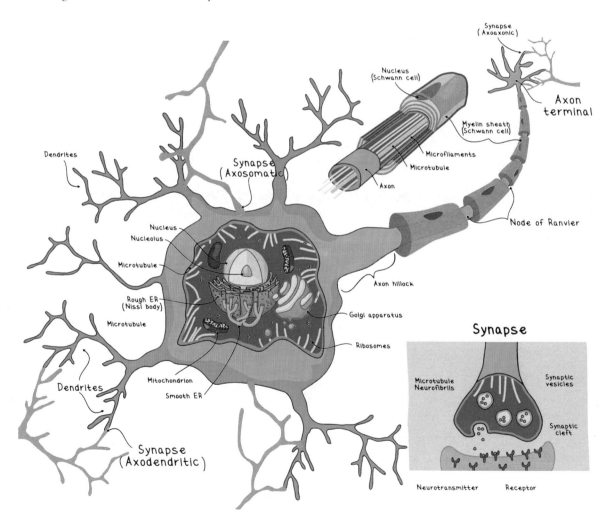

Figure 7. Anatomy of a PNS neuron

5. Action Potentials

In order to understand how neurons send signals through action potentials, we have to set the stage. As the membrane of living cells is nonpolar, it's fairly impervious to ions, although specific transporters can regulate the entry and exit of specific ions. The ability of cells to regulate the intracellular concentration of specific ions results in the presence of a **membrane potential**, or a difference in electric potential on each side of the membrane. The most intuitive way to think of an electric potential difference is as a difference in the distribution of charged particles between two locations. If there are more positively charged particles on the outside of a cell than on the inside, then by convention, this is referred to as a negative membrane potential, and reflects the deficit of positive charge between inside and outside.

Although the extracellular environment is, in some sense, more "positive" than the intracellular environment, the concentrations of specific ions are dramatically different inside and outside of the cell. For instance, in mammals, the intracellular concentration of K^+ is about 140 mM, while the concentration in the blood is about 5 mM. In contrast, Na^+ shows the opposite pattern, with an extracellular concentration that is more than 10 times higher than the intracellular concentration. Finally, the extracellular concentration of Cl^- ions is many times higher than the intracellular concentration. This may seem surprising as it was stated the intracellular environment is more "negative," but the cell interior is also much richer in negatively-charged proteins, and the extracellular environment is much richer in Ca^{2+} ions, by multiple orders of magnitude. There's no need to memorize the precise numbers, but it is important to know that the intracellular environment is relatively rich in K^+, and relatively poor in Na^+, Cl^-, and Ca^{2+}. The key takeaway is that the membrane potential is maintained by differences in the concentration of several ions.

	INTRACELLULAR CONCENTRATION	EXTRACELLULAR CONCENTRATION
Sodium	5-20 mM	145 mM
Potassium	140 mM	5 mM
Chloride	4 mM	110 mM
Calcium	0.0001 mM	1 mM

Table 3. Normal physiological concentrations of major ionic species in humans

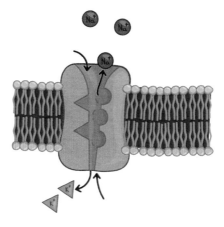

Figure 8. The sodium-potassium pump

These concentration differences are regulated by transmembrane ion transporters. Perhaps the most important of these transporters is **Na⁺/K⁺ ATPase**, or the **sodium-potassium pump**, which is an enzyme that hydrolyzes ATP to pump three sodium ions at a time to the outside of the cell while bringing in two potassium ions. It is constitutively expressed in all cells and always active, so much so that it accounts for a large portion of most cells' ATP hydrolysis. However, the cell membrane is somewhat permeable to potassium, so some of the work of Na⁺/K⁺ ATPase is constantly undone by the outward diffusion of potassium. Regardless, this system stabilizes at a **resting membrane potential** of about -70 mV. Any changes in the activity of transmembrane ion transporters that have the effect of destabilizing this potential difference—that is, by bringing it closer to 0 mV—result in **depolarization**. Inversely, **hyperpolarization** occurs in response to changes making the potential difference more negative.

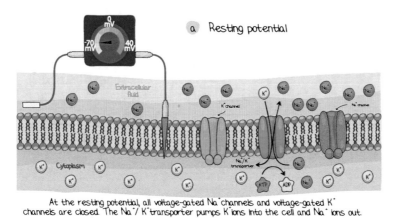

At the resting potential, all voltage-gated Na⁺ channels and voltage-gated K⁺ channels are closed. The Na⁺/K⁺ transporter pumps K⁺ ions into the cell and Na⁺ ions out.

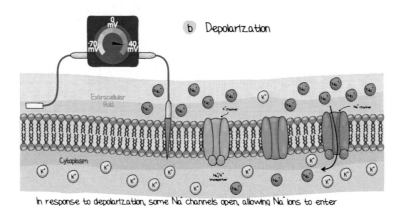

In response to depolarization, some Na⁺ channels open, allowing Na⁺ ions to enter the cell. As the membrane starts to depolarize, the charge across the membrane lessens.

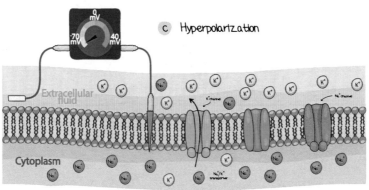

At the peak action potential, Na⁺ channels close while K⁺ channels open. K⁺ leaves the cell, and the membrane eventually becomes hyperpolarized.

Figure 9. Depolarization and hyperpolarization of the neural membrane

Now that we've established these foundational concepts, let's look at how a signal is transmitted. First, **neurotransmitters** are released into the **synaptic cleft**, the small space between the terminal of one neuron and the dendrites of another neuron. On the plasma membrane of dendrites, there are many different receptors, each specific for a different type of neurotransmitter. When a neurotransmitter binds to an appropriate receptor, that receptor will allow a specific ion to flow inside. This ion flow slightly changes the membrane potential, an effect called a graded potential. Most graded potentials are excitatory, meaning that they raise the membrane potential, making it more positive. Therefore, these are known as **excitatory postsynaptic potentials (EPSPs)**. However, **inhibitory postsynaptic graded potentials (IPSPs)** are also possible—these make the membrane more negative, resulting in hyperpolarization. Graded potentials can add up together, if they are either located close to each other or happen within a very short time span—phenomena that are technically referred to as spatial summation and temporal summation, respectively. They can also propagate to some extent, along the soma and towards the axon hillock.

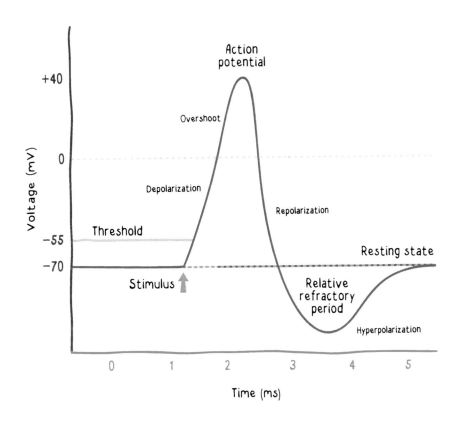

Figure 10. Depolarization and hyperpolarization of the neural membrane

Immediately past the axon hillock, numerous **voltage-gated sodium channels** can be found. By definition, voltage-gated channels open or close in response to a change in membrane potential. If enough graded potentials occur in a short enough time, they can add up to the threshold potential that causes voltage-gated sodium channels to open. When that happens, the first few voltage-gated sodium channels open up. Like a flood, sodium comes rushing in from the outside, down both its concentration gradient and its electrical gradient. This causes the membrane potential to increase even further, becoming even more positive than the threshold, and the neighboring voltage-gated sodium channels begin to open up as well. A chain reaction is set in motion, since voltage-gated sodium channels are present in large quantities all along the axon. This cascade of **depolarization** traveling down the axon, towards the terminal, is what forms the action potential itself.

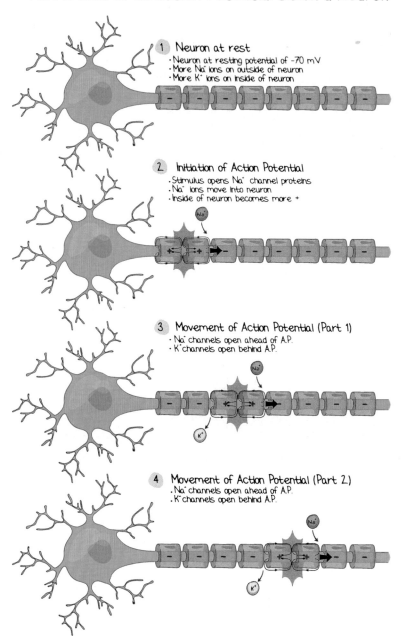

Figure 11. Propagation of an action potential

So far, so good—but it is also important to account for how the neuron repolarizes, or returns to its resting potential, as the action potential doesn't just keep traveling back and forth. **Repolarization** starts when voltage-gated potassium channels open up. At the same time, the voltage-gated sodium channels close, at about +35 mV, after only being open a very short time. Once the sodium channels are closed, and the potassium channels are open, Na⁺ isn't rushing *in* anymore—instead, K⁺ is rushing *out*. This loss of cations quickly makes the membrane potential negative again. In fact, it becomes so negative that **hyperpolarization** occurs. Once the voltage-gated potassium channels close, Na⁺/K⁺ ATPase is sufficient to bring both the membrane potential and concentration gradient back to normal.

After the sodium channels close, depolarization hits its peak at around +40 mV, and they cannot open again for a certain period of time, known as the **absolute refractory period**. This serves as a safety check, by preventing the signal from traveling backwards. In contrast to the absolute refractory period, there's also a **relative refractory**

period, which occurs when the sodium channels are able to open again, but the membrane remains hyperpolarized. This refractory period is called "relative" because it is possible, just more difficult, to generate another action potential during this time.

Our next concern is the fate of this wave of depolarization traveling towards the terminal. At the end of the axon, instead of voltage-gated Na⁺ channels, we encounter **voltage-gated Ca²⁺ channels**. These channels open in response to the change in membrane potential caused by the arriving wave of depolarization. Their opening results in an influx of Ca²⁺, which causes a chemical signaling cascade that ends with the exocytosis of neurotransmitters from vesicles—storage structures that fuse with the plasma membrane of the terminal. The neurotransmitters previously contained in the vesicle spill out into the synaptic cleft, where they can bind with receptors on the dendrites of the next neuron, starting the process all over.

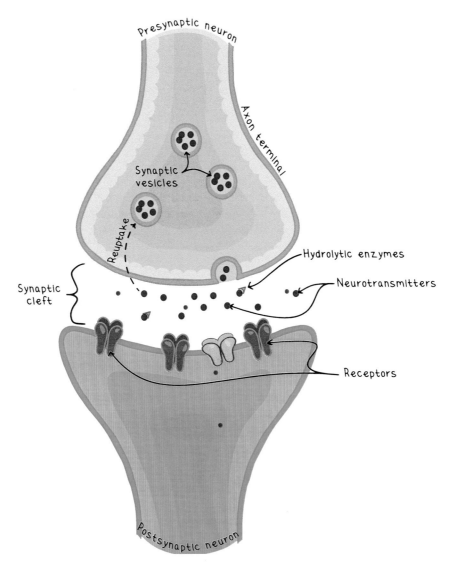

Figure 12. A chemical synapse

We're now faced with one more big question: what happens to those neurotransmitters after they're spilled into the synaptic cleft? If left alone, we can imagine how they might keep binding, dissociating, and re-binding to receptors, thereby continuing to cause graded potentials. That would not be very effective for creating a short-term, controlled response. While some neurotransmitters diffuse away, other neurotransmitters in the synapse undergo either degradation or reuptake.

In **degradation**, hydrolytic enzymes rapidly break the neurotransmitter apart, thereby preventing it from binding to receptors any further. The most well-known example of this is the enzyme acetylcholinesterase, a protein located on the postsynaptic membrane—that is, on the membrane of dendrites. This enzyme is highly efficient at catalyzing the breakdown of the ester linkage that holds the neurotransmitter acetylcholine together, thereby ensuring that the effect of acetylcholine in the synapse is very brief. Chemical agents inhibiting such enzymes have strong and nearly immediate effects, and have been used both in the treatment of disorders of the nervous system and in chemical warfare.

In contrast, **reuptake** occurs when neurotransmitters are moved out of the synaptic cleft either by presynaptic neurons or by astrocytes. Neurotransmitters are moved out of the cleft by various transport proteins in the membrane of the presynaptic neuron. In some cases, reuptake is followed by breakdown. This is the case for monoamines, such as norepinephrine and dopamine. After being removed from the synaptic cleft, these neurotransmitters are often further broken down and recycled by monoamine oxidases, a class of enzymes located on the outer membrane of mitochondria. As you can imagine, each of these steps can also be regulated by exogenous chemicals. For instance, serotonin reuptake inhibitors, or SSRIs, were introduced in the 1980s for the treatment of depression.

NEUROTRANSMITTERS	
Acetylcholine	Activates muscle contraction at the neuromuscular junction. Used in all autonomic outputs from the brain to autonomic ganglia. Used in the parasympathetic nervous system for post-ganglionic connections.
Dopamine	Used in reward pathways and motor pathways. Particularly associated with Parkinson's disease and the loss of dopaminergic neurons in the substantia nigra.
Endorphin	Suppresses pain and can produce euphoria.
Epinephrine	Stimulates fight-or-flight response.
GABA	Main inhibitory neurotransmitter of the CNS that hyperpolarizes cells to reduce action potential firing. Associated with many of the physiological effects of alcohol intoxication.
Glutamate	Excitatory neurotransmitter and most common neurotransmitter (90% of brain cells are glutaminergic).
Glycine	Inhibitory neurotransmitter of the spinal cord and brainstem.
Norepinephrine	Used in post-ganglionic connections in the sympathetic division of the autonomic nervous system. Increases arousal, alertness, and focuses attention.
Serotonin	Regulates intestinal movement in the GI tract as well as mood, appetite, and sleep in the brain. Low levels particularly associated with depressive mood disorders.

Table 4. Common neurotransmitters.

To summarize this process, neurotransmitters first bind to receptors in the dendrites, causing graded potentials that travel to the axon hillock. If enough graded potentials are present to reach the threshold, voltage-gated sodium channels open and start a cascade called an action potential. This action potential travels down the axon, until it reaches the terminal, where voltage-gated calcium channels open up in response to depolarization. Calcium now flows into the cell and ultimately causes the release of neurotransmitters into the synapse. These neurotransmitters then bind to receptors on the postsynaptic membrane and the process continues. Finally, neurotransmitters either diffuse away, are degraded, or are taken back up.

With this in mind, there are a couple special cases to consider. First, we just described what happens at a *chemical* synapse. At an electrical synapse, the sending and receiving neurons are even closer to each other, to the point that they're linked through structures called gap junctions. **Gap junctions** allow ions to diffuse between the two neurons, enabling the membrane potential of one to directly and immediately influence that of the other. This speeds up signal transmission, but removes the possibility of amplifying or modulating signals at all.

The other major special case involves the way a signal is triggered in sensory neurons specifically. We presented this as occurring in response to stimuli from other neurons, in the form of neurotransmitters, but sensory neurons generate signals through a different mechanism, in which some other stimulus triggers a graded potential. The specific details vary across the broad category of sensory neurons, with each type of sensory neuron specializing in responding to a specific type of stimulus. For instance, photoreceptors respond to light, baroreceptors respond to pressure, and so on. Everything else that we've discussed about how action potentials work still holds true for sensory neurons; the only difference is how the process gets started.

	CHEMICAL SYNAPSE	ELECTRICAL SYNAPSE
Signaling method	Neurotransmitter binding to transmembrane receptor protein	Direct, cell-to-cell diffusion of ions through gap junctions
Speed	Fast	Very fast
Direction of signaling	Unidirectional	Bidirectional
Advantages	Amplification of signal, highly modifiable	Response speed

Table 5. Chemical and electrical synapses

6. Electrochemistry of Neurons

Moving beyond the anatomy of neurons and the sequence of steps involved in the generation and transmission of action potentials, it's helpful to take a deeper dive into the electrochemical principles underlying action potential transmission. For instance, what determines how fast a wave of depolarization can travel, or why some neurons are easier to depolarize than others?

As a brief review, in any electrical system, capacitance is the ability to store charge, while resistance is the ability to resist the flow of charge. The cell membranes of neurons are characterized by both **capacitance**, as reflected by the difference in charge between both sides of the membrane, and **resistance**. Capacitance, as you may recall from physics, is just a function of how much charge is on both sides of an insulator and the thickness of that insulation. The insulator in this case is just the plasma membrane, so this phenomenon is called membrane capacitance. The higher the membrane capacitance, the more difficult it will be to change the membrane potential. This both slows down conduction and makes a neuron harder to depolarize. Since larger neurons have larger surfaces, they have more area to store charge along their membranes, and therefore, they have a higher membrane capacitance, making them harder to depolarize.

When it comes to resistance, we should be careful to distinguish membrane resistance, which is the ability of the membrane to keep charges separate, from cytoplasmic resistance, which is how much the cytoplasm itself impedes the flow of ions. Cytoplasmic resistance is more straightforward: the more the cytoplasm impedes the flow of ions, the slower and more difficult conduction will be. Thus, cytoplasmic resistance makes a major contribution to how well a neuron conducts. More specifically, the larger the neuron, the lower the cytoplasmic resistance.

Next, since **membrane resistance** reflects the ability of a membrane to effectively separate charge, it follows that high membrane resistance promotes the effective transmission of an action potential. For visualization purposes, imagine a leaky membrane, with low membrane resistance. Ions that should be in the cytoplasm would leak into the extracellular space, and vice versa, thereby interfering with the delicate machinery of ion transport involved in how depolarization spreads down the axon. In contrast, *high* membrane resistance makes the transmission of action potentials more effective.

To tie all these concepts together, larger neurons have lower cytoplasmic resistance than smaller ones and significantly higher capacitance. This makes them overall faster at conducting signals, but harder to depolarize in the first place.

CABLE PROPERTIES	
Membrane resistance	Opposition to the flow of ions across the membrane
Membrane capacitance	Charged stored across the membrane
Cytoplasmic resistance	Opposition to the flow of ions through the cytoplasm

Table 6. The cable properties of a neuron

Although these properties apply everywhere in the neuron, **conduction speed** along the axon is of particular interest, because axons can be quite long. Speed of communication in the nervous system is vital for an organism to be able to react promptly to the environment, so how exactly does an action potential move reasonably quickly along a 1-meter long axon in a human? Or the nearly 15-meter axon of a giant squid?

Although membrane resistance, membrane capacitance, and cytosolic resistance always influence conduction speed, myelination drastically decreases membrane capacitance and increases membrane resistance. As mentioned above, this involves insulating large portions of the axon.

Myelinating a portion of the axon largely prevents the efflux, or outflow, of ions in that region. Since membrane resistance reflects the degree to which the membrane keeps certain groups of ions separate, myelination dramatically increases membrane resistance. Myelin layers tend to be fairly thick, introducing a large separation between the cytoplasm and the extracellular fluid. This significantly decreases capacitance, as capacitance is inversely proportional to the distance of charge separation. As a result of these two properties, conduction is extremely rapid along any myelinated segment.

The charge difference between inside and outside of the membrane does decay as the depolarization travels along a myelinated portion of the axon. If an axon were myelinated without interruption along its entire length, depolarization would certainly fizzle out before it reaches the terminal. That's where nodes of Ranvier come in: intermittent, very short, unmyelinated regions in which all our usual players—Na^+ channels, K^+ channels, and Na^+/K^+ ATPase—are highly abundant. An action potential begins in the axon hillock and axon initial segment. The depolarization wavefront is then conducted down the axon very quickly along the myelinated portion, decaying a little bit in the process. As the depolarization reaches a node of Ranvier, it again causes voltage-gated sodium channels to open, 'replenishing' it to full intensity. It then rapidly conducts down the next myelinated region, towards the next **node of Ranvier**. Overall, this increases conduction speed massively, making the existence of very large or very agile vertebrates possible. Clinical pathology also emphasizes the importance of myelination, as partial failures to maintain myelination are the hallmark of debilitating neurological diseases such as multiple sclerosis and other degenerative neuropathologies.

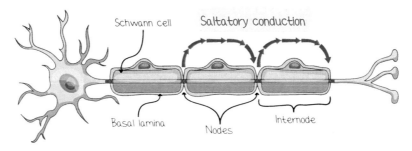

Figure 13. Myelination

As a final note on the electrochemistry of neurons, let's return to the fundamental idea of a **resting membrane potential**. Recall that the *resting* membrane potential is the potential that is present when the influx and efflux of ions through the membrane equalizes. That is, it's the membrane potential that the system "balances out" at when it's not actively depolarizing.

Equation 1.

$$E_{cell} = E^\circ_{cell} - \frac{RT}{nF} \ln Q$$

Let's apply what we know from electrochemistry to this idea, by treating the neuron as a concentration cell. If we wanted to determine the cell potential with respect to just one ion, for example potassium, we could use the Nernst equation. The Nernst equation tells us that the cell potential of any electrochemical cell is the standard cell potential minus the natural log of Q, the reaction quotient, multiplied by a few constants and adjusted for *n*, or moles of electrons. For now, we can ignore both *n* and the constants and instead focus on two quantities: the standard cell potential and the reaction quotient.

Equation 2.

$$E_{cell} = E^\circ_{cathode} - E^\circ_{anode}$$

Recall that the standard cell potential is defined as the difference between the cell potential of the cathode, $E^\circ_{cathode}$, and the cell potential of the anode, E°_{anode}. Since in this case, both our anode and our cathode have the exact same ion, our standard cell potential, E°_{cell}, is simply 0. This is an arrangement called a **concentration cell**.

For our reaction quotient, the definition is the concentration of products over reactants.

Equation 3. Nernst Equation

$$E = \ln \left(\frac{ion_{out}}{ion_{in}} \right) \frac{RT}{zF}$$

$[ion]_{in}$	= ion concentration inside the cell
$[ion]_{out}$	= ion concentration outside the cell
R	= gas constant
T	= temperature (degrees Kelvin)
z	= valence of ion
F	= Faraday's constant

Let's use the actual approximate values for extra- and intracellular potassium concentration here. We input those values and get $\ln \left(\frac{5}{140} \right)$, which we can already estimate to be a negative number, as the log of numbers less than one will always be negative. If we then input that product into the equation, we will calculate the equilibrium potential for potassium as about -89 mV.

MEMBRANE POTENTIALS	
Sodium	+66 mV
Potassium	-89 mV
Resting membrane potential	-70 mV

Table 7. Membrane potentials of individual species and the resting membrane potential

Note that these equations, particularly our simplified form, imply a few things. First, concentrations drive membrane potential. In other words, if the concentration of a given ion was equal inside and outside the cell, its equilibrium potential would 0. In the same vein, if the concentrations for *all* relevant ions were equal on both sides of the cell membrane, the membrane potential would also be 0, since ln(1) = 0. This matches up well with what we know about diffusion: once concentrations are equal, no net diffusion should occur. To sum this up, it can be said that membrane potential is an electric potential difference caused by unequal concentrations of various charged ions on each side of the cell membrane. Thus, these concentration gradients are a way for the cell to store potential energy that can be rapidly released later for signal transmission.

Now that all is said and done, with this comprehensive grounding in the anatomical structure, electrophysiology, and electrochemistry of neurons, you'll be well-equipped for any passage that you encounter about neurons.

6. Must-Knows

> The nervous system serves to take in and integrate information from the environment and allows the organism to respond appropriately.

> The central nervous system includes both the brain and the spinal cord. The various components of the brain are associated with key functions.

> The peripheral nervous system is divided into the autonomic and somatic nervous systems.
  - The somatic nervous system controls voluntary responses via skeletal muscle.
  - The autonomic nervous system controls involuntary responses through the sympathetic (fight or flight) and the parasympathetic (rest and digest) systems.

> The functional unit of the nervous system is the neuron, and all neurons require supporting glial cells to function correctly.
  - Glial cells include oligodendrocytes, Schwann cells, ependymal cells, satellite cells, astrocytes, and microglia.
  - Neurons come in several types, including sensory cells that are bipolar and pseudounipolar, and motor and interneurons that are multipolar.

> Neurons maintain a resting potential of -70 mV by pumping sodium out and potassium into the cell. They maintain selective permeability that does not allow sodium cells or proteins bearing negatively charged residues to pass through the membrane.

> Neurons transmit information via action potentials.
  - An action potential begins with a depolarization phase during which sodium rushes into the cell.
  - After peaking at +40 mV, the cell closes sodium channels and opens potassium channels. Potassium rushes out of the cell, repolarizing it.
  - The cell briefly hyperpolarizes with a potential below -70 mV. During this phase, it is much more difficult to stimulate a new action potential.
  - The sodium-potassium pump re-establishes the resting state.

> When the action potential reaches the end of the axon, the signal is transmitted to the post-synaptic membrane via a neurotransmitter.
  - Calcium rushes in to the pre-synaptic axon terminal, which sends vesicles containing neurotransmitter into the synaptic cleft. The neurotransmitter binds to the post-synaptic membrane and serves as a catalyst for its effect.

> Neurons can be modeled both as concentration cells and as capacitors. The MCAT will want you to be familiar with these concepts from chemistry and physics and be able to apply them even if you're working through a biology passage.

End of Chapter Practice

The best MCAT practice is **realistic**, with a focus on identifying steps for further improvement. For those reasons, we recommend completing practice questions in an online setting that simulates the real MCAT interface, and taking advantage of advanced analytic features to help you determine how best to move forward in your MCAT study journey.

With that in mind, **online end-of-chapter** questions for Biology, Biochemistry, Chemistry + Organic Chemistry, Physics, and Psychology/Sociology are available through your Blueprint MCAT account.

As a further supplement, given the importance of active learning for effective studying, we also suggest that you consult the Must-Knows at the end of each chapter as a basis for creating a study sheet, in which you list out key terms and test your ability to briefly summarize them.

The Endocrine System

0. Introduction

The endocrine system refers to the organs that secrete hormones, which are signal molecules secreted into the bloodstream that are used for communication and the regulation of physiological parameters.

The endocrine system is a high-yield topic. First, the current MCAT places an emphasis on information flow and regulation, which is precisely the function of the endocrine system. Second, a solid understanding of the endocrine system is important for understanding how other organ systems function, which also has implications for psychology. Third, the chemical concept of polarity is crucial for understanding how different hormones work. Whenever you see an intersection between a biological system and a core concept from chemistry or physics, pay close attention! Such intersections are likely to come up on the exam. Fourth, as the single largest skill category of MCAT questions is Skill 2 (Scientific Reasoning and Problem-Solving), the communicative and regulatory functions of the endocrine system make it a promising target for passage-based questions testing this skill.

As you're studying, it's important for you to learn how to approach the endocrine system through multiple conceptual lenses, as this chapter contains a tremendous amount of information that can be organized and approached in many different ways. On the exam, you will have to apply information about the endocrine system in the context of a specific passage or question. It is crucial for you to know the material from multiple different angles in order to do so efficiently and accurately—just like, as a future physician. At a minimum, you should understand (1) how the chemical structure of hormones influences their effects on the body, (2) the physiological effects of hormones and how they are regulated, and (3) the organs that make up the endocrine system and which hormones they secrete. These goals are reflected in this chapter, which begins with a discussion of the mechanisms and regulatory principles of the endocrine system, presents an overview of the physiological effects of hormones, and concludes with a review of the organs involved in the endocrine system.

1. Mechanisms and Regulation

Terminology

A reasonable first question about the endocrine system would be "why do they call it that?" In fact, a first step in studying the endocrine system is to give a good answer to this question, and in particular, to be able to define what it means to say that something is an **endocrine gland**.

Let's start with the difference between exocrine and endocrine glands. The primary difference is that **exocrine glands** secrete their products into ducts, whereas endocrine glands secrete hormones directly into the circulatory system. Exocrine glands are found in a few organ systems, and are generally responsible for secreting bodily fluids: sweat (sweat glands), skin oil (sebaceous glands), earwax (ceruminous glands), breastmilk (mammary glands), saliva (salivary glands), and tears (lacrimal glands). The most important **endocrine glands** discussed are the hypothalamus, pituitary gland, thyroid gland, parathyroid, adrenal cortex and medulla, pancreas, and gonads. An organ can have both exocrine and endocrine components. The best-known example of this is the pancreas, which releases digestive enzymes through ducts (exocrine function) and releases key hormones such as insulin and glucagon (endocrine function). The liver is also an example of this, as it secretes bile through the bile duct (exocrine function) and also secretes hormones such as angiotensinogen (endocrine function).

Although the definition of an endocrine gland is the most important aspect of this discussion of terminology, it's helpful to have an understanding of all the other terms describing signaling and secretion that end in "-crine," in order to eliminate potential sources of confusion.

MCAT STRATEGY >>>

These terms can be difficult to keep separate, but a careful study of their prefixes can help with these and other medical terms. For exocrine, think of the same "ex-" as in "external"—exocrine glands secrete something *out* through ducts. The prefix "endo-" means "inside," so think of endocrine glands as secreting things into your bloodstream, which runs *inside* of you. "Para" means "close to or next to," so paracrine signaling is signaling to nearby cells. "Auto-" means "self-," so autocrine signaling is when a cell affects itself. "Juxta-" is less common, but you can think of words like *juxtaposition* or even being *just next to* something.

One set of "-crine" terms refers to the physical scope of a signaling pattern. **Paracrine signaling** occurs when a cell secretes a signaling molecule that acts on nearby cells, and is heavily involved in differentiation in embryonic development. In contrast, endocrine signaling has long-distance effects throughout the entire organism. **Autocrine signaling** takes place when a cell releases a molecule that acts on itself, and is thought to play a role in the development of cancer. Less commonly, you may encounter **juxtacrine signaling**, which refers to signaling that requires cells to be in close contact with each other—juxtacrine signaling is even more local than paracrine signaling.

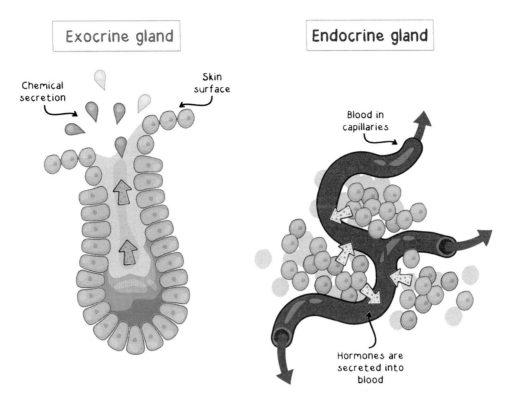

Exocrine gland

Chemical secretion

Skin surface

Endocrine gland

Blood in capillaries

Hormones are secreted into blood

Figure 1. Endocrine versus exocrine signaling

Another set of "-crine" terms is used to classify ways in which exocrine glands release substances. These terms are relatively low-yield for the MCAT, and are very unlikely to be the primary focus of a question, but are worth being able to recognize if they appear among the answer choices. If a cell releases its secretions through exocytosis, it is known as a **merocrine cell**; the term **eccrine** refers more specifically to merocrine cells in the sweat glands. **Apocrine cells** release their secretions through membrane-bound vesicles. Some examples include the cells of the mammary gland and certain sweat glands in the human body. Be sure not to confuse "apocrine" with "autocrine"! Finally, **holocrine secretion** results from rupture of the plasma membrane, destroying the cell and releasing its product from the cytoplasm into the lumen. Examples include the sebaceous glands of the skin.

Structure and Mechanisms of Action

Hormones can be classified according to their chemical structure as **peptide hormones**, **steroid hormones**, or **amino acid derivatives**. The distinction between peptide and steroid hormones is particularly important because their difference in chemical structure causes peptide and steroid hormones to function differently.

So, what's the difference? As the name implies, **peptide hormones** are composed of a polypeptide chain (an amino acid chain). **Steroid hormones** are derivatives of the lipid cholesterol, and have a characteristic four-ring structure. The most important distinction between peptide and steroid hormones is that peptide hormones are hydrophilic, and steroid hormones are hydrophobic. This explains why peptide and steroid hormones have different mechanisms of action and tend to have different physiological effects.

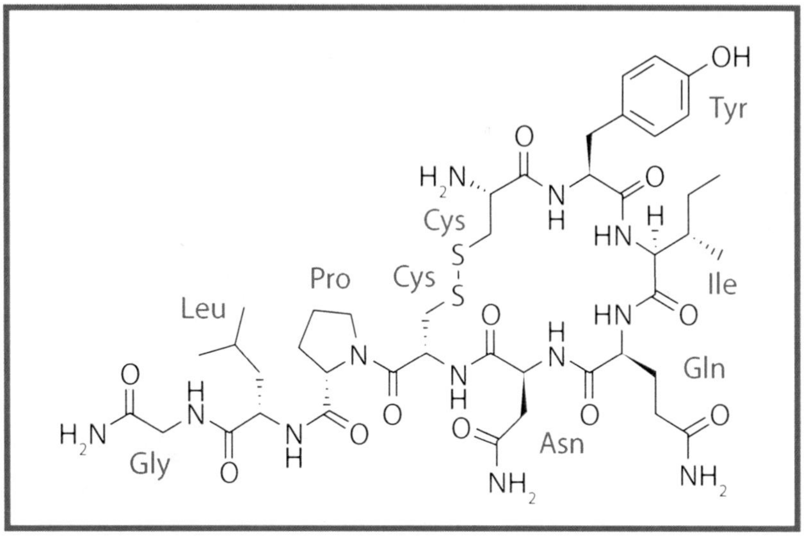

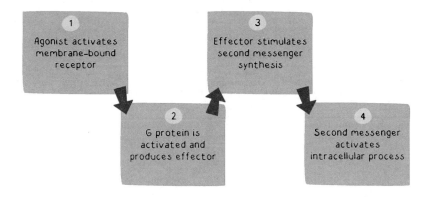

Figure 2. Structure of oxytocin, a peptide hormone

>> CONNECTIONS <<

Chapter 1 of Biology

First, let's explore the hydrophilic nature of **peptide hormones**. Because they're hydrophilic, they diffuse freely in the blood, but cannot freely cross the lipid bilayer membrane of their target cells. This means that they have to exert their effects through **receptors** embedded on the plasma membrane's outer surface. These receptors then change their conformation to produce an effect in the target cell (also known as the effector), often through a second messenger, such as cyclic AMP (cAMP), cyclic GMP (cGMP), or inositol triphosphate (IP$_3$). **Second messenger systems** (the hormone itself is referred to as the first messenger) result in a signal cascade that allows the signal to undergo rapid amplification within the cell, which can cause a rapid and intense impact on cellular function. Therefore, peptide hormones are typically associated with rapid, short-term changes in physiological function. We will see several examples of this below when we discuss the endocrine control of blood chemistry.

Figure 3. Second messenger systems

How does this picture change for steroid hormones, which are hydrophobic and therefore have a solubility profile opposite that of peptide hormones? First, **steroid hormones** are not soluble in the bloodstream, and therefore require transport proteins to reach their targets. These **transport proteins** may be relatively specific (for example, sex hormone-binding globulin transports estradiol and testosterone) or relatively non-specific (for example, albumin). Once steroid hormones reach their target cells, their small size and hydrophobicity allow them to diffuse directly through the lipid bilayer membrane and enter the cell. The location for most steroid hormone receptors is the nucleus or cytoplasm, but there are also plasma membrane receptors. In the nucleus, the receptor-hormone complex binds directly to DNA and affects gene transcription. Since steroid hormones work by modulating gene transcription, they are associated with slower-onset and longer-lasting physiological effects.

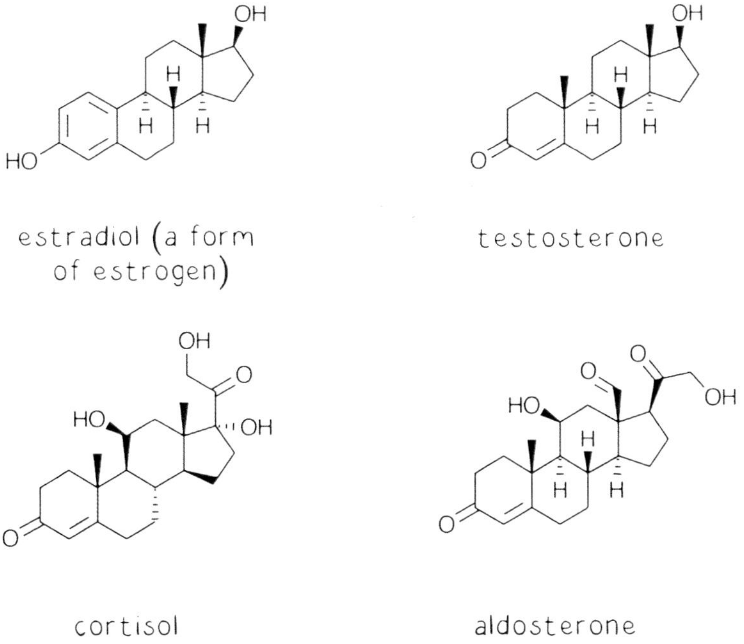

estradiol (a form of estrogen)

testosterone

cortisol

aldosterone

Figure 4. Structure of steroid hormones

Another important distinction between peptide hormones and steroid hormones is how they are synthesized and released into circulation. **Peptide hormones** are produced in stages. They are first translated as **preprohormones**, early precursors that are transferred to the rough ER, and modified into **prohormones**, inactive immediate precursors of the hormones. Prohormones are processed in the Golgi apparatus. It is there that they are cleaved by endopeptidases and may be modified by the addition of carbohydrates to generate the final, active form of the hormone. The hormones are then packaged into vesicles to be released through **exocytosis**. In contrast, **steroid hormones** are synthesized from **cholesterol** in the smooth ER and diffuse directly through the cell membrane.

MCAT STRATEGY >>>

The connection between hormone structure and function is a prototypical example of how the MCAT tests the interplay between biochemical structures and physiological outcomes. Walk through this line of reasoning a couple of times and then be alert to other instances where it could be applied, both while studying and eventually on the exam itself.

These points, as well as some other distinctions between peptide and steroid hormones, are summarized below in Table 1.

	PEPTIDE HORMONES	STEROID HORMONES
Biochemical precursor	Amino acids	Cholesterol (lipid)
Size	Relatively large but variable	Small
Polarity	Polar	Nonpolar
Hydrophilic or hydrophobic?	Hydrophilic	Hydrophobic
Location of synthesis	Rough ER → Golgi → vesicles → exocytosis	Smooth ER
Intermediate stages?	Yes (preprohormones, prohormones, hormones)	No
Solubility in blood	Soluble; freely diffuse	Insoluble; require transport protein
Type of receptor	Membrane-bound receptor	Usually cytoplasmic or nuclear receptors
Interaction with lipid membrane of target cell	Cannot diffuse	Diffuse through membrane
Mechanism of effect	Second messenger system in cytosol	DNA transcription in nucleus
Physiological effects	Fast onset, short-term	Slow onset, longer-term
Typical functions	Regulation of other hormones, short-term responses	Sex, sugar [glucocorticoids], and salt [mineralocorticoids] (the three S's)
Examples	Thyroid-stimulating hormone, oxytocin, insulin, calcitonin	Estrogen, testosterone, cortisol, aldosterone

Table 1. Key differences between peptide and steroid hormones.

MCAT STRATEGY >>>

Most of the hormones you have to know for the MCAT are peptide hormones. Learn the steroid hormones and amino acid-derived hormones separately, and assume that anything else is a peptide hormone unless a passage or question stem tells you differently.

Finally, **amino acid-derived hormones** are small hormones derived from individual amino acids. The **thyroid hormones** (T_3, triiodothyronine and T_4, thyroxine) are tyrosine derivatives that are lipid-soluble and behave much like steroid hormones, with powerful and long-lasting effects on metabolism. In contrast, the catecholamines **epinephrine** and **norepinephrine** are also derived from tyrosine. However, they are water-soluble and act similarly to peptide hormones, exerting powerful short-term effects in response to stress. **Melatonin**, which plays a major role in regulating wakefulness cycles, is both lipid-soluble and water-soluble and derived from tryptophan.

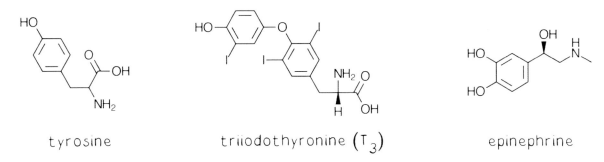

Figure 5. Structures of tyrosine, T_3, and epinephrine

Regulation

So far, we've been talking about hormones in terms of their physiological effects, but it's also possible for hormones to affect the release of other hormones. Such hormones are known as tropic hormones. Nontropic hormones target other cell types and directly induce physiological effects.

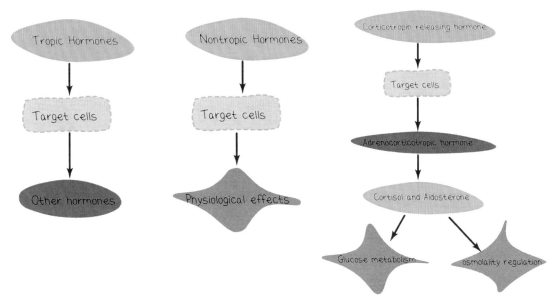

Figure 6. Tropic vs. nontropic hormones and a sample pathway

It is vital to understand the broad principles underlying endocrine regulation, and in particular the distinction between negative and positive feedback. **Negative feedback** loops are by far the most common regulatory mechanism in the endocrine system, and can be examined in several ways. From a functional point of view, negative feedback systems serve to maintain homeostasis—that is, to maintain a relatively constant value of a physiological parameter despite external stimuli. From a technical point of view, negative feedback refers to a phenomenon in which a "downstream" product of a pathway inhibits the pathway itself.

A classic example of a negative feedback loop is the **hypothalamus-anterior pituitary-adrenal cortex (HPA)** axis. The hypothalamus secretes a tropic hormone known as corticotropin-releasing hormone (CRH), which acts on the anterior pituitary gland and stimulates the release of another tropic hormone known as adrenocorticotropic hormone (ACTH). ACTH then acts on the adrenal cortex, causing the release of cortisol, a steroid hormone that plays a role in long-term responses to stress. Elevated levels of cortisol then inhibit the release of both CRH and

ACTH. As always, when studying a synthetic or regulatory pathway, the initial question is: what's the function of this feature from a physiological point of view? In this case, the negative feedback exerted by cortisol on CRH and ACTH inhibits further cortisol production, which prevents levels of cortisol from skyrocketing out of control and inducing an overly intense long-term stress response.

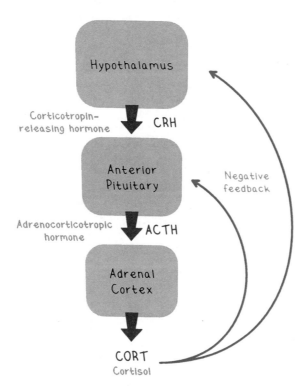

Figure 7. Hypothalamus-anterior pituitary-adrenal cortex (HPA) axis

Positive feedback loops in the endocrine system are rare. From a functional perspective, a positive feedback loop works to push a system out of its normal limits. From a technical standpoint, positive feedback means that the "downstream" product of a pathway stimulates its own production. A common example of a positive feedback system is **oxytocin**, a small peptide hormone secreted by the posterior pituitary gland. Oxytocin has several effects, as we'll discuss in more detail later in this chapter, but one of its most important effects is that it stimulates contractions of the uterus at the end of pregnancy. Uterine contractions stimulate the release of more oxytocin, which stimulates stronger uterine contractions, and the process continues to amplify itself through labor and childbirth (also known as parturition). Note that this process has a well-defined external physiological endpoint. Without such an endpoint, positive feedback loops would tend to spiral out of control, resulting in dangerously extreme physiological states.

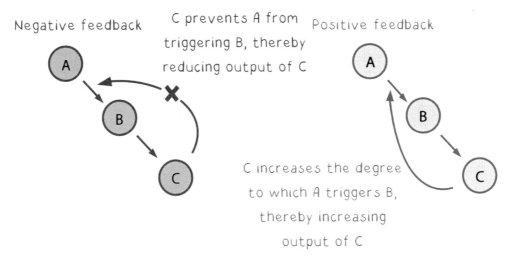

Figure 8. Negative vs. positive feedback loops

Another concept related to regulation you should be aware of is **neuroendocrinology**, a term that refers to the fact that the nervous and endocrine systems "talk to" each other. From a big picture perspective, this is necessary because the nervous and the endocrine systems can be thought of as the two communication networks of the body, and they have to interact to make sure that the body responds appropriately to stimuli. An example of how this occurs is provided by the HPA axis, which we presented above as starting with the release of CRH by the hypothalamus to stimulate ACTH secretion in the anterior pituitary. A natural follow-up question would be: why does the hypothalamus release CRH? The answer is that it does so in response to signaling from the nervous system regarding stressful stimuli. Neuronal signaling allows the body to quickly integrate information about external stimuli and new developments in the body, which can then be relayed to the endocrine system. For this reason, the hypothalamus is often considered the bridge between the nervous and endocrine systems.

> **MCAT STRATEGY >>>**
>
> You should be *very* careful about choosing "positive feedback" as the answer to any question on the MCAT. A passage may point you in that direction, but in general, when thinking about endocrine regulation (and, for that matter, the regulation of biochemical pathways), your default assumption should always be negative feedback.

2. Physiological Effects of Hormones

Now that we've covered the basic principles governing the endocrine system, let's move on to discuss the specific physiological effects of various hormones.

Glucose Levels

Glucose can be thought of as the body's main source of fuel under most circumstances, and the regulation of blood glucose levels is therefore critically important in maintaining overall metabolic function. The two main hormones associated with glucose regulation are **insulin** and **glucagon**, although **growth hormone (GH)**, **epinephrine**, and **cortisol** also affect glucose levels.

Insulin is a peptide hormone released by the beta cells of the pancreas in response to high blood glucose levels, and its basic function is to reduce blood glucose levels by promoting the transport of glucose into cells via **insulin receptors**. This activates membrane-bound **glucose transporters** and increases the transport of glucose into the cell. Let's evaluate the consequences of increased glucose uptake in cells. First, the cells have to decide what to do with all of this glucose. They are faced with three options: cells can use the glucose immediately through **glycolysis**, muscle and liver cells can store the glucose as **glycogen**, and adipocytes (fat cells) can store downstream byproducts of glucose metabolism in the form of **triglycerides**. Insulin upregulates all of those processes, as well as **protein synthesis**. Insulin also reduces the rate of glycogenolysis, lipolysis, fatty acid oxidation in the muscle and liver, and protein breakdown in the muscles. The effects of insulin are numerous, but they are all linked intuitively in that they reflect the presence of excess available energy in the form of glucose.

Glucagon is a peptide hormone released by the alpha cells of the pancreas and is essentially insulin's opposite. It is released in low glucose levels and increases blood glucose levels by promoting glycogenolysis and gluconeogenesis in liver cells.

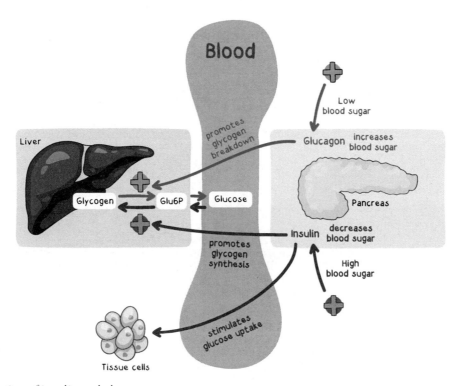

Figure 9. Regulation of insulin and glucagon

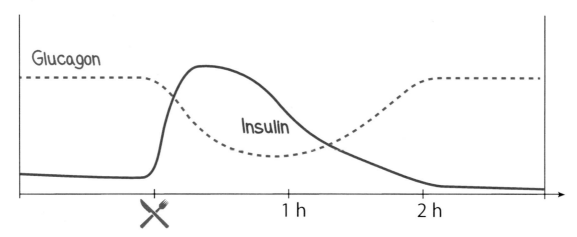

Figure 10. Effects of insulin and glucagon over time in response to a high carbohydrate meal

As important as insulin and glucagon are, they are not the only hormones that increase blood glucose levels. **Cortisol** (the main example of the hormone class glucocorticoids) is released by the adrenal cortex. It is associated with long-term responses to stress, and it increases blood glucose levels. **Epinephrine**, which is released by the adrenal medulla and plays a major role in the fight-or-flight response to immediate stress, also raises blood glucose levels. In addition, under conditions of intense physical stress, as well as during periods of physical growth, **growth hormone (GH)** can be released. **GH** has many functions, including increasing blood glucose levels due to its antagonistic effects on insulin. Nonetheless, if you see a question about blood glucose levels, you should immediately think of the insulin-glucagon pair, unless the passage or question points you specifically in the direction of other hormones that may affect blood glucose levels.

Calcium Levels

Calcium plays a key role in multiple physiological functions: most notably in bones, neurotransmitter release, muscle contractions, and as a second messenger within the cell. The body must maintain serum Ca^{2+} levels within very tight ranges, and the primary hormones that perform this maintenance are **parathyroid hormone (PTH)**, **calcitonin** and **calcitriol**.

PTH is secreted from the parathyroid glands in response to low blood calcium levels. It elevates blood calcium levels by stimulating increased activity in **osteoclasts**, which are cells that break down bone, releasing calcium into the blood. **Calcitonin** has the opposite effect; it is released by the C cells of the thyroid gland and inhibits osteoclast activity. Just as a review, **osteoblasts** are cells that help build bone—and therefore reduce blood calcium levels by "storing" calcium in bone tissue—whereas osteoclasts are cells that break down bone, releasing calcium into the bloodstream.

CLINICAL CONNECTIONS >>>

Diabetes mellitus (DM) is one of the most important diseases to be aware of for the MCAT. Diabetes is commonly associated with elevated glucose levels (hyperglycemia), but fundamentally it is a disorder of insulin metabolism. Type 1 DM is an autoimmune disorder in which the beta cells of the pancreas are destroyed; as a result, insulin is not produced. Patients with type 1 DM require treatment in the form of insulin injections. Type 2 DM involves insulin resistance that develops as a result of chronically elevated blood sugar levels. In its initial stages, type 2 DM can be treated with drugs that improve insulin response, such as metformin, but patients with type 2 DM may also eventually require insulin injections.

MCAT STRATEGY >>>

You can remember what glucagon does by recalling that it is released when *glucose* is *gone*.

>>CONNECTIONS <<

Chapter 12 of Biology

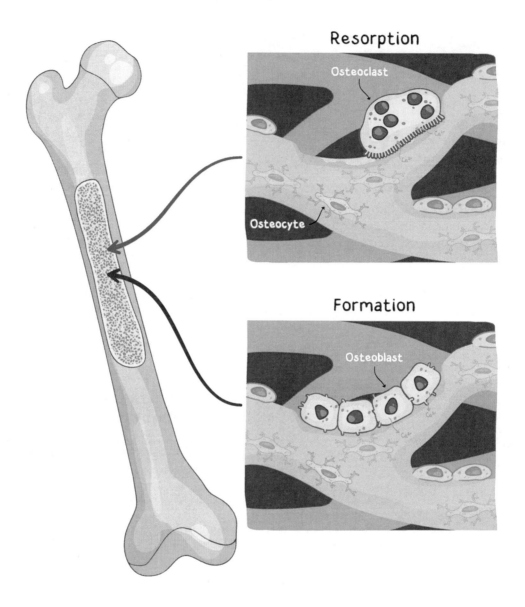

Figure 11. Osteoblasts and osteoclasts

Vitamin D plays a crucial role in the regulation of serum calcium and phosphate levels. Vitamin D exists in multiple forms. Cholecalciferol is the inactive form of vitamin D_3, which is processed to form calcitriol and is the biologically active form that affects calcium and phosphate levels. Calcitriol increases serum calcium levels, similarly to PTH, but it does so primarily through a different mechanism: it promotes the absorption of Ca^{2+} from the gastrointestinal tract. It promotes an increase in serum calcium by a few other mechanisms as well.

>> **CONNECTIONS** <<

Chapter 10 of Biology

Fluid Regulation

Another crucial task performed by the endocrine system is the fluid level regulation. For the purposes of the MCAT, you can think of this as blood volume and optimal blood osmolarity. There are two dilemmas that the body can encounter: too little fluid and too much fluid. Let's first think through how these conditions manifest physiologically as this is a prerequisite to correctly applying the information described in this section. Having **too little fluid** in one's system manifests in a few ways: reduced blood volume (because relatively little water is present in the blood plasma) and **reduced blood pressure** (a consequence of reduced blood volume—less liquid is present to exert pressure against the walls of the blood vessels). Depending on the cause of the fluid loss, blood osmolarity can also be affected. Correspondingly, **increases in the amount of fluid** present in the system manifest as **increased blood volume** and **increased blood pressure**. Blood osmolarity can also be affected by changes in the volume of fluid, but the change depends on the cause of the increased fluid volume.

> **MCAT STRATEGY >>>**
>
> Practice working through these causal relationships until they become second nature. If given information about relative levels of fluid, you should immediately be able to predict the consequences for blood volume and pressure.

Two major hormones respond to low fluid levels by increasing fluid retention: **aldosterone** (the main example of a class of steroid hormones known as mineralocorticoids) and **antidiuretic hormone (ADH)**, a peptide hormone that is also known as vasopressin. However, these two hormones have different mechanisms. **Aldosterone** works by increasing sodium absorption in the distal convoluted tubule and collecting duct of the nephron, which, in conjunction with ADH, drives water absorption. Aldosterone also increases excretion of potassium and hydrogen ions in the urine. In contrast to aldosterone, **ADH** increases the permeability of the collecting duct to water, thereby increasing water absorption. The result is that ADH acts to reduce the osmolarity of blood by increasing the amount of water present without changing the solute levels, whereas aldosterone does not affect osmolarity because sodium reabsorption drives water absorption.

> **MCAT STRATEGY >>>**
>
> The presence of an *s* in aldosterone can help you remember that its mechanism involves sodium reabsorption.

ADH is released by the **posterior pituitary gland** in response to low blood pressure and high plasma osmolarity. Aldosterone is released by the **adrenal cortex** in response to low blood pressure, but is regulated by the renin-angiotensin-aldosterone system, as illustrated in Figure 13. In response to low blood pressure, the juxtaglomerular cells of the kidney release an enzyme known as **renin**. Renin converts **angiotensinogen**, which is an inactive plasma protein, into **angiotensin I**. In the lungs and in blood vessels elsewhere in the body, angiotensin-converting enzyme converts angiotensin I to angiotensin II, which is the immediate stimulus of aldosterone release. Aldosterone restores blood pressure, which in turn inhibits the release of renin, in another example of a negative feedback loop.

> **MCAT STRATEGY >>>**
>
> Why does drinking alcohol dehydrate you? It turns out that one of the many effects of ethanol on the body is the inhibition of ADH production. ADH promotes water retention, so less ADH means more water excretion (that is to say, increased urination) and therefore dehydration.

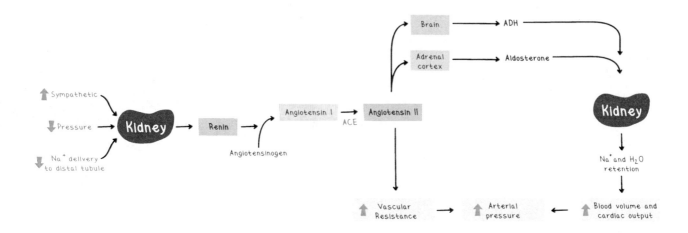

Figure 12. Renin-angiotensin-aldosterone system

Although less high-yield for the MCAT, it is worth learning about **atrial natriuretic peptide ANP**, which is a hormone used to combat excess blood volume. It is released in response to high blood volume and decreases sodium reabsorption in the kidney, as well as increasing the glomerular filtration rate (GFR) and inhibiting aldosterone release.

Stress

We've already discussed stress to some extent in the section on blood glucose regulation, since the elevation of blood glucose levels is one element of the body's response to stress. The most important differentiation for the MCAT is between long-term and short-term responses to stress.

The steroid hormone **cortisol** is associated with **long-term responses to stress**. Cortisol is released from the adrenal cortex and is a member of the class of hormones known as glucocorticoids (other examples include cortisone and prednisone). Cortisol has two main effects to review. First, it increases blood glucose levels by stimulating gluconeogenesis and acting as an insulin antagonist, facilitating insulin resistance. Second, it reduces inflammation by inhibiting certain inflammatory immune responses.

Short-term responses to stress (the **"fight or flight" response**) are associated with **epinephrine** and **norepinephrine**, which are hormones (although norepinephrine and epinephrine also function as neurotransmitters) derived from tyrosine. Epinephrine and norepinephrine belong to a family of hormones known as **catecholamines** and are released from the adrenal medulla. They increase blood glucose levels through a variety of mechanisms, including glycogenolysis, gluconeogenesis, and glucagon release. These hormones also lead to a broad range of systematic responses, including an increased heart rate, respiratory rate, lipolysis, and vasodilation of the blood vessels supplying skeletal muscles combined with vasoconstriction of most other blood vessels.

The effects of epinephrine and norepinephrine presented here are very similar to those of the sympathetic nervous system, as discussed in Chapter 6. Some terminological clarification is in order to reveal why this topic needs to be discussed in the context of the endocrine system as well. We briefly mentioned that norepinephrine is both a neurotransmitter and a hormone— how is this possible? Norepinephrine is a neurotransmitter when it is used to relay signals between neurons in the sympathetic nervous system, but when it is released into the blood to induce systemic effects in other organ systems, it functions as a hormone. Analogously, sympathetic nervous system signaling triggers the release of epinephrine and norepinehrine into the blood, at which point they function as hormones to exert their downstream effects. Another way of thinking about this might involve a division of labor between the nervous system and the endocrine system in response to stress.

Metabolic Rate

The thyroid hormones **triiodothyronine (T_3)** and **thyroxine (T_4)** regulate the body's general metabolic rate. T_4 contains four iodine atoms and is the prohormone, or precursor, of T_3, which contains three iodine atoms. Beyond this structural difference, T_3 and T_4 can be thought of as synonymous for the purposes of the MCAT. They are released in response to **thyroid-stimulating hormone (TSH)**. Insufficient levels of thyroid hormones, often caused by an iodine deficiency, leads to hypothyroidism: a clinical condition characterized by fatigue, cold intolerance, weight gain, and reductions in body temperature, heart rate, and respiratory rate. Hyperthyroidism, which may be caused by a tumor, an autoimmune disease, or other causes, results in the opposite set of symptoms.

Reproduction and Secondary Sex Characteristics

These topics are discussed in greater detail in Chapter 8, which focuses on the reproductive system, but it is nonetheless useful to briefly review the hormonal regulation of reproduction and secondary sex characteristics in the context of the endocrine system as a whole. This will allow you to gain an appreciation of how high-level themes such as the contrast between peptide and steroid hormones and the concepts of negative and positive feedback can be applied.

Estrogen and **testosterone**, which are steroid hormones secreted by the ovaries and testes, respectively, are the two most important hormones involved in reproduction and the development of secondary sex characteristics. For the MCAT, you should be aware that estrogen is involved in the regulation of the menstrual cycle and contributes to the development of female secondary sex characteristics, while testosterone contributes to the development of male secondary sex characteristics. In reality, both hormones have a complex profile of systemic effects, but a full discussion of the effects of these hormones can wait for medical school. Another steroid hormone involved in the reproductive system that you should be aware of is **progesterone**, which prepares the uterus for implantation and maintains it throughout pregnancy. Note how all three of these hormones have

CLINICAL CONNECTIONS >>>

Anti-hypertensive medications are a mainstay of the everyday practice of medicine, and physicians must understand the different mechanisms of blood pressure medications in order to prescribe them appropriately. The renin-angiotensin-aldosterone system is an area that scientists have targeted with this goal in mind. Inhibitors of angiotensin-converting enzyme (ACE inhibitors) prevent the formation of angiotensin II, which reduces blood pressure by inhibiting aldosterone secretion and counteracting the tendency of angiotensin II itself to raise blood pressure.

MCAT STRATEGY >>>

Information about the function of a substance is often reflected in its nomenclature. Imagine you had never before heard of atrial natriuretic peptide and wanted to know what it does. Well, "atrial" tells you that it's secreted from the heart muscles, and "peptide" tells you that it's a peptide. For the "natriuretic" part of the name, "uretic" might point you towards thinking about urine! This doesn't give you the whole story about its function, but it at least gives you somewhere to start. Leveraging information like this can be very helpful in tackling passages.

CLINICAL CONNECTIONS >>>

Cortisone is a glucocorticoid with anti-inflammatory effects that is often directly injected to treat inflamed muscles or joints.

>>CONNECTIONS <<

Chapter 6 of Biology

relatively long-term effects, as is typical for steroid hormones.

The release of estrogen and testosterone is stimulated by **luteinizing hormone (LH)**, which is a peptide hormone secreted in response to low levels of these hormones. LH is released in response to **gonadotropin-releasing hormone (GnRH)**. An LH surge leads to ovulation. Another peptide hormone released in response to GnRH that plays an important role in reproduction is **follicle-stimulating hormone (FSH)**, which, as the name suggests, promotes the growth of ovarian follicles in females. It also has the effect of promoting spermatogenesis in males. During pregnancy, **human chorionic gonadotropin (hCG)** maintains the corpus luteum and induces it to secrete progesterone during the first trimester.

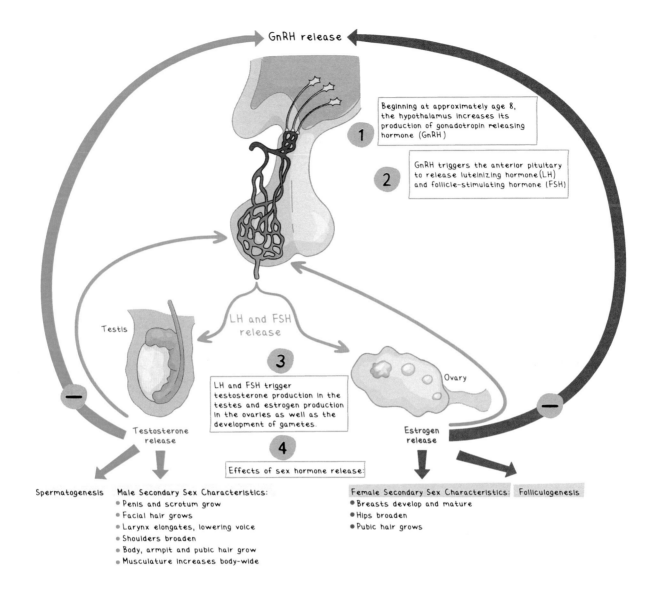

GnRH release

Beginning at approximately age 8, the hypothalamus increases its production of gonadotropin releasing hormone (GnRH)

1

GnRH triggers the anterior pituitary to release luteinizing hormone (LH) and follicle-stimulating hormone (FSH)

2

Testis

LH and FSH release

3

LH and FSH trigger testosterone production in the testes and estrogen production in the ovaries as well as the development of gametes.

Ovary

4

Testosterone release

Estrogen release

Effects of sex hormone release:

Spermatogenesis

Male Secondary Sex Characteristics:
- Penis and scrotum grow
- Facial hair grows
- Larynx elongates, lowering voice
- Shoulders broaden
- Body, armpit and pubic hair grow
- Musculature increases body-wide

Female Secondary Sex Characteristics: Folliculogenesis
- Breasts develop and mature
- Hips broaden
- Pubic hair grows

Figure 13. Regulation of reproductive hormones

A final hormone related to reproduction that you should be aware of is **prolactin**, which acts on the mammary glands to enable milk production. Prolactin is released in response to the reduced levels of dopamine that occur after the placenta is expelled during childbirth. Dopamine secretion from the hypothalamus is also reduced in response to an infant latching onto the breast, thereby facilitating milk production.

Regulation of Other Hormones (Tropic Hormones)

Finally, **tropic hormones** have the function of regulating other hormones, thereby contributing to the exquisitely fine-tuned ability of the endocrine system to respond to various stimuli.

Several crucial tropic hormones are released by the anterior pituitary gland. **Thyroid-stimulating hormone (TSH)** promotes the release of the thyroid hormones T_3 and T_4, while **adrenocorticotropic hormone (ACTH)** stimulates the adrenal cortex to release mineralocorticoids and glucocorticoids (which belong to the class of hormones known as corticosteroids). As discussed in the previous section on reproduction, **Luteinizing hormone (LH)** is a tropic hormone that stimulates the release of estrogen and testosterone, as discussed in the section dealing with reproduction, and follicle-stimulating hormone (FSH) activates further signaling pathways to promote the development of ovarian follicles and spermatogenesis.

Although the above tropic hormones are the most important for the MCAT, it is worth being aware that tropic hormones can be regulated by other tropic hormones. Many such hormones are secreted from the hypothalamus, which can be thought of as the bridge between the nervous and endocrine system. Examples of tropic hormones secreted from the hypothalamus include: **gonadotropin-releasing hormone (GnRH)**, which stimulates the release of LH and FSH; **thyrotropin-releasing hormone (TRH)**, which stimulates the release of TSH; **corticotropin-releasing factor (CRF)**, which stimulates the release of ACTH; and **growth hormone-releasing hormone (GHRH)**, which stimulates the release of growth hormone.

A final tropic hormone to be aware of is **human chorionic gonadotropin (hCG)**, which stimulates the release of progesterone to maintain the uterus throughout the first trimester of pregnancy.

The following table summarizes the hormones essential for the MCAT according to function. Since some hormones are involved in multiple functions, this table contains some duplication of hormones.

FUNCTION	HORMONE	STRUC-TURAL TYPE	STIMULUS	EFFECT	LOCATION OF SECRETION
Glucose levels	Insulin	Peptide	↑ Glucose	↓ Glucose	Pancreas (beta cells)
	Glucagon	Peptide	↓ Glucose	↑ Glucose	Pancreas (alpha cells)
	Cortisol	Steroid	Stress	↑ Glucose (& other systemic effects)	Adrenal cortex
	Epinephrine and norepinephrine	AA-derived (polar)			Adrenal medulla
	Growth hormone (GH)	Peptide	Stress, puberty, and other stimuli	↑ Glucose	Anterior pituitary
Calcium levels	Parathyroid hormone (PTH)	Peptide	↓ Ca^{2+}	↑ Ca^{2+}	Parathyroid
	Calcitonin	Peptide	↑ Ca^{2+}	↓ Ca^{2+}	Thyroid
	Calcitriol (bioactive vitamin D)	Steroid	PTH promotes activation of vitamin D in the kidney	↑ Ca^{2+}	Kidney

FUNCTION	HORMONE	STRUCTURAL TYPE	STIMULUS	EFFECT	LOCATION OF SECRETION
Fluid regulation	Aldosterone	Steroid	↓ BP, ↑ osmolarity, angiotensin II	↑ Na⁺ reabsorption in DCT and collecting ducts, ↑ K⁺ and H⁺ secretion	Adrenal cortex
	Antidiuretic hormone (ADH, vasopressin)	Peptide	↓ BP, ↑ osmolarity	↑ H_2O reabsorption in collecting duct, vasoconstriction	Posterior pituitary
	Atrial natriuretic peptide (ANP)	Peptide	↑ Blood volume	↓ Na⁺ reabsorption in the kidney, ↓ fluid levels, increase GFR	Heart muscle cells
Stress	Cortisol	Steroid	Stress (long-term)	↑ Glucose, ↓ inflammation	Adrenal cortex
	Epinephrine	Amino acid-derived (polar)	Stress (short-term)	↑ Glucose, sympathetic nervous system/ fight-or-flight response	Adrenal medulla
	Norepinephrine	Amino acid-derived (polar)			
Metabolic rate	T_3 and T_4	Amino acid-derived (nonpolar)	TSH	↑ Basal metabolic rate	Thyroid

FUNCTION	HORMONE	STRUC-TURAL TYPE	STIMULUS	EFFECT	LOCATION OF SECRETION
Reproduction and development	Estrogen	Steroid	LH	Female secondary sex characteristics, menstrual cycle regulation	Ovaries
	Testosterone	Steroid		Male secondary sex characteristics	Testes
	Progesterone	Steroid	LH, hCG	Prepares and maintains uterus for pregnancy	Ovaries, placenta
	Luteinizing hormone (LH)	Peptide	GnRH, ↓ estrogen or testosterone, ↑ estrogen triggers LH surge	↑ Estrogen or testosterone	Anterior pituitary
	Follicle-stimulating hormone (FSH)	Peptide	GnRH	Follicle development, spermatogenesis	Anterior pituitary
	Human chorionic gonadotropin (hCG)	Peptide	Released by placenta	↑ Progesterone	Placenta
	Prolactin	Peptide	↓ Dopamine, nipple stimulation	Milk production	Anterior pituitary
	Oxytocin	Peptide	Neural signaling (uterine stretching, nipple stimulation)	Smooth muscle contraction (uterine contractions in labor, milk release in breastfeeding)	Posterior pituitary

FUNCTION	HORMONE	STRUCTURAL TYPE	STIMULUS	EFFECT	LOCATION OF SECRETION
Tropic hormones	Thyroid-stimulating hormone (TSH)	Peptide	TRH	↑ Thyroid hormones	Anterior pituitary
	Adreno-corticotropic hormone (ACTH)	Peptide	CRF	↑ Adrenal cortex activity (↑ corticosteroids)	Anterior pituitary
	Luteinizing hormone (LH)	Peptide	GnRH, ↓ estrogen or testosterone, ↑ estrogen triggers LH surge	↑ Estrogen or testosterone	Anterior pituitary
	Follicle-stimulating hormone (FSH)	Peptide	GnRH	Follicle development, spermatogenesis	Anterior pituitary
	Human chorionic gonadotropin (hCG)	Peptide	Released by placenta	↑ Progesterone	Placenta
	Gonadotropin-releasing hormone (GnRH)	Peptide	Neural signaling	↑ LH, ↑ FSH	Hypothalamus
	Thyrotropin-releasing hormone (TRH)	Peptide	Neural signaling	↑ TSH	Hypothalamus
	Corticotropin-releasing hormone (CRH)	Peptide	Neural signaling in response to stress	↑ ACTH	Hypothalamus
	Growth hormone-releasing hormone (GHRH)	Peptide	Neural signaling	↑ GH	Hypothalamus

Table 2. Hormones involved in crucial functions of the endocrine system

3. Organs of the Endocrine System

Although MCAT passages are likely to focus on the physiological and systemic effects of hormones, it is also necessary to understand the function of each organ of the endocrine system and identify which hormones they release. This section breaks down hormones according to their associated organ and provides information about those organs. Some information is repeated from the previous section that focused on key endocrine functions; in such cases, a more detailed discussion is presented in the previous section. However, this section also presents some other hormones that have isolated effects less closely linked to crucial general functions of the endocrine system. A complete list of MCAT-relevant hormones is presented in Table 3 at the end of this chapter.

Hypothalamus

As we've discussed, the endocrine system ultimately relies on signaling from the nervous system in order to properly respond to external stimuli. The **hypothalamus** plays a crucial role in this process and can be thought of as the bridge between the nervous system and the endocrine system. It is located in the forebrain, directly above the pituitary gland, and receives input from several sources elsewhere in the brain. It then secretes several tropic hormones into the **hypophyseal portal system**, which connects the hypothalamus to the anterior pituitary. The hypophyseal portal system allow the hormones secreted by the hypothalamus to be conveyed quickly and directly to the anterior pituitary, facilitating the fine-tuned control of downstream endocrine responses. Another portal system in the body is the hepatic portal system, discussed in Chapter 10.

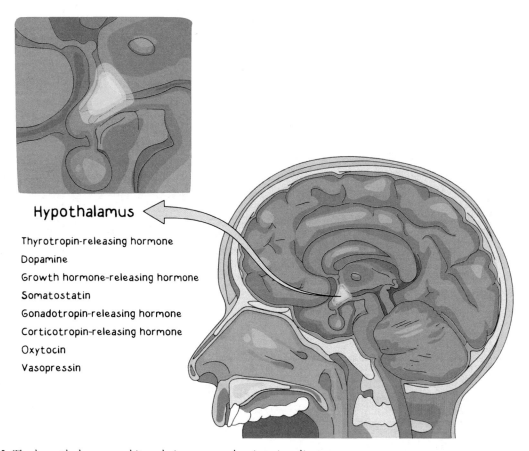

Hypothalamus

Thyrotropin-releasing hormone
Dopamine
Growth hormone-releasing hormone
Somatostatin
Gonadotropin-releasing hormone
Corticotropin-releasing hormone
Oxytocin
Vasopressin

Figure 14. The hypothalamus and its role in neuroendocrine signaling

For the most part, the tropic hormones secreted by the hypothalamus regulate the secretion of other tropic hormones. This is the case for gonadotropin-releasing hormone (GnRH), which promotes the secretion of luteinizing hormone (LH) and follicle-stimulating hormone (FSH) from the anterior pituitary. It is also true for thyrotropin-releasing hormone (TRH), which stimulates the anterior pituitary to release thyroid-stimulating hormone (TSH) and corticotropin-releasing hormone (CRH), which promotes the secretion of adrenocorticotropic hormone (ACTH) from the anterior pituitary. The hypothalamus secretes growth hormone-releasing hormone (GHRH) as well, which stimulates the secretion of growth hormone, a nontropic hormone released from the anterior pituitary gland.

Anterior and Posterior Pituitary

The pituitary gland is divided into two parts: the anterior and posterior pituitary gland. These two sections have drastically different functions, to the point that you should treat them as two distinct endocrine organs. One point of commonality, however, is that all of the hormones secreted by the pituitary are peptide hormones.

As discussed above, the **anterior pituitary** receives input from the hypothalamus via the hypophyseal portal system, and secretes both tropic and direct hormones.

> **MCAT STRATEGY >>>**
>
> Mnemonic: FLAT PEG stands for **F**SH, **L**H, **A**CTH, and **T**SH (all tropic) and **P**rolactin, **E**ndorphin, and **G**rowth hormones (all nontropic).

The tropic hormones released by the anterior pituitary include luteinizing hormone (LH) and follicle-stimulating hormone (FSH), which are released in response to gonadotropin-releasing hormone (GnRH) release from the hypothalamus. In males, LH stimulates Leydig cells to release testosterone. In females, LH stimulates the release of estrogen and a surge of LH stimulates ovulation. FSH stimulates the growth of ovarian follicles in females and promotes spermatogenesis in males. The anterior pituitary releases adrenocorticotropic hormone (ACTH), which acts on the adrenal cortex to induce the secretion of corticosteroids, most notably cortisol and aldosterone. Thyroid-stimulating hormone (TSH) is released by the anterior pituitary and acts on the thyroid to stimulate the release of the thyroid hormones.

The direct hormones released by the anterior pituitary are prolactin, endorphin, and growth hormones. Prolactin acts on the mammary glands to stimulate milk production in response to reduced dopamine levels. Endorphins are a family of hormones that reduce the perception of pain. Growth hormone is released both in response to stress and when the body is undergoing periods of accelerated growth. It exerts a range of systemic effects associated with growth, and also, when released in response to stress, has the effect of raising blood glucose levels.

The **posterior pituitary gland** releases hormones in direct response to signaling from the hypothalamus. It is responsible for the release of two hormones: antidiuretic hormone (ADH), also known as vasopressin, and oxytocin. ADH plays a major role in regulating fluid balance in the body, and is released in response to low blood volume and high blood osmolarity, both of which are signals of dehydration. It promotes water reabsorption directly by increasing the permeability of the collecting duct, resulting in increased blood pressure, increased blood volume, and decreased blood osmolarity. ADH also causes vasoconstriction. Oxytocin has two main functions that you should be aware of: it promotes uterine contractions leading up to childbirth and milk ejection resulting from the contraction of smooth muscle tissues in the milk ducts. The role of oxytocin in promoting uterine contractions is a well-known example of a positive feedback loop, as discussed earlier in the chapter. In addition to this, oxytocin plays an important role in promoting social bonding.

Parathyroid and Thyroid

The **thyroid gland** is located on the anterior (front) surface of the trachea and the **parathyroid glands** are four small glands, roughly the size of peas, located on the posterior (back) of the thyroid. The thyroid produces T_3 and T_4, often referred to simply as thyroid hormone, which act to increase an individual's basal metabolic rate. The thyroid produces calcitonin as well, which decreases plasma Ca^{2+} levels by increasing Ca^{2+} storage in the bones (if Ca^{2+} is locked up in bone tissue, it's not in the blood) and increasing Ca^{2+} excretion from the body.

> **MCAT STRATEGY >>>**
>
> This is a good example of the various ways the body can handle an excess of something: absorb less of it, utilize it in some way, avoid the negative effects of having it in excess, and/or get rid of it.

The parathyroid glands release parathyroid hormone (PTH), which has the opposite effect of calcitonin on serum calcium levels. PTH increases Ca^{2+} absorption from the intestine indirectly by promoting the activation of vitamin D, decreases Ca^{2+} storage in the bones, and in the kidneys promotes Ca^{2+} retention instead of excretion.

Adrenal Cortex and Medulla

The **adrenal glands** sit on top of the kidney. Each adrenal gland consists of two anatomically and functionally distinct areas: the cortex and the medulla.

The **adrenal cortex** secretes steroid hormones known as corticosteroids, which are further subclassified into glucocorticoids (the main example of which is cortisol), mineralocorticoids (the main example of which is aldosterone), and the cortical sex hormones. Cortisol is involved in long-term responses to stress and has the effect of increasing blood glucose and decreasing inflammatory immune responses. Aldosterone promotes fluid retention by increasing Na^+ reabsorption in the distal convoluted tubules and collecting ducts. Cortical sex hormones are a category of hormones including various androgens and estrogens, such as testosterone. Generally speaking, cortical sex hormones do not play a major role in the regulation of secondary sex characteristics due to the larger quantity of sex hormones produced in the gonads, but they are worth reviewing.

The **adrenal medulla** secretes the amino-acid derived hormones epinephrine and norepinephrine, which are involved in short-term stress responses. They are members of a larger class of compounds known as catecholamines; practically speaking, all this means is that you should be able to associate the term "catecholamine" with these hormones if prompted. They have the effect of increasing blood glucose levels and mediating many of the responses involved in the fight-or-flight stress response induced by the sympathetic nervous system.

Pancreas

The **pancreas** is located behind the stomach in the abdominal cavity, and is noteworthy as it plays an important role in both the endocrine and digestive systems. The endocrine cells of the pancreas you have to be aware of for the MCAT are referred to using Greek letters: alpha (α) cells, beta (β) cells, and delta (δ) cells.

The **alpha cells** of the pancreas secrete glucagon, which is secreted in response to low blood glucose levels and increases blood glucose levels. The **beta cells** secrete insulin. High glucose levels trigger insulin release that reduce blood glucose levels by promoting glucose uptake into cells. **Delta cells** secrete somatostatin, which slows down the rate of digestive hormone secretion in response to high levels of glucose and amino acids (i.e., it tells the body to be less efficient about processing food when plenty of nutrients are already present). It also inhibits the secretion of insulin and glucagon. The layout of this paragraph looks a little bit off to me. "insulin and glucagon" should be left flush, not centered.

Gonads

The reproductive system and its anatomy are discussed in more detail in Chapter 8. For the endocrine system, it is most important to be aware that both the **ovaries** (in females) and **testes** (in males) respond to the gonadotropins luteinizing hormone (LH) and follicle-stimulating hormone (FSH), and release estrogen and testosterone, respectively. These steroid hormones have a range of effects; for the purposes of the MCAT, their most important effect is stimulating the development of secondary sex characteristics.

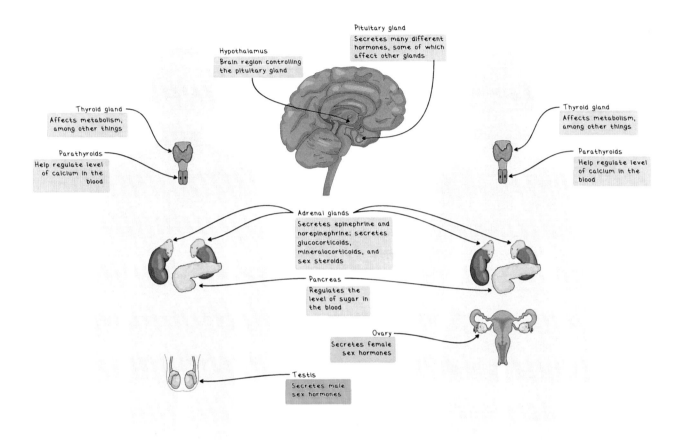

Figure 15. Key endocrine organs of the body

Others

Not all endocrine cells are located in the major endocrine organs or are deeply interwoven into the major physiological functions of the endocrine system discussed in Section 2. This section briefly presents select other hormones to be aware of for the MCAT.

> **>> CONNECTIONS <<**
>
> Chapter 10 of Biology

In the brain, the **pineal gland** secretes an amino-acid derived hormone known as melatonin. Melatonin has a variety of functions, including the regulation of circadian rhythms.

Muscle cells of the heart release atrial natriuretic peptide (ANP), which has effects opposite to those of aldosterone: that is, it is released in response to high blood volume and has the net effect of decreasing blood volume by promoting fluid excretion. Its mechanisms are discussed in more depth above, in Section 2.

The **thymus** is an immune organ where T cells mature, and it secretes thymosin, which is a hormone important for the development and maturation of T cells.

The **digestive system** includes endocrine cells involved in the release of digestive hormones, such as gastrin, secretin, and cholecystokinin. These are discussed in more detail in Chapter 10 on the digestive system, and are not usually included in discussions of the endocrine system because they do not exert systemic effects.

Table 3 summarizes all MCAT-relevant hormones sorted by the organ they are secreted from. Be sure to study both this and Table 2, which sorts the hormones by important physiological functions. Being able to approach the hormones through both lenses will prove very advantageous on the MCAT.

ORGAN	HORMONE	STRUCTURAL TYPE	STIMULUS	EFFECT	NOTES
Hypothalamus	Gonadotropin-releasing hormone (GnRH)	Peptide	Neural signaling	↑ LH, ↑ FSH	Not highest-yield for the MCAT; be aware of these hormones but they should not be your highest priority
	Thyrotropin-releasing hormone (TRH)	Peptide	Neural signaling	↑ TSH	
	Corticotropin-releasing hormone (CRH)	Peptide	Neural signaling in response to stress	↑ ACTH	
	Growth hormone-releasing hormone (GHRH)	Peptide	Neural signaling	↑ GH	

ORGAN	HORMONE	STRUCTURAL TYPE	STIMULUS	EFFECT	NOTES
Anterior pituitary	Thyroid-stimulating hormone (TSH)	Peptide	TRH	↑ Thyroid hormones	
	Adrenocorticotropic hormone (ACTH)	Peptide	CRH	↑ Adrenal cortex activity (↑ corticosteroids)	
	Luteinizing hormone (LH)	Peptide	GnRH, ↓ estrogen or testosterone, ↑ estrogen triggers LH surge	↑ Estrogen or testosterone	
	Follicle-stimulating hormone (FSH)	Peptide	GnRH	Follicle development, spermatogenesis	
	Prolactin	Peptide	↓ Dopamine, nipple stimulation	Milk production	
	Endorphins	Peptide	Pain, exercise	↓ Pain	
	Growth hormone (GH)	Peptide	Stress, puberty, and other stimuli	↑ Glucose	
Posterior pituitary	Oxytocin	Peptide	Neural signaling (uterine stretching, nipple stimulation)	Smooth muscle contraction (uterine contractions in labor, milk release in breastfeeding)	Example of positive feedback
	Antidiuretic hormone (ADH, vasopressin)	Peptide	↓ BP, ↑ osmolarity	↑ H_2O reabsorption in collecting duct; vasoconstriction	
Parathyroid	Parathyroid hormone (PTH)	Peptide	↓ Ca^{2+}	↑ Ca^{2+}	
Thyroid	T_3 and T_4	Amino acid-derived (nonpolar)	TSH	↑ Basal metabolic rate	Contain 3 and 4 iodine atoms, respectively
	Calcitonin	Peptide	↑ Ca^{2+}	↓ Ca^{2+}	

ORGAN	HORMONE	STRUCTURAL TYPE	STIMULUS	EFFECT	NOTES
Adrenal cortex	Cortisol	Steroid	Stress (long-term)	↑ Glucose, ↓ inflammation	Most important glucocorticoid; also classified as corticosteroid
	Aldosterone	Steroid	↓ BP, ↑ osmolarity, angiotensin II	↑ Na⁺ reabsorption in DCT and collecting ducts, ↑ K⁺ and H⁺ secretion	Most important mineralo-corticoid; also classified as a corticosteroid
Adrenal medulla	Epinephrine	Amino acid-derived (polar)	Stress (short-term)	↑ Glucose, fight-or-flight response	
	Norepinephrine	Amino acid-derived (polar)			Also a neurotransmitter with major role in sympathetic nervous response
Pancreas	Insulin	Peptide	↑ Glucose	↓ Glucose	Secreted by the beta cells of pancreas
	Glucagon	Peptide	↓ Glucose	↑ Glucose	Secreted by the alpha cells of pancreas
	Somatostatin	Peptide	Neural signaling, ↑ glucose, ↑ amino acids	Inhibits digestive hormones, inhibits the secretion of insulin and glucagon, slows digestion	Secreted by the delta cells of pancreas
Reproductive organs	Estrogen	Steroid	LH	Female secondary sex characteristics, menstrual cycle regulation	Secreted by the ovaries
	Testosterone	Steroid		Male secondary sex characteristics	Secreted by the testes
	Progesterone	Steroid	LH, hCG	Prepares and maintains uterus for pregnancy	Secreted by the ovaries, placenta
	Human chorionic gonadotropin (hCG)	Peptide	Released by the placenta	↑ Progesterone	Secreted by the placenta

ORGAN	HORMONE	STRUCTURAL TYPE	STIMULUS	EFFECT	NOTES
Others	Melatonin	Amino acid- derived	Neural signaling	Circadian rhythms	Pineal gland
	Atrial natriuretic peptide (ANP)	Peptide	↑ Blood volume	↓ Na⁺ reabsorption in the kidney, ↓ fluid levels, ↑ GFR	Heart muscle cells
	Digestive hormones	Peptides	Various (see Chapter 10)	Various (see Chapter 10)	Endocrine cells in the digestive system
	Thymosin	Peptide	Various	T-cell development	Thymus

Table 3. Important hormones for the MCAT by organ of secretion

4. Must-Knows

> High-level points about the endocrine system:
> - "Endocrine" refers specifically to ductless glands that release signaling molecules (hormones) into the circulation.
> - Its role is communication among organ systems.
> - Endocrine signaling is slower than neural signaling.
> - Many endocrine functions are ultimately controlled by the nervous system (through intermediaries).
> The structural differences between peptide hormones, steroid hormones, and amino acid hormones, and how they contribute to the function of these hormone types:
> - Peptide hormones are made up from amino acid chains and are hydrophilic. Steroid hormones are derived from cholesterol, have a four-ring structure, and are lipophilic.
> - Peptide hormones cannot diffuse through the plasma membranes of their target cells, so they interact with transmembrane receptors that activate second messenger signaling systems in the cytosol.
> - Steroid hormones can and do diffuse through the plasma membranes of their target cells, bind with receptors, and influence gene expression in their target cells.
> - Peptide hormones typically have quick-onset, short-acting effects. Steroid hormones typically have a delayed onset and long-lasting effects.
> - Steroid hormones affect sex (estrogen, testosterone, progesterone), salt (aldosterone, a mineralocorticoid), and sugar (cortisol, a glucocorticoid). Amino acid-derived hormones include T_3/T_4 and (nor)epinephrine. All other high-yield hormones are peptides.
> Negative feedback: common in the body; downstream product inhibits upstream steps; maintains homeostasis.
> Positive feedback: unusual in body; downstream product upregulates upstream steps; pushes the body towards an extreme state; example is oxytocin in labor/childbirth.
> Major functions of the endocrine system:
> - Glucose: Insulin decreases glucose, glucagon increases glucose.
> - Serum calcium concentration: PTH & vitamin D_3 increase Ca^{2+}, Calcitonin decreases Ca^{2+}.
> - Fluids: Aldosterone & ADH increase fluid retention, ANP increases fluid excretion.
> - Stress:
>   - Cortisol: increases glucose, long-term stress.
>   - Epinephrine: increases glucose and fight or flight response, short-term stress.
> - Metabolic rate: T_3 and T_4 increase basal metabolic rate.
> - Reproduction and development: Estrogen & testosterone initiate secondary sex characteristics.
> - Tropic hormones play a role in multi-step signaling pathways.

End of Chapter Practice

The best MCAT practice is **realistic**, with a focus on identifying steps for further improvement. For those reasons, we recommend completing practice questions in an online setting that simulates the real MCAT interface, and taking advantage of advanced analytic features to help you determine how best to move forward in your MCAT study journey.

With that in mind, **online end-of-chapter** questions for Biology, Biochemistry, Chemistry + Organic Chemistry, Physics, and Psychology/Sociology are available through your Blueprint MCAT account.

As a further supplement, given the importance of active learning for effective studying, we also suggest that you consult the Must-Knows at the end of each chapter as a basis for creating a study sheet, in which you list out key terms and test your ability to briefly summarize them.

This page left intentionally blank.

Reproduction and Development

0. Introduction

Reproductive health is a tremendously diverse and important domain of medicine, which you will explore in more depth in medical school. The MCAT does not expect you to be aware of everything regarding reproductive health, but you are expected to have a grounding in the anatomical and physiological basics that will provide a scaffold for you to expand upon later. As always for the MCAT, it is important to focus on areas where anatomical/physiological information can be approached with an eye towards building connections with signaling systems, as well as interactions with the environment, and other areas of testable content. The reproductive system also has abundant examples of such intersections. In this chapter, we start by presenting the basic anatomy and physiology of the male and female reproductive systems, including spermatogenesis and oogenesis, then proceed to discuss embryogenesis, development, and pregnancy, and conclude with an overview of the hormonal control of reproduction that builds upon the material presented in Chapter 7 on the endocrine system.

1. Male Reproductive System

For both the female and male reproductive systems, it is helpful to distinguish between the terms "**genitalia**" and "**gonads**." Gonads are specifically the organs in which gametes are made: that is, the testes in males and the ovaries in females. The term "genitalia" refers more broadly to the reproductive organs, and can be subdivided into the internal genitalia and external genitalia. The external organs can be classified as the external genitalia. In the male reproductive system, the external genitalia are the penis and scrotum.

The **scrotum** is a pouch that hangs behind the **penis**. Its main function is to contain the **testes**. The testes (singular = testis) are where sperm is produced, but also secrete hormones, most notably **testosterone**. An interesting aspect of spermatogenesis is that it operates optimally a few degrees below body temperature, and the scrotum therefore contains musculature to regulate the temperature of the testes. When the external temperature is cold, the testes should be closer to the body to keep them at the correct temperature; to do so, the cremaster muscle pulls the scrotum up and closer to the body, while the dartos muscle contracts and makes the scrotum wrinkly, which has the effect of reducing the surface area through which heat can be lost. The opposite changes happen in hot environments where the testes need to be cooled instead of warmed.

The core of the testis is made up by **seminiferous tubules** that are separated by septa (singular = septum; "septum" is the anatomical term for a barrier or partition between two spaces, and is used in many different contexts in anatomy). The seminiferous tubules are where meiosis and spermatogenesis take place. **Germ cells** are present within the seminiferous tubules, and **Sertoli cells**, which constitute the epithelium of the seminiferous tubules, help germ cells develop into **spermatozoa**. Additionally, **Leydig cells** are found adjacent to the seminiferous tubules. These cells are linked to the endocrine function of the testes and secrete androgens (male sex hormones) such as testosterone.

Immature spermatozoa made in the seminiferous tubules move to the **epididymis**, a structure attached to the rear of the testes that is used for the storage and further maturation of spermatozoa. When spermatozoa enter the epididymis, they are non-motile (unable to move independently), but they gain this ability over the period of two to three months they are stored in the epididymis. The life cycle of spermatozoa splits at the epididymis: either spermatozoa proceed through ejaculation or are broken down and reabsorbed.

In the event of ejaculation, spermatozoa move from the epididymis to the **vas deferens**, a tube that connects the epididymis to the ejaculatory ducts. The ejaculatory ducts are formed by a fusion of the vas deferens with the **seminal vesicles**, which are glands located below the urinary bladder that generate the majority of the liquid component of semen. In particular, the seminal vesicles secrete fructose, vitamins, enzymes, and other proteins necessary for spermatozoa to stay alive after ejaculation. The ejaculatory ducts run through the **prostate gland**, and then join with the prostatic **urethra**. Secretions from the **bulbourethral glands** (also known as Cowper's glands) lubricate the urethra before ejaculation and neutralize any remaining acidic urine that is present. The semen then travels through the urethra and is released from the penis upon **ejaculation**.

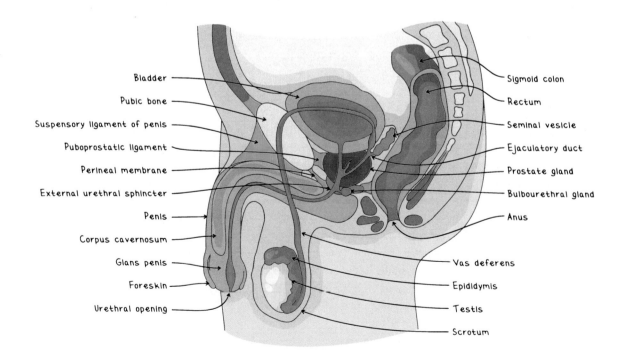

Figure 1. Male reproductive system

An important point to remember is the distinction between sperm (or spermatozoa) and semen. Sperm are the haploid gametes with flagella that can fertilize an egg, while semen consists of the sperm and the secretions of the male accessory glands. Semen is alkaline (weakly basic), while the female reproductive tract is acidic. Vaginal pH normally ranges between 3.8 and 4.5. For reference, the skin maintains a pH of approximately 4.7-5.2. It is entirely possible for ejaculated semen not to contain any sperm. This is caused by a condition known as azoospermia, which is associated with male-factor infertility. It has multiple causes and affects approximately 1% of the population.

2. Female Reproductive System

The female reproductive system can also be subdivided into internal and external genitalia. The **internal genitalia** include the ovaries, fallopian tubes, uterus, cervix, and vagina. The **external genitalia** are collectively known as the vulva. Some important structures of the vulva include the labia majora, labia minora, clitoris, and vaginal opening.

The **ovaries** are the female gonads, and are where **oogenesis** takes place, resulting in egg cells. The interior of the ovaries contains many follicles, and when puberty begins, there are approximately 400,000 follicles are present. Each follicle contains an oocyte (immature egg cell), which is supported by various other cells that provide nutrients and hormonal support to the oocytes. During each **menstrual cycle**, one follicle releases a secondary oocyte (egg) into the fallopian tube (also known as the oviduct), in a process known as ovulation. The ovaries are also endocrine organs, and secrete estrogen and progesterone.

The **fallopian tubes** connect the ovaries to the uterus. They have a smooth muscle layer that carries out peristalsis (patterns of automatic muscle contraction that push contents through a tube. See Chapter 10.) and an abundance of ciliated cells; both of these anatomical structures help move the egg from the ovaries to the uterus.

> **>> CONNECTIONS <<**
>
> Chapter 10 of Biology

The **uterus** is where a fetus develops during pregnancy. Its innermost layer, composed of epithelial cells and a lamina propria, is known as the endometrium. Its middle layer consists of smooth muscle, and is known as the myometrium (the prefix "myo-" is often used for structures involving muscles). The lower part of the uterus is known as the **cervix** (from a Latin term meaning "neck". Etymologically, the name of this structure means "neck of the uterus"). The cervix is cylindrical, and the cervical canal connects the uterine cavity with the vaginal canal. Sperm deposited in the vagina during intercourse must travel through the cervical canal for fertilization to take place. For this reason, mechanically blocking the cervical canal has historically been one approach to contraception. The **vagina** runs from the cervix to the vaginal opening. The vaginal canal is elastic and muscular, and can stretch to accommodate a fetus during childbirth. The vagina is also home to a rich population of bacteria, and the maintenance of healthy vaginal microbiota is an important aspect of reproductive health.

As mentioned above, the external female genitalia are collectively known as the **vulva**. The **urethral opening** is located anterior (front) to the vaginal opening, and both structures are flanked by the **labia minora**, or inner lips. The labia minora are in turn located between the **labia majora**, or outer lips. The labia minora in particular help protect the sensitive areas of the urethral opening and vaginal opening from irritations and infections. The **clitoris** is a complex, highly innervated sex organ. The visible area of the clitoris is located anterior to the urethral opening, with the clitoral hood formed by the junction of the labia minora. The clitoral hood covers the clitoral glans.

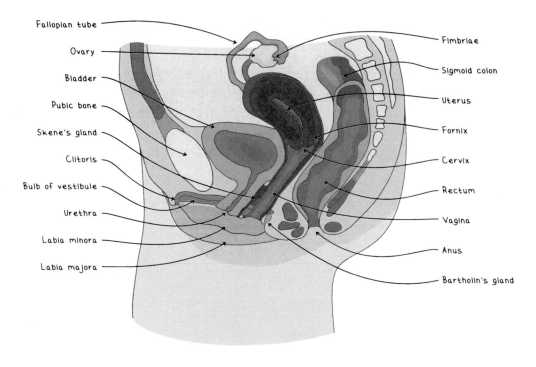

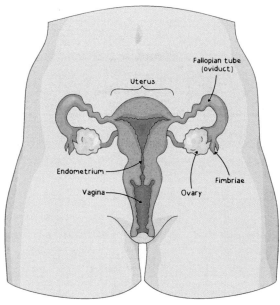

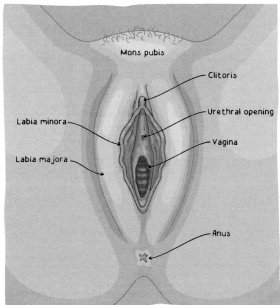

Figure 2. Female reproductive system

3. Spermatogenesis and Oogenesis

Spermatogenesis and oogenesis refer to the processes through which gametes (spermatozoa and ova, respectively) are generated. They are similar in that both involve meiosis, but have several important differences.

Spermatogenesis begins with spermatogonial stem cells and ends with mature spermatozoa, but there are several intermediate stages that you should be familiar with. First, spermatogonial stem cells can either divide into descendent spermatogonial stem cells (thereby maintaining the supply) or differentiate into spermatogonia. Spermatogonia divide through mitosis into two primary spermatocytes. Primary spermatocytes go through meiosis

184

I and divide into two secondary spermatocytes. This is where the transition from diploid (2n) to haploid (n) happens. Secondary spermatocytes then go through meiosis II, forming spermatids. A total of four spermatids are formed from each primary spermatocyte. This process corresponds fairly closely with how meiosis is generally shown in textbook chapters on cell biology.

Spermatids initially lack some of the most important features of the mature sperm cells that are released during ejaculation, and they gain those features in a process known as **spermiogenesis**. The main events of spermiogenesis are as follows: (1) formation of the acrosomal cap, which facilitates the ability of a sperm to fertilize an egg; (2) formation of a tail, and (3) loss of excess cytoplasm. Spermiogenesis results in non-mature spermatozoa that are incapable of independent movement, and are transferred to the epididymis to undergo maturation.

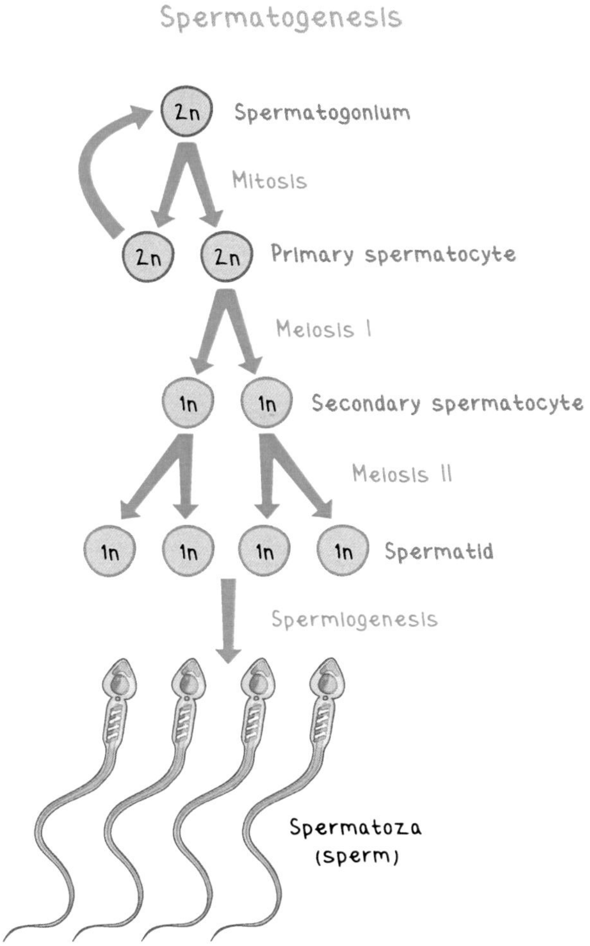

Figure 3. Spermatogenesis

As suggested by the fact that spermatids must lose excess cytoplasm, mature **sperm cells** are compact and contain the bare minimum of structures necessary for their functionality. A mature sperm cell has a head, a mid-piece, and a tail. The head contains the cell's DNA and is surrounded by the acrosomal cap. The mid-piece contains abundant mitochondria, which are necessary because sperm cells require quite a bit of energy throughout their life cycle, and the tail provides motility.

Spermatogenesis is initiated during puberty and continues throughout the lifespan. The process of spermatogenesis takes approximately three months, and approximately 100 million viable sperm are produced daily. As mentioned above in section one, spermatogenesis is highly sensitive to temperature. In particular it is most effective a few degrees Celsius below body temperature, which is reflected in the ability of the scrotum to retract and contract in order to regulate its temperature. Spermatogenesis is actually a very sensitive process in general, and can be adversely affected by factors as diverse as hormones, vitamin deficiencies, oxidative stress, and exposure to toxins.

Oogenesis begins with oogonia, which are formed from primordial germ cells in a process known as gametogenesis. At least some oogonia are present by approximately weeks four to five of fetal development, and they continue to develop through the first five months of fetal development. At that point, oogonia differentiate into primary oocytes. The next stage of development is for primary oocytes to undergo meiosis I and become secondary oocytes, but this process is halted in fetuses in prophase I. Thus, female babies are born with the full set of oocytes necessary for their lifetime: approximately 1-2 million are present at birth, which decreases to 300,000 at the time of puberty.

Once primary oocytes are frozen at prophase I, oogenesis is essentially halted until puberty. **Menarche**, or the first menstrual cycle, marks the resumption of oogenesis, but only in a few cells at a time. Each month, one primary oocyte completes meiosis I, but instead of resulting in two identical secondary oocytes, one secondary oocyte is generated, along with one polar body. Meiosis I in oogenesis is an unequal division: the secondary oocyte receives the vast majority of the cytoplasm from the primary oocyte, while the polar body essentially withers away. Similar to what we saw with primary oocytes, secondary oocytes start undergoing meiosis II, but freeze at metaphase II until fertilization. Since fertilization is involved in the next step, we will cover it in more detail in the next section, but the essential point is that after fertilization the secondary oocyte completes meiosis II, generating a mature ovum and another polar body.

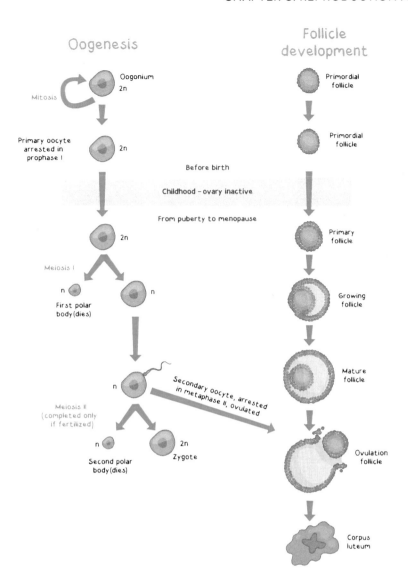

Figure 4. Oogenesis

4. Embryogenesis, Development, and Pregnancy

Fertilization takes place in the fallopian tube, and the first step is for a **sperm cell** to encounter a **secondary oocyte**. To understand what happens next, we need to take a closer look at the anatomy of the secondary oocyte, and to keep in mind the big-picture goal here: a mechanism needs to be in place to ensure that *one and only one,* sperm cell can fertilize an egg. If this process fails, and more than one sperm cell fertilizes an egg (known as polyspermy), a viable zygote will not be created.

> ### CLINICAL CONNECTIONS >>>
>
> In an interesting side note, researchers in 2007 reported a pair of viable twins that appear to have developed through this mechanism, but for the purposes of the MCAT, polyspermy can be assumed to lead to no pregnancy or a non-viable pregnancy.

As the sperm cell approaches the secondary oocyte, it passes through area known as the **corona radiata**, which comprises a layer of follicular cells surrounding the oocyte. Next, it passes through the **zona pellucida**, which is a layer of glycoproteins between the corona radiata and the oocyte. One of the glycoproteins in the zona pellucida binds with the sperm head and triggers the acrosome reaction, in which digestive enzymes are released that allow the nucleus of the sperm cell to enter the egg.

At this point, two major events occur. The glycoproteins in the zona pellucida form cross-linked structures that prevent another sperm cell from fertilizing the egg. The steps leading to this outcome are known as the cortical reaction. Additionally, the secondary oocyte completes meiosis II, creating a second polar body and a mature ovum. Then, the haploid nuclei of the sperm cell and the ovum merge, creating a diploid one-cell zygote.

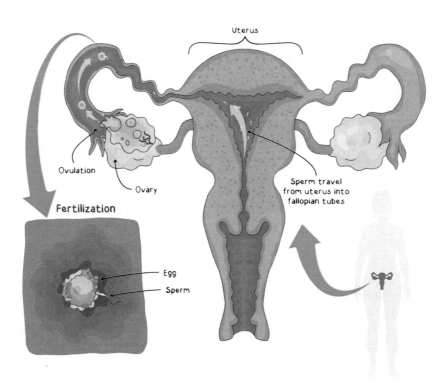

Figure 5. Fertilization

The **zygote** now travels from the fallopian tubes to the uterus for future development. If this does not occur, the result is known as an **ectopic pregnancy**. More specifically, a **tubal pregnancy** occurs if development occurs in the fallopian tube, while the broader category of ectopic pregnancy also includes zygotic/embryonic development within the abdomen, cervix, or ovaries. Ectopic pregnancies almost never lead to viable fetuses, and are associated with poor maternal outcomes if not properly treated.

As the zygote travels to the uterus, it undergoes a series of mitotic cell divisions known as **cleavage**. Since the zygote is defined by unicellularity, as soon as cleavage takes place, the zygote is considered to be transformed into an **embryo**. Also, note that we have now left meiosis behind: the zygote (and embryo) is diploid, and all subsequent cell divisions that take place during embryonic development are mitotic. This holds true for the entire life cycle of the embryo, with the exception of meiotic divisions in the next generation of gametogenesis. During cleavage, the overall size of the embryo does not change. More and more cells are created, but they are smaller than the original zygote and thus the **nuclear-to-cytoplasmic (N:C) ratio** increases.

Once the zygote has cleaved into a mass of 16 cells three to four days after fertilization, it is known as the **morula** (Latin for "little mulberry")—the zygote appears like a compact ball here. By three to five days after fertilization, the morula develops some degree of internal structure and becomes a **blastocyst.** The blastocyst is characterized by a fluid-filled cavity in the middle that is known as the **blastocoel**. As you can see in Figure 6, the blastocoel is not perfectly round. A U-shaped protrusion pokes into part of the blastocoel. This is known as the **inner cell mass**

(ICM), and the ICM is what will eventually develop into the fetus. The other cells surrounding the blastocoel are known as the **trophoblast**, and eventually generate the placenta.

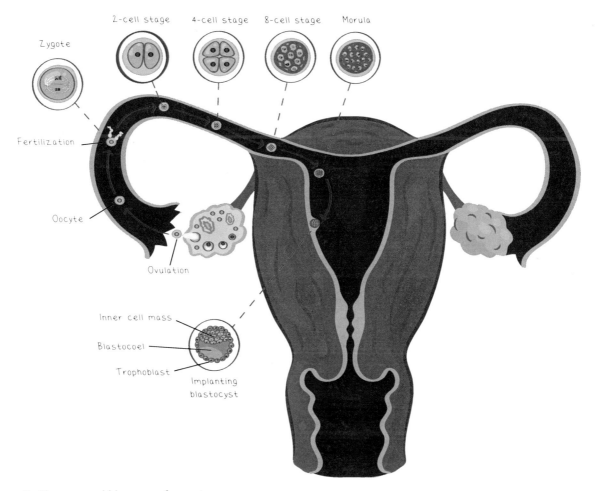

Figure 6. Cleavage and blastocyst formation

The blastocyst then implants in the **uterine endometrium**. **Implantation** is a multi-stage process that involves close communication and adaptation between the embryo and the uterine tissue. In particular, the trophoblast cells develop into the chorion and eventually the placenta, while the inner cell mass develops into the embryo. The chorion and amnion go on to form the amniotic sac, which envelops the embryo/fetus throughout pregnancy.

Once implanted, the embryo further differentiates into the **gastrula**. The gastrula has three layers: the **ectoderm**, the **mesoderm**, and the **endoderm**. These layers eventually go on to form specific organs and components in the body.

The **ectoderm** primarily gives rise to the nervous system and epidermis (skin), as well as related structures like hair, nails, and sweat glands. It is also worth noting that the linings of the mouth, anus, and nostrils are also derived from the ectoderm, although the MCAT tends to primarily focus on the nervous system and the skin. The process through which the nervous system is formed from the ectoderm is known as **neurulation**. The first step in

MCAT STRATEGY >>>

You can remember the stages of embryonic development using the following mnemonic: **Z**ach's **m**other is a **b**ig **g**iant **n**erd, for zygote → morula → blastula/blastocyst → gastrula → neurulation.

neurulation is the formation of a rod of mesodermal cells known as the **notochord**, which induces the formation of the neural plate in the ectodermal tissue located above it. The neural plate folds upward, with the neural folds on the side and the neural groove in the middle. The folding process continues, and the neural folds eventually meet, at which point they form the neural tube. The **neural tube** goes on to form the central nervous system, while **neural crest cells**—initially located on the neural folds form the peripheral nervous system. At the end of this process, the surface ectoderm surrounds the neural tube, such that the central nervous system can develop within the body.

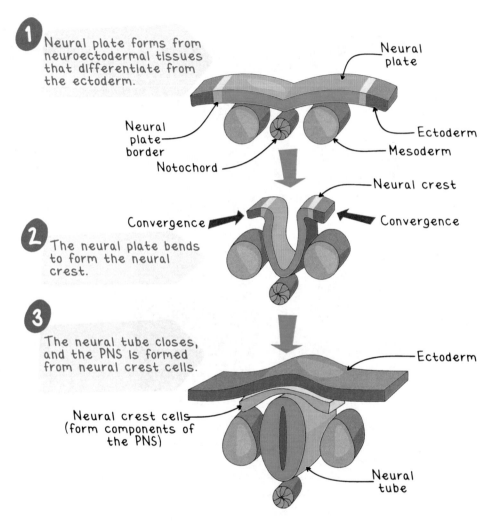

Figure 7. Neurulation

CLINICAL CONNECTIONS >>>

The ectoderm basically describes the external layer of organs, the mesoderm describes what's in the middle, and the endoderm develops into the most internal layer (internal linings).

The **mesoderm** generates many of the structures present within the body, including the musculature, connective tissue (blood, bone, and cartilage), the gonads, the kidneys, and the adrenal cortex. The **endoderm** is responsible for interior linings of the body, including the linings of the gastrointestinal system, the pancreas and part of the liver, the urinary bladder and part of the urethra, and the lungs.

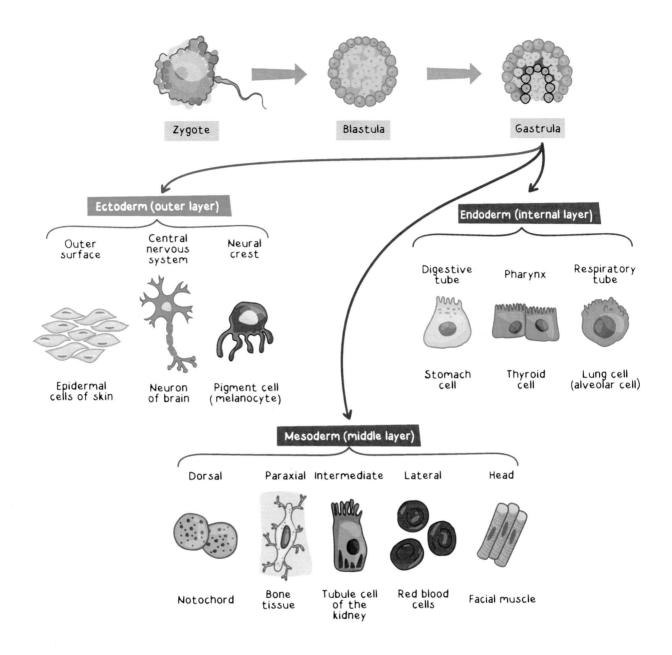

Figure 8. Germ cell layers and their respective developmental paths

Throughout the first trimester of pregnancy, the major organs develop in a process known as **organogenesis**. Then, in the second and third trimesters, the fetus grows larger and develops further, however, the details of fetal development are beyond the scope of the MCAT. Throughout pregnancy, the fetus obtains nutrients via the **placenta**, which is an organ that allows nutrient and gas exchange between the mother and the fetus. Maternal blood and fetal blood, however, do not co-mingle. Instead, maternal blood comes extremely close to the fetal circulation so that nutrients, gases, and waste products can be exchanged through a combination of passive and active transport. The placenta is also an endocrine organ. Early in pregnancy, it secretes human chorionic gonadotropin (hCG), and later in pregnancy it secretes progesterone and estrogen. Both hCG and progesterone have the effect of maintaining the pregnancy. One interesting fact to be aware of for the MCAT is that fetal hemoglobin has a higher affinity for oxygen than adult hemoglobin. This fact allows oxygen to be passed more efficiently from the maternal circulation to the fetal circulation. The fetus is connected to the placenta through the umbilical cord.

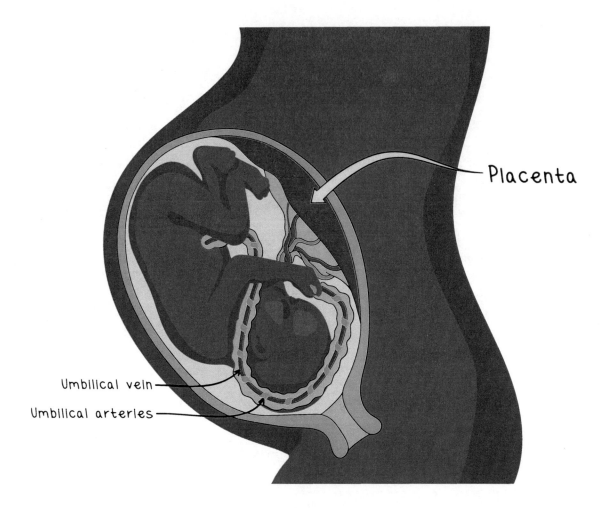

Figure 9. Placenta and umbilical cord

Sexual differentiation takes place before birth in fetuses. This process is complex, and the MCAT does not expect you to be familiar with all of its details. However, you should know that the female developmental pattern can be thought of as more or less the default, whereas the development of male sex organs is induced by genes on the Y chromosome, in particular the sex-determining region of the Y chromosome (the *SRY* gene).

Pregnancy most commonly lasts between 37 and 41 weeks, and comes to an end with labor and childbirth (also known as **parturition**). The details of labor and delivery will be covered in medical school, but for the MCAT you should be aware that uterine contractions play a major role in labor, and that they are driven by the hormone oxytocin in a rare example of a physiological **positive feedback loop**; oxytocin causes uterine contractions, which stimulate more oxytocin release, which then stimulates more and stronger uterine contractions, and so on until the fetus is delivered through the vaginal canal.

5. Hormonal Control of Reproduction

Many aspects of the reproductive system are controlled by hormones. We will start by reviewing reproductive development, and then discuss the menstrual cycle.

As discussed above, the sexual differentiation of fetuses takes place before birth. Throughout childhood, little happens in this regard until puberty, when wide-ranging hormonal changes take place. This facilitates the development of children into sexually mature adults capable of reproduction. Pulses of **gonadotropin-releasing** hormone (GnRH) set puberty in motion. GnRH stimulates the release of **luteinizing hormone (LH)** and **follicle-stimulating hormone (FSH)**. It's at this point that we see differences emerge between males and females. LH and FSH affect the ovaries in females and the testes in males, and trigger the release of other downstream hormones. In males, LH causes the Leydig cells of the testes to produce testosterone, while FSH affects Sertoli cells, causing them to produce factors necessary for sperm maturation. In females, FSH stimulates follicular growth in the ovary and the production of estrogen. Meanwhile, LH stimulates ovulation, the transformation of the follicle into the corpus luteum and the production of progesterone.

> ## MCAT STRATEGY >>>
>
> A systematic approach is key for successfully studying the menstrual cycle (and many other topics!) for the MCAT, so be sure that you have a solid grasp of the basic anatomical changes involved in the menstrual cycle before moving on to its hormonal regulation—otherwise, you run the risk of memorizing without understanding, which makes you prone to errors if asked to apply your knowledge in a new context.

Estrogen and **testosterone** are the main sex hormones in females and males, respectively. Their release during puberty stimulates the development of the reproductive tract as well as **secondary sexual characteristics**, which are typical markers of biological sex that are not directly involved in reproductive function. For females, the development of secondary sexual characteristics includes changes in the pattern of fat distribution, widening of hips, the growth of body hair, and the growth of breasts. For males, they include the development of facial and body hair, a deeper voice, and so on.

Estrogen and **progesterone** are also involved in the menstrual cycle, which is a regular hormonal cycle in women of reproductive age, although considerable variability exists in the timing of menstruation. The menstrual cycle starts at puberty, and continues through menopause, which usually takes place between 45 and 55 years of age and marks the end of the reproductively active period of a woman's life. Advances in assisted reproductive technology, however, especially the use of donor eggs, have allowed some women to conceive later in life.

The terms **ovarian cycle** and **uterine cycle** are used to reflect the fact that we can focus on how the menstrual cycle plays out either in the ovaries or in the uterus. We'll focus first on the ovarian cycle and then analyze the uterine cycle because doing so better reflects the underlying logic of the biological processes at hand. Keeping careful track of which terminology applies to the ovarian cycle and the uterine cycle will also help avoid some common sources of terminological confusion.

The **ovarian cycle** begins with the follicular phase, followed by **ovulation**, which is in turn followed by the luteal phase. As discussed earlier, one secondary oocyte is released every menstrual cycle, and the ovarian phase simply reflects the logic of what this process entails. A follicle matures in the follicular phase and releases the egg at ovulation. The luteal phase refers to what happens after the secondary oocyte is released: the follicle is transformed into a structure known as the **corpus luteum**. The corpus luteum secretes progesterone, helping to maintain the uterine lining. The corpus luteum decays towards the end of this phase, and another cycle begins.

The **uterine cycle** begins with **menstruation**, which overlaps with the first part of the follicular phase of the ovarian cycle. During menstruation, the uterine lining that was built up in the previous cycle is sloughed off. Menstruation typically lasts from three to five days, although variation within the range of two to seven days is also common. As mentioned above, considerable variability exists among individuals regarding the timing of the menstrual cycle. Once menstruation is complete, the **uterine endometrium** is built up again during the **proliferative phase**. The final phase of the uterine cycle is known as the **secretory phase**,

> ## MCAT STRATEGY >>>
>
> The MCAT likes to ask about the menstrual cycle because it is a complex, multi-staged physiological process with important real-world implications.

and this overlaps with the luteal phase of the ovarian cycle. During the secretory phase, the uterine endometrium continues to build up and undergoes various changes to make it more receptive for implantation, under the influence of the progesterone secreted by the corpus luteum.

Given a solid understanding of the anatomical steps involved in ovulation and implantation, the stages of the ovarian and uterine cycle are quite logical, because you can think of them as simply reflecting the steps that must happen for this system to work. The next step is to understand how hormonal regulation shapes the various steps of the menstrual cycle. Since hormones can affect both the ovaries and uterus, it is difficult to firmly separate the ovarian and uterine cycles when discussing the hormonal regulation of the menstrual cycle. This underscores the importance of mastering the basic anatomical processes involved.

At the beginning of the follicular phase, there is a moderate rise in **follicle-stimulating hormone (FSH)**, which induces follicular development before gradually dropping off. Throughout most of the follicular phase, **estrogen** levels gradually increase, stimulating the development of the uterine endometrium. After estrogen levels reach a certain threshold close to ovulation, it stimulates a brief surge in **luteinizing hormone (LH)** and **FSH** levels; the spike in LH levels is particularly notable and is what triggers ovulation. As a side note, this is essentially why LH is called *luteinizing* hormone: by inducing ovulation, it induces the transformation of the follicle into the corpus *luteum*. The luteal phase is characterized by high levels of progesterone, which help maintain the readiness of the uterine endometrium for implantation.

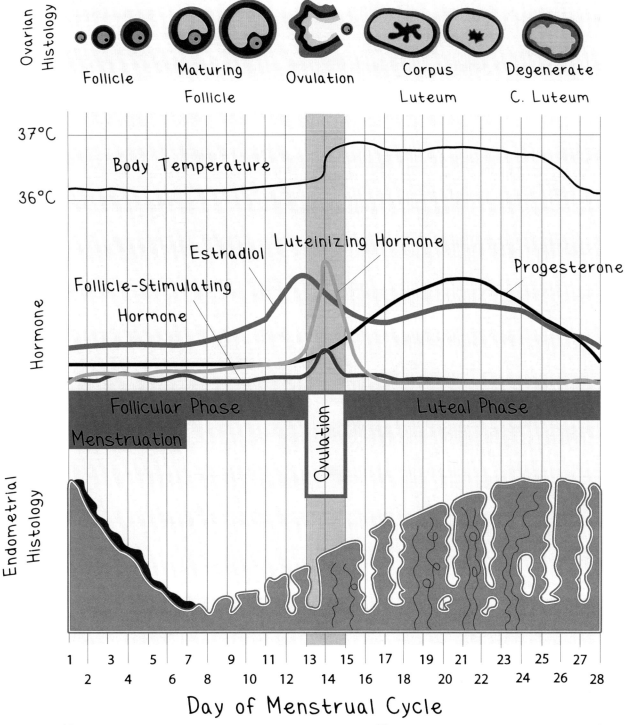

Figure 10. The menstrual cycle

Finally, it's worth taking a look at how the body "knows" whether or not implantation has taken place, and therefore whether to transition into another menstrual cycle or into pregnancy. In the absence of implantation, successive

negative feedback loops keep the cycle moving. Progesterone exerts negative feedback on LH, and eventually, as LH declines, the corpus luteum will degenerate. Remember the close connection between LH and the corpus luteum that is implied by the fact that they essentially share the same name. As the corpus luteum degenerates, it no longer secretes progesterone. Recall that progesterone keeps the endometrium ready for implantation. If progesterone declines, then so does the ability of the endometrium to undergo implantation, and the stage is set for menstruation and for the next menstrual cycle to happen.

In contrast, if implantation *does* happen, the body has to have a mechanism of preventing the endometrium from being sloughed away. The key here is that the embryo secretes a hormone known as human chorionic gonadotropin (hCG), which allows the corpus luteum to be maintained and for progesterone levels to be sustained. By the second trimester, hCG levels drop because they are no longer necessary. By this point, the placenta can function as an endocrine organ and independently secrete progesterone (as well as estrogen).

6. Must-Knows

> Path of sperm through the male reproductive tract: seminiferous tubules → epididymis → vas deferens → ejaculatory duct → urethra → penis.
   – Mnemonic: SEVEN UP, where "N" stands for "nothing".
> Path of eggs through female reproductive tract: ovaries → fallopian tube, then:
   – If fertilization occurs → zygote/morula/blastocyst goes to uterus → pregnancy → childbirth through vaginal canal.
   – If no fertilization occurs → uterine lining shed during menstruation.
> Spermatogenesis:
   – Takes place in testes, which are maintained a few degrees Celsius cooler than body temperature.
   – Spermatogonial stem cells → spermatogonia (2n) → primary spermatocytes (2n) → secondary spermatocytes (n) → spermatids → spermatozoa.
   – Sperm mature and gain motility in epididymis.
   – Spermatogenesis is a constant process from puberty throughout rest of lifespan.
> Oogenesis:
   – Oogonia → primary oocyte → secondary oocyte + polar body → ovum + polar body.
   – Oogenesis is *not* a constant process. Primary oocytes are halted at prophase I at birth, meiosis I completed in the ovary to form secondary oocyte, which is then arrested at metaphase II. Meiosis II is completed at fertilization.
> Fertilization: takes place in fallopian tube.
   – Acrosome reaction allows sperm cell to enter egg. Results in cortical reaction that prevents polyspermy.
> Stages of embryonic development:
   – Morula (16-cell ball) → blastocyst (fluid-filled sac in the middle) → gastrula (three germ cell layers present).
   – Ectoderm → skin, nervous system, sweat glands, hair, nails.
   – Mesoderm → connective tissue (including blood and bone), muscles, gonads.
   – Endoderm → internal linings of GI tract, lungs, urinary bladder.
> Menstrual cycle: takes place every ~28 days in reproductive-age women.
   – Ovarian cycle: follicular phase (follicle develops), ovulation (egg is released), luteal phase (follicle → corpus luteum).
   – Uterine cycle: menstruation (uterine endometrium from previous cycle is shed), proliferative phase (endometrium develops again), secretory phase (endometrium is ready for implantation).
   – Estrogen gradually rises throughout follicular phase, triggering LH surge, which causes ovulation. Progesterone, secreted by corpus luteum, maintains uterine endometrium for implantation.
   – If implantation happens, human chorionic gonadotropin (hCG) maintains corpus luteum, thereby maintaining progesterone and maintaining pregnancy.

End of Chapter Practice

The best MCAT practice is **realistic**, with a focus on identifying steps for further improvement. For those reasons, we recommend completing practice questions in an online setting that simulates the real MCAT interface, and taking advantage of advanced analytic features to help you determine how best to move forward in your MCAT study journey.

With that in mind, **online end-of-chapter** questions for Biology, Biochemistry, Chemistry + Organic Chemistry, Physics, and Psychology/Sociology are available through your Blueprint MCAT account.

As a further supplement, given the importance of active learning for effective studying, we also suggest that you consult the Must-Knows at the end of each chapter as a basis for creating a study sheet, in which you list out key terms and test your ability to briefly summarize them.

This page left intentionally blank.

This page left intentionally blank.

Respiratory and Circulatory Systems

0. Introduction

This chapter deals with aspects of our physiology that sustain life on a minute-to-minute basis. Namely, it addresses how we get oxygen from the atmosphere to our tissues, and how we remove some waste products from our body. The closely interwoven respiratory and circulatory systems are responsible for these tasks, although the excretory system also plays a major role in waste removal. As you may have seen already in work or volunteering experiences, acute problems with the respiratory and circulatory systems can cause major medical emergencies, while chronic respiratory and circulatory problems also have major impacts on quality of life and mortality.

From the standpoint of the MCAT, as you study these topics, you should always have gas exchange at the back of your mind. How does oxygen enter the body? Once it enters the body, how does it get to the tissues where it is needed? When carbon dioxide is generated, how does it leave the body? The MCAT places a major emphasis on how biological systems function. This is also underscored by how important oxidative respiration is for the MCAT as a biochemistry topic, although what happens to oxygen within a cell is outside of the scope of this chapter. You will find that focusing on this unifying theme will help you make sense of the details of these physiological systems and to apply them successfully on Test Day.

1. Mechanisms of Breathing

In this section, we'll attempt to answer what may initially seem to be a simple question: how do we breathe? The mechanism of breathing is elegant but intricate, so let's get started.

First, let's review some anatomy. As air enters our body, it travels either through the **nostrils** (also known as the nares) or the oral cavity. The **nasal cavity** is located behind the external nostrils, and contains mucous membranes and hairs known as vibrissae that filter out particulate matter. The air then travels down through the **pharynx**, which is located at the back of the mouth. It's important to note that the pharynx is also part of the digestive system because food passes through it as well as air. The next structure of the respiratory tract, the **epiglottis**, can be thought of as a switch-point that separates the respiratory and digestive systems. The epiglottis is a cartilaginous tissue that covers the larynx during the act of swallowing, shunting food into the esophagus. Otherwise, air continues into the larynx. The **larynx** contains the vocal cords, which vibrate to produce sounds when air is pushed through them and are consciously controlled during speaking.

The air then moves down through the **trachea**, also known as the windpipe. The epithelium of the trachea is lined with goblet cells, which produce mucus, and the epithelial cells themselves are ciliated. Particulate matter and microbes that are still present in the air are trapped in the mucus. The cilia then push the mucus upwards, where it becomes phlegm that can either be expelled or swallowed. The **bronchi** (singular bronchus) then split off from the bottom of the trachea. The transition from the trachea to the bronchi is where the respiratory system becomes bilateral (i.e., has both left and right sides). The epithelium of the bronchi is also lined with goblet cells and ciliated epithelial cells, much like the trachea. The bronchi then divide again into successively smaller segments. The first division from the trachea are the primary (main) bronchi, then the secondary bronchi, tertiary bronchi, and then, after numerous divisions, the bronchioles. The **bronchioles** continue to divide, ultimately leading to alveoli. This process ends in the formation of very small structures known as **alveoli**, which are where gas exchange occurs. Alveoli are sacs coated with surfactant, a film that reduces surface tension, allowing the alveoli to remain inflated when the lung is compressed during exhalation. Each alveolus is surrounded by tiny capillaries. An average pair of lungs contains something on the order of 500 million alveoli, resulting in a collectively tremendous surface area available for gas exchange.

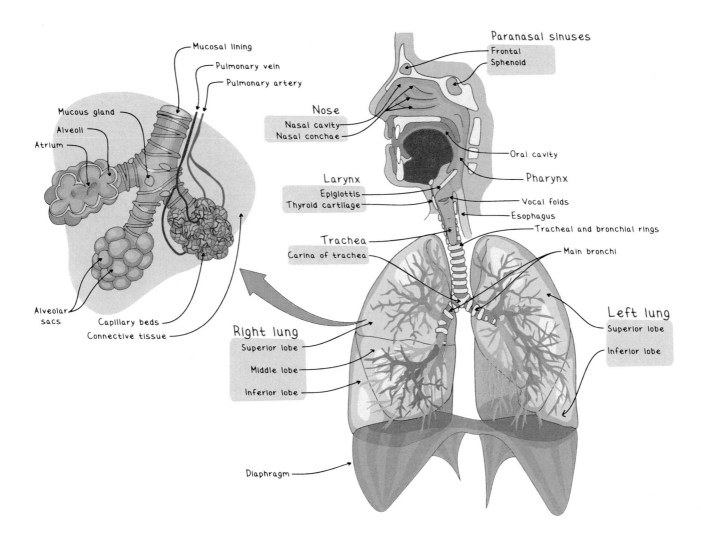

Figure 1. Anatomy of respiratory tract and lungs

The **thoracic cavity** contains the lungs as well as the heart, and is protected by the rib cage. However, the lungs do not adhere directly to the thoracic wall. Instead, the lung is covered by a serous membrane known as the **pleura**. The inner layer, known as the visceral (pulmonary) pleura, covers the lung. The outer layer, known as the parietal pleura, adheres to the thoracic wall. Between the two pleurae is the pleural cavity, which, under normal conditions, contains just a very thin layer of liquid that lubricates movements between the two pleurae. As a result of certain pathological conditions, fluid can accumulate in the pleural space, resulting in **pleural effusion**. If air enters the pleural space, the resulting condition is known as **pneumothorax**. Both pleural effusion and pneumothorax are serious medical conditions that can result in emergencies.

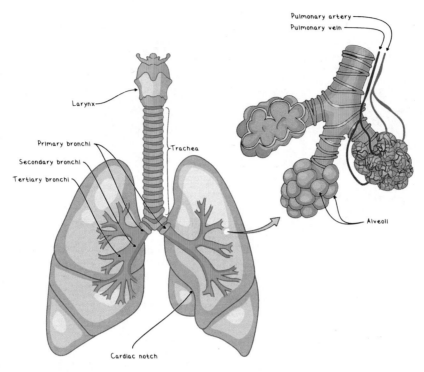

Figure 2. Structure of lungs and alveoli

Now that we've covered the basic anatomy of the respiratory system, we can make sense of the mechanism of breathing. The main driver of breathing is the **diaphragm**, the muscle at the bottom of the thoracic cavity that separates it from the abdominal cavity below. When the diaphragm contracts, the thoracic cavity expands. This causes the parietal pleura to expand, which in turn causes expansion of the pulmonary pleura and the lungs. When the lungs expand, the pressure within them decreases. Remember Boyle's law from general chemistry: pressure and volume are inversely related at a constant temperature. The decreased pressure compared to the external environment causes air to rush into the respiratory tract. This mechanism is known as **negative-pressure respiration**.

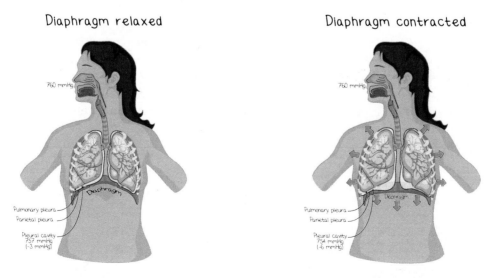

Figure 3. Mechanism of breathing

Exhalation can be either passive or active. In **passive exhalation**, the simple relaxation of the diaphragm is sufficient to increase the pressure in the lungs to expel the air. However, the muscles between the ribs (internal intercostal muscles) and abdominal muscles can be used to force air out more intensely and quickly. This frequently occurs during exercise, but increased reliance on **active exhalation** even at rest can be a sign of respiratory disease.

The final part of breathing is **gas exchange**. The mechanism of gas exchange is actually fairly simple. Blood runs through the alveolar capillaries and is separated by a wall only one cell thick from the breathed-in air. The deoxygenated blood being returned to the lungs is rich in carbon dioxide (see Sections 2 and 6 for more details regarding this point) and poor in oxygen, while the air breathed in is rich in oxygen and relatively poor in carbon dioxide. Therefore, oxygen and carbon dioxide can simply diffuse down their respective concentration gradients through the cell wall separating the alveolar capillaries and the blood flow. Oxygen and carbon dioxide are carried by hemoglobin, which is described in more detail in Section 6.

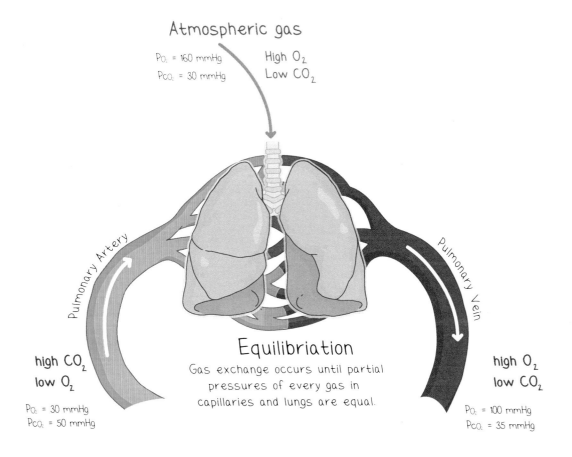

Figure 4. Mechanism of gas exchange

Several measures of lung capacity are used in clinical practice. They are not as important as the fundamental physiology of respiration for the MCAT, but they may be worth being aware of. **Tidal volume (TV)** is the volume of air contained in a normal breath. The additional air amount that can be exhaled after a normal exhalation is known as the **expiratory reserve volume (ERV)**. Finally, the amount of additional air that can be inhaled after a normal inhalation is the **inspiratory reserve volume (IRV)**. There are three other measures that you should be aware of that are not linked to a normal breath. **Total lung capacity (TLC)**, as the name implies, is the most air that can possibly be present in the lungs after inhaling as deeply as possible. The **residual volume (RV)** is the air that remains in the lungs after breathing out as much as possible, and the **vital capacity (VC)** is the difference between the TLC and the RV.

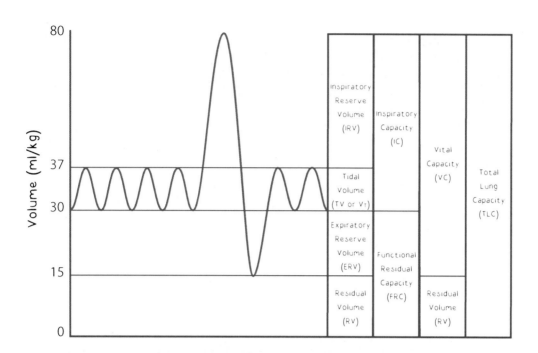

Figure 5. Measurements of respiratory volume

2. Physiology of Respiration

While it is important to be aware of the basic anatomy of the respiratory tract and the mechanism of breathing, it is even more important to understand the physiology of respiration. The MCAT loves to focus on how physiological systems operate, interact with each other, and respond to external stimuli.

As already mentioned, the ciliated cells and mucus produced throughout the respiratory tract help trap particulate matter and pathogens. Additionally, antibiotic proteins known as defensins are secreted in the respiratory tract, which means that the respiratory system plays a role in the **innate immune system**.

>> CONNECTIONS <<

Chapter 11 of Biology

The respiratory system also plays a role in **thermoregulation**, although sweating and shivering are the main physiological responses to hyperthermia and hypothermia, respectively. Extensive capillary beds are present in the nasal cavity and the trachea. Regulation of the amount of blood flowing through the capillary beds will allow for differing amounts of heat transfer. When more blood passes through vessels close to an interface with the external environment (i.e., the skin or the nasal/tracheal epithelium), more heat can be radiated. Conversely, when less blood is circulated through such vessels, heat is conserved. These processes are known as **vasodilation** and **vasoconstriction**, respectively. Their role in thermoregulation is not limited to the respiratory system. Their other functions are discussed more below in Section 4. Although the respiratory system does not play a major role in thermoregulation in humans, it does in many mammals that cannot sweat or can only sweat to a limited extent and therefore must rely on the respiratory system to disperse surplus heat through a pattern of rapid breathing known as panting. In panting, evaporation from the moist surfaces of the tongue and the lungs cools the body.

Of course, the most fundamental function of the respiratory system is **gas exchange**. Recall that oxygen is used as the final electron acceptor in aerobic respiration, and that carbon dioxide is produced as a byproduct of aerobic respiration. This means that you can think of carbon dioxide as a waste product. **Carbon dioxide** participates in an equilibrium with **carbonic acid** and the **bicarbonate ion**, as shown below:

$$CO_2 + H_2O \rightleftharpoons H_2CO_3 \rightleftharpoons HCO_3^- + H^+$$

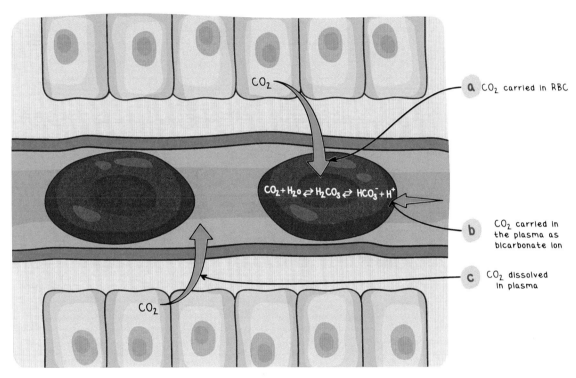

Figure 6. Bicarbonate equilibrium

This equilibrium is a **buffer system** that maintains the pH of the blood between 7.35 and 7.45. If the pH of the blood leaves this range, the resulting conditions of **acidemia/acidosis** (if the pH goes below 7.35) or **alkalemia/alkalosis** (if the pH goes above 7.45) can have catastrophic consequences. As a quick note on terminology, acid*emia* and alkal*emia* refer specifically having blood that is too acidic or basic, respectively, while acid*osis* and alkal*osis* refer to the disease processes that result in acidemia or alkalemia. For the purposes of the MCAT, it is worth being able to recognize both sets of terms that you will need to distinguish between them. Too much carbon dioxide in the blood both indicates that the body needs more oxygen to power aerobic respiration and makes the blood too acidic (acidemia).

MCAT STRATEGY >>>

The bicarbonate equilibrium equation is an absolute must for the MCAT. Don't just memorize it, though—work to understand why Le Châtelier's principle means that the various components of this equation are essentially synonymous in biological processes. For example, all things being equal, more H^+ means more CO_2, and vice versa. Similarly, removing H^+ from the blood is a way to reduce CO_2 concentration in the blood by pushing this reaction to the right.

The nervous system detects this through **chemoreceptors** that detect acidic conditions. When these chemoreceptors are stimulated, they increase the respiratory rate. As the respiratory rate increases, the body expels more carbon dioxide and brings in more oxygen. This shifts the balance of the bicarbonate equilibrium away from H^+, and thereby increases the pH of the blood. Similarly, if the pH of the blood is too high (alkalemia), reducing the rate of respiration allows carbon dioxide to build up, thereby lowering the pH of the blood.

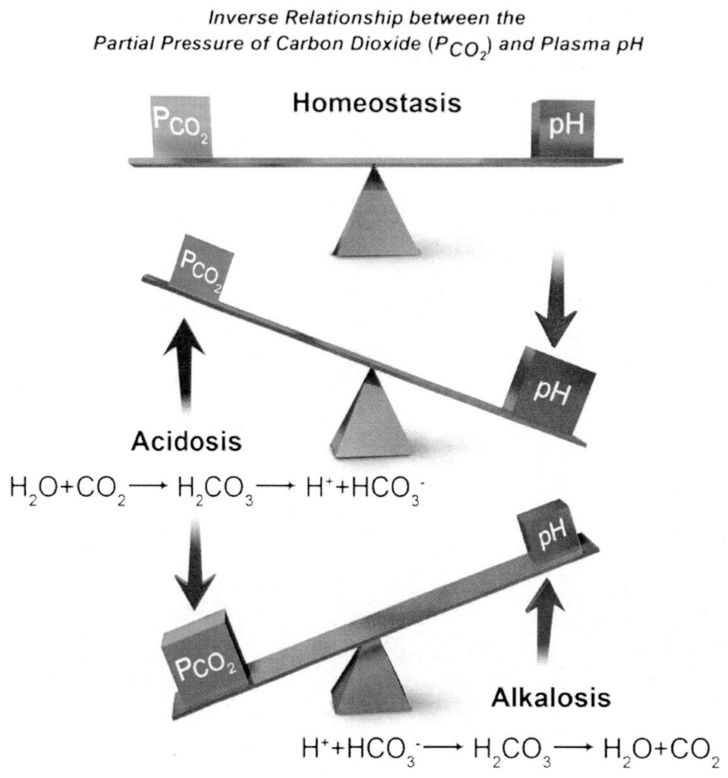

Inverse Relationship between the
Partial Pressure of Carbon Dioxide (P_{CO_2}) and Plasma pH

Acidosis

$$H_2O + CO_2 \longrightarrow H_2CO_3 \longrightarrow H^+ + HCO_3^-$$

Alkalosis

$$H^+ + HCO_3^- \longrightarrow H_2CO_3 \longrightarrow H_2O + CO_2$$

Figure 7. Carbon dioxide and pH control

3. Blood

The human body contains four to six liters of blood, which consists of two parts: cellular material and plasma. The cellular components of blood are all made in the bone marrow before their release into the circulatory system, while **plasma** is the aqueous solution in which these cells are found. Although textbooks tend to focus on the cellular components of blood, plasma is essential to life. Blood plasma is composed of water, nutrients, hormones, proteins, salts, gases, and amino acids. Plasma is so complex that it is near impossible to create in a laboratory, and many people can make money by selling their plasma to blood banks. When clotting proteins are removed from the plasma, as is common when laboratory tests are performed, the resulting material is known as the **serum**, and the various substance concentrations are given in terms of serum concentrations. For the MCAT, you can think of this as equivalent to the level of a substance in the bloodstream.

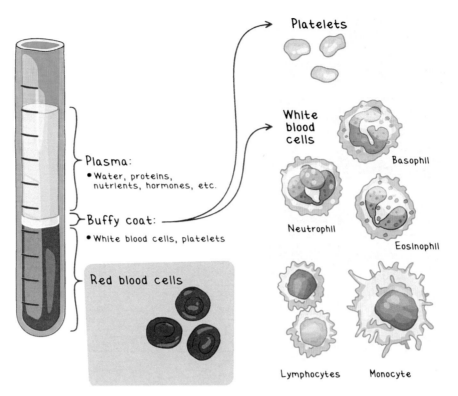

Figure 8. Blood composition

Plasma is also important as **plasma volume** is connected both to **hydration** and **blood pressure**. Greater plasma volume correlates to higher blood pressure levels. On an intuitive level, this makes sense because, if more liquid is contained by the vessel walls, it will exert more pressure. Correspondingly, less plasma volume lowers blood pressure. Since fluctuations in the amount of water present in plasma can cause plasma volume to vary, hydration status is linked to plasma volume. In particular, dehydration is associated with low plasma volume and low blood pressure.

Plasma volume is regulated by the endocrine system, jointly with the excretory system. **Aldosterone** and **anti-diuretic hormone** (**ADH**) are two hormones that are involved in the regulation of fluid balance. Aldosterone increases sodium absorption in the distal convoluted tubule and collecting duct of the nephron, which in the presence of ADH, drives water reabsorption through osmosis. ADH acts directly on the collecting duct in the nephron to increase water absorption. In contrast, **atrial natriuretic peptide** (**ANP**) is essentially the opposite of aldosterone as it decreases plasma volume by decreasing sodium absorption. For more details about these hormones, see Chapter 7 on the endocrine system, and if you need a review of the nephron, see Chapter 10.

The formed elements of blood are divided into three categories: leukocytes, platelets, and erythrocytes. **Leukocytes** are also known as white blood cells, and are a major component of the immune system. They are covered in depth in Chapter 11 on the immune system.

MCAT STRATEGY >>>

Review the material in this paragraph until you can recall it with ease. If a question stem or a passage tells you that an individual has (for instance) less plasma volume, can you predict the consequences for blood pressure? Hydration status? You want to invest time in developing this reflex now, rather than when taking the exam.

Platelets are not whole cells. Rather, they are cell fragments that are involved in hemostasis. If a blood vessel ruptures, the process of hemostasis will occur preventing blood from continuously leaking out of the vessel. One

>> CONNECTIONS <<

Chapter 7 of Biology

>> CONNECTIONS <<

Chapter 10 of Biology

>> CONNECTIONS <<

Chapter 11 of Biology

of the initial events that occur with hemostasis is the formation of the platelet plug a process known as clotting. The events that lead to **clotting**, known as the clotting cascade, are quite complicated. The details of the full pathway go beyond the scope of the MCAT, but you should be aware that the clotting cascade must be tightly regulated in order to keep an appropriate level of clot formation, preventing either an overgeneration or undergeneration of clot formation. For example, a blood clot can become dislodged and get stuck in a blood vessel, causing a serious medical condition known as thromboembolism. Some of the major events of the clotting cascade include the conversion of prothrombin into thrombin, which then converts fibrinogen to fibrin. As the name implies, **fibrin** forms a fibrous structure that can be thought of as the skeleton of the clot.

Erythrocytes (also known as **red blood cells** or **RBCs**) are responsible for carrying oxygen to the different tissues of the body, and aid in carrying carbon dioxide to the lungs, where it is exhaled. Erythrocytes can do this because they are packed full of hemoglobin, a polymer of 4 proteins and iron that binds oxygen. Erythrocytes are created in the bone marrow in response to **erythropoietin**, a hormone that is released from the kidney whenever erythrocyte levels are low. During development in the bone marrow, erythrocytes lose their membrane-bound organelles, including their mitochondria and nucleus. As such, they only engage in anaerobic metabolism and have a limited lifespan of only about 120 days. Their lack of internal organelles contributes to their characteristic biconcave shape, which helps them travel more efficiently through capillaries and maximizes their surface area, which assists in gas exchange. Erythrocytes are degraded by the spleen, which is located in the left upper quadrant of the abdomen. In a clinical context, hematocrit refers to the percentage of a blood sample that is composed by red blood cells.

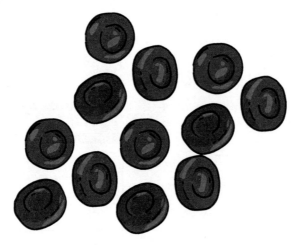

Figure 9. Erythrocytes

Erythrocytes also express a variety of glycoproteins on their surface, some of which are antigens that play a role in blood typing. A surprising number of blood typing systems exist, but the most relevant ones for the MCAT are the ABO blood type system and the Rh factor system.

The **ABO blood type system** is especially important for the MCAT as it is an example of codominance, where two dominant phenotypes are expressed simultaneously. In an individual with type A blood, the erythrocytes express the A antigen on their surface, while in an individual with type B blood the erythrocytes express the B antigen. Similarly, in someone with type AB blood, both the A antigen and the B antigen are present on the surface of the erythrocyte. The recessive phenotype, in which neither the A antigen nor the B antigen is present, is referred to as O.

By convention, the gene responsible for the ABO system is referred to using the letter "I": the dominant alleles are denoted as I^A and I^B, while the recessive allele is indicated with a lowercase "i."

The practical importance of blood typing stems from the fact that individuals develop antibodies against the antigens that they *do not* have and the body then attacks blood cells that have the antigens that the body considers as foreign. This can be very dangerous when a blood transfusion is performed, because an individual must receive blood that they will not produce antibodies to. In other words, an individual must receive the same type of blood (A, B, AB, or O) during a transfusion, otherwise their body will attack the newly introduced blood as a foreign body. This is why blood typing is so important from a medical point of view. As an interesting historical sidebar, the discovery of blood typing was crucial (along with antiseptic techniques and antibiotics) for routine surgery to become practicable. Table 1 below summarizes the ABO system and its implications for blood donation.

CLINICAL CONNECTIONS >>>

The hemoglobin present in erythrocytes undergoes a slow but predictable process of glycation by glucose present in the blood stream. Therefore, the fraction of glycosylated hemoglobin molecules (HbA1c) can be used as a proxy indicator for blood glucose levels on average over approximately the last three months (three months being the average life span of erythrocytes). HbA1c levels, in addition to fasting blood glucose readings, are commonly used to monitor the status of patients with diabetes.

GENOTYPE	BLOOD TYPE	ANTIBODIES PRODUCED	CAN RECEIVE BLOOD FROM:	CAN DONATE BLOOD TO:
$I^A i$	A	Anti-B	A, O	A, AB
$I^A I^A$				
$I^B i$	B	Anti-A	B, O	B, AB
$I^B I^B$				
$I^A I^B$	AB	None	A, B, AB, O	AB
ii	O	Anti-A Anti-B	O	A, B, AB, O

Table 1. ABO blood types and blood donation.

You'll notice that the **Rh factor** is caused by a different gene and does not exhibit codominance. Instead, it involves a single antigen that is either present (+) or absent (-). The Rh factor is completely independent from the ABO typing system, so an individual's blood type is characterized both by their ABO status and by their Rh status: for example, someone's blood type could be A⁺ or AB⁻ or O⁺, among others. Combining both systems, we can observe that someone with AB⁺ blood is a universal acceptor, because they will not produce anti-A, anti-B, or anti-Rh antibodies, and therefore can accept any type of blood. In contrast, people with type O⁻ blood are universal donors, because their blood contains none of the relevant antigens.

4. Cardiovascular Anatomy

The **heart** provides the driving force for the blood within the body. It has four chambers: the **left and right atria** are found at the top of the heart, and the **left and right ventricles** are found below. Let's review the path of blood as it moves through the heart. Deoxygenated blood returns to the right atrium via the superior and inferior venae cavae and the coronary sinus, which drains the coronary veins. From there, it is pumped into the right ventricle through the tricuspid valve. From the right ventricle, it goes to the pulmonary arteries through the pulmonary semilunar valves. After becoming oxygenated, blood returns to the heart via the pulmonary veins, and enters the left atrium. It is pumped through the bicuspid valve from the left atrium to the left ventricle, and then the left ventricle pushes the blood into circulation (more specifically, through the aortic semilunar valves into the ascending aorta).

The valves in the heart function to ensure that blood only flows in one direction. They can be subdivided into the **atrioventricular (AV) valves** and the **semilunar valves**. As the name suggests, the AV valves are found between the atria and ventricles. The **bicuspid valve**, which regulates blood flow from the left atrium to the left ventricle, is also known as the mitral valve because it was thought to be shaped like a bishop's hat, known as a "mitre." However, the names "bicuspid" and "tricuspid" are arguably more useful, because this helps reinforce the distinction that the bicuspid valve has two leaflets, while the tricuspid valve has three. The semilunar (SL) valves are located between the ventricles and the systemic circulation: the pulmonary SL valve prevents backflow of blood from the pulmonary circulation back into the right ventricle, while the aortic SL valve prevents backflow of blood from the ascending aorta back into the left ventricle. Both the pulmonary and aortic SL valves have three leaflets. The valves are also responsible for the heart sounds. The closure of the AV valves produces the first heart sound ("lub") and the closure of the SL valves produces the second heart sound ("dub").

> **MCAT STRATEGY >>>**
>
> A mnemonic you can use to help remember the AV valves is LAB RAT: **l**eft **a**trium = **b**icuspid, **r**ight **a**trium = **t**ricuspid.

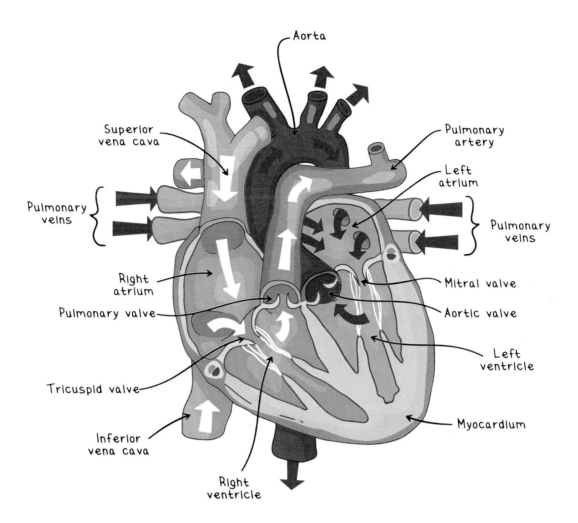

Figure 10. Heart anatomy and blood flow

The atria have thinner walls and are much less muscular than the ventricles, because their job is to receive blood returning to the heart and to pump blood into the ventricles, whereas the ventricles are very muscular because they pump blood away from the heart throughout the various vessels. In particular, the left ventricle is the most muscular, as it must pump blood throughout the body, whereas the right ventricle must only pump blood to the lungs. The term "**systole**" is used to refer to when the heart contracts, pushing blood into circulation, and the term "**diastole**" refers to when the heart relaxes, in between heartbeats. The corresponding blood pressure readings are known as systolic and diastolic, respectively; they are measured in units of mmHg (although this is frequently omitted in clinical contexts) and the systolic blood pressure reading is used first. Low blood pressure (**hypotension**) can be a sign of shock or other serious medical problems, while high blood pressure (**hypertension**) can be a transient response to stress or a chronic condition.

Next, let's move on to track how blood moves throughout the body. There are three types of blood vessels: arteries, capillaries, and veins. **Arteries** are defined as vessels

CLINICAL CONNECTIONS >>>

Hypertension affects almost one in three adults in the United States, making it a mainstay of everyday clinical practice. Hypotension, in contrast, is a common problem encountered in patients who are in shock or undergo trauma. One way or the other, you will become very familiar with blood pressure in the future as you enter into the practice of medicine!

that move blood *away* from the heart, **capillaries** are tiny blood vessels where gas exchange takes place, and **veins** move blood back towards the heart. Students often learn that arteries carry oxygenated blood, while veins carry deoxygenated blood, but this is an oversimplification. In reality, arteries are defined by carrying blood away from the heart (which you can remember by associating "<u>a</u>rteries" with "<u>a</u>way"), while veins carry blood back to the heart. In the systemic circulation, which supplies blood to the tissues of the body, arteries do indeed supply oxygenated blood. However, in the pulmonary circulation, which specializes in gas exchange, the pulmonary artery carries deoxygenated blood away from the heart to get reloaded with oxygen in the lungs, and then the pulmonary vein returns the newly oxygenated blood to the body.

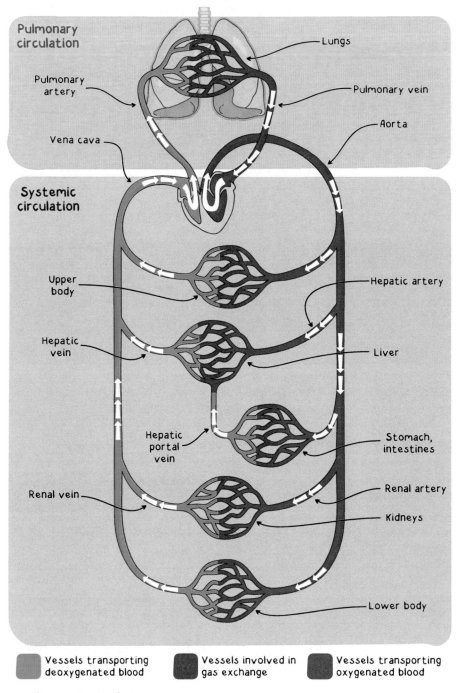

Figure 11. Pulmonary and systemic circulation

Arteries carry high-pressure blood and therefore have thick, muscular walls. Arteries and arterioles can also constrict and dilate, depending on the needs of the body. As discussed above, this can be used in **thermoregulation**, in which vasoconstriction of the arterioles near the skin is used to conserve heat in a cold environment, while vasodilation of those arterioles is used to dissipate excess heat. **Vasodilation** can be used to supply more oxygenated blood (and more energy) to specific body tissues in response to neurological control. For example, the sympathetic nervous system response ("fight or flight") causes the vessels supplying the muscles to dilate, allowing an influx of oxygenated blood to these tissues, while constricting most other arterial vessels, including those that supply the digestive tract. This essentially allows the body to shunt metabolic resources towards an immediate reaction, while postponing functions that are essential but can wait until the immediate danger has passed.

As arteries branch off from each other, they develop into smaller, more numerous **arterioles**. The blood pressure drops quickly between the arterioles and capillaries. **Capillaries** are tiny, thin vessels through which erythrocytes move one at a time and are where gas exchange occurs. After moving through the capillaries, deoxygenated blood (in the systemic circulation) moves into **venules**, which drain into **veins**, which then gather into the venae cavae before returning to the heart.

The blood pressure in veins is much lower and therefore they have much thinner walls. However, they have an interesting anatomical quirk of their own, due to the fact that they need to get blood back to the heart without the heart being able to provide a push. This is difficult in the lower limbs, where the veins must counteract the downward-pulling effects of gravity. This problem is solved by **valves** that allow blood to flow in only one direction.

MCAT STRATEGY >>>

Knowing that arteries and veins are defined by directionality, not oxygenation, and that the pulmonary arteries carry deoxygenated blood while the pulmonary veins carry oxygenated blood, can help answer trick questions and/or eliminate tricky answer choices on Test Day, so make sure it becomes a familiar fact!

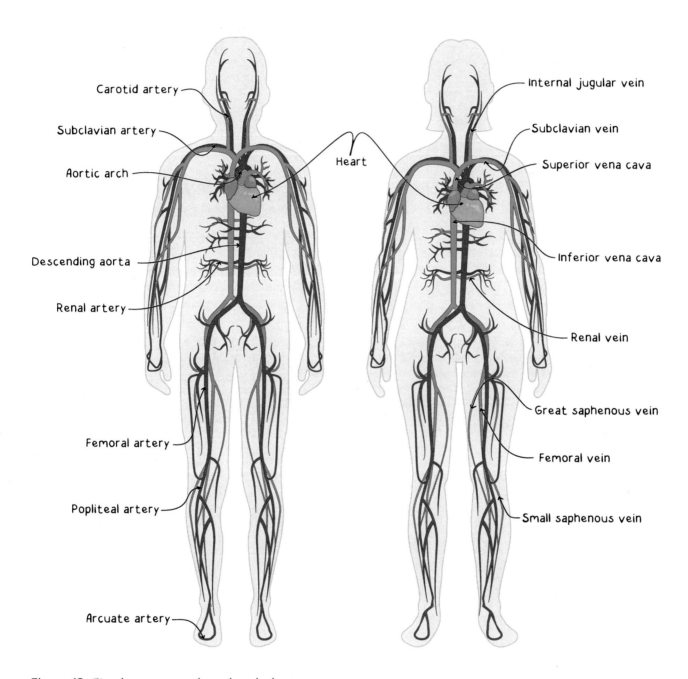

Figure 12. Circulatory system throughout body

Blood vessels are lined with **endothelial cells**, which are structurally similar to epithelial cells, except that they contain the protein vimentin, rather than keratin. Endothelial cells play a major role in vascular physiology, including functioning as a selective barrier between blood vessels and the rest of the tissue of the body, as well as mediating inflammation, vasodilation and vasoconstriction, blood clotting, and angiogenesis (the development of new blood vessels). Endothelial dysfunction has been implicated in a range of serious diseases, such as hypertension, atherosclerosis, and some of the negative complications of diabetes mellitus. The details go beyond the scope of the

MCAT, but endothelial physiology is an area of active research with direct clinical implications, and so the MCAT expects you to be aware of its general importance.

5. Cardiovascular Physiology

In this section, we'll move beyond the simple anatomy of the circulatory system to consider some of the ways in which it intersects with other systems of the body.

First, let's review how the heart **contracts**. It can set its own rhythm, which is controlled by the **sinoatrial (SA) node**, found at the roof of the right atrium. The cells in the SA node periodically send out **action potentials**, much like nerve cells. **Gap junctions** between the cardiac muscle cells allow the action potential to propagate throughout the tissue, causing contractions. The action potential flows from the SA node into the atria, but not into the ventricles because of a layer of insulating tissue. This causes both atria to contract, pushing the blood forward into the ventricles.

The **atrioventricular (AV) node** allows the action potential to pass through to the ventricles after the atria have contracted. At this point, the ventricles must contract to push the blood out of the heart. The signal is sent through the **bundle of His**, right and left bundle branches, and **Purkinje fibers** to all the muscle cells of the ventricles.

The heart rate is regulated by both the nervous and endocrine systems. The **autonomic nervous system**, which is subdivided into the sympathetic and parasympathetic nervous systems, regulates heart rate. The **parasympathetic nervous system**, which is responsible for the "rest and digest" response, slows the heart rate. In contrast, the **sympathetic nervous system** response ("fight or flight") raises the heart rate. The heart rate is also increased by the hormones epinephrine and norepinephrine, which are released by the adrenal medulla.

One of the reasons why the circulatory system is important for the MCAT is because it provides a way to test the physics of fluids in a biological context. With that in mind, it is important to review how the fundamental topics of fluid dynamics apply to the circulatory system. Let's start off with a high-level perspective on how flow throughout the circulatory system works on the most basic level: a **pressure differential** is used to drive flow through a network of tubes that provide **resistance**. In particular, we can formalize this intuition by saying that $Q = \Delta P/R$, where Q is the flow through the system (equivalent to cardiac output for the systemic circulation), ΔP is the overall change in pressure, and R is peripheral resistance (i.e., the resistance provided by the blood vessels).

Equation 1. $$Q = \frac{\Delta P}{R} \text{ or } RQ = \Delta P$$

Simply rearranging this equation to $RQ = \Delta P$ provides us with an important conclusion: given constant flow, resistance and ΔP are proportional to each other. This means that if we increase resistance, ΔP goes up as well (if we maintain the same flow). With this fundamental equation in mind, let's take a closer look at resistance. Note that this is analogous to the equation $V = IR$ for circuits, where V for electric potential is analogous to ΔP (both are forms of potential energy), I for electrical current is analogous to Q (blood flow), and R is used for resistance in both contexts.

Resistance in blood vessels can be modeled using a form of Poiseuille's law that is modified to focus on resistance:

Equation 2. $$R = \frac{8L\eta}{\pi r^4}$$

You may note that the r^4 term in Equation 2 is in the denominator, not the numerator unlike the form of Poiseulle's law that is most commonly given in discussions of fluids. This is because Equation 2 is an adaptation of Poiseulle's law that focuses on resistance, rather than laminar flow, which is given by $Q = \pi\Delta Pr^4/8\eta L$. In Equation 2, R again refers to resistance. L refers to the length of the artery, η to the viscosity of the blood, and r to the radius of the blood vessel. Let's work through the physiological implications of these variables.

The first variable we mentioned, L, is the most straightforward. The length of a blood vessel generally cannot be altered, so it is not a parameter used to regulate resistance/blood pressure physiologically. The viscosity of blood (η) is related to the proportion of erythrocytes in the blood, or hematocrit (as discussed above). All things being equal, the greater the hematocrit, the greater the resistance, which can either correspond to less flow or greater pressure, according to Equation 1. Of note, increased hematocrit is an adaptation to higher altitudes due to the lower availability of oxygen at higher pressures. The MCAT could ask you to combine those insights and ask how adaptation to high-altitude conditions could affect blood flow and/or pressure. However, in normal circumstances, our final variable (r, the radius of the blood vessel) is the most important for explaining how pressure decreases as blood moves along its path through the circulatory system. Resistance is not only inversely related with radius, but the relationship is to the fourth power! This means that as the total radius increases as the blood moves from arteries to arterioles to capillaries, the resistance (and therefore pressure) drops dramatically.

Wait a minute, you might say: what do you mean that the total radius increases as you go from arteries to arterioles to capillaries? Aren't capillaries much narrower than arteries? That is correct, but it's important to understand that this equation can be applied *both* to a simple system consisting of a single vessel, in which narrowing the vessel would increase the pressure, *and* to the more complex system present in the body, where one artery may branch out into thousands of capillaries. The total cross-sectional area, and therefore the total radius, increases dramatically when evaluating the capillary *system* as a whole in comparison to the artery or arteries supplying it.

The **continuity equation** can also be applied to the circulatory system, with the same need to be clear about whether it is used to analyze a single vessel or a more complex system in which a single larger vessel branches into multiple smaller vessels. For a given volume of fluid, the continuity equation relates the velocity of blood flow to the cross-sectional area through which flow takes place.

Equation 3.
$$A_1v_1 = A_2v_2$$

Care must be taken when applying this equation to think through the anatomical and physiological context correctly. As discussed above, this equation could be applied directly to modeling the effect of, for example, narrowing a blood vessel through a plaque. However, what if we were apply it to predicting the rate of blood flow in the arteries compared to in the capillaries? We might be tempted to solve this problem by saying that the cross-sectional area of a capillary is much smaller than that of an artery. While that is true, it fails to adequately account for the assumptions of the continuity equation: namely, we have to hold the volume constant. This means that we have to consider *all* of the capillaries fed by a given artery. The total cross-sectional area of these capillaries is much greater than that of the artery. This means that blood flow slows down dramatically in the capillaries compared to the arteries located "upstream," which is physiologically useful because it provides adequate time for the necessary gas and solute exchange to take place.

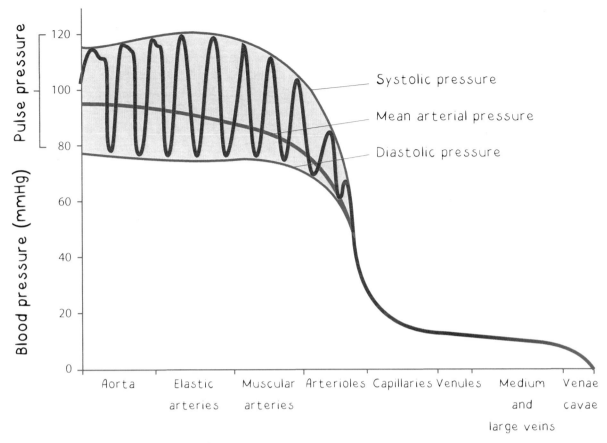

Figure 13. Blood pressure throughout body

If you have already carefully reviewed your content on fluids, you may wonder whether the **Bernoulli equation** can be applied here. It is given below as Equation 4, for reference.

Equation 4.
$$P_1 + \frac{1}{2}\rho v_1^2 + \rho g h_1 = P_2 + \frac{1}{2}\rho v_2^2 + \rho g h_2$$

As a brief review, the Bernoulli equation is essentially **conservation of energy** applied to fluids. The terms $\frac{1}{2}\rho v^2$ and $\rho g h$ are the fluid equivalents of kinetic energy and gravitational potential energy respectively, while the term P refers to the potential energy corresponding to pressure. Essentially, the Bernoulli equation is conservation of energy for fluids. As such, it's theoretically applicable to blood (after all, no exceptions to conservation of mass and energy exist in the universe). However, the Bernoulli equation is defined for *ideal* fluids, and we have to be careful about what assumptions that entails. In particular, ideal fluids lack viscosity. We also neglect frictional interactions with the walls of the container. For an analogy, note that the familiar $KE_1 + PE_1 = KE_2 + PE_2$ equation that we use for conservation of energy in problems involving objects in motion also requires us to neglect friction. It's one thing to neglect viscosity and friction when dealing with water flowing through metal pipes, but that's more dubious when it comes to blood, which *is* viscous to a meaningful extent and *does* interact with the surrounding vessels, especially in narrow vessels like capillaries, where there may only be enough room for literally a single red blood cell to move through at a time. When applying Bernoulli's

MCAT STRATEGY >>>

What's the takeaway point for the MCAT? Be extremely cautious about using Bernoulli's law for blood unless a question either tells you to assume that blood is an ideal liquid, or you have a good reason to think that it would be OK to neglect viscosity and friction.

law to blood flow, care must also be taken to compare the entire *system* at different points, and to avoid committing the error we discussed above for the continuity equation of trying to compare a single artery to a single capillary, neglecting the fact that virtually countless capillaries are supplied by a single artery.

In addition to viewing the system of vessels through the lens of fluid dynamics, the proper balance of fluid must be maintained between the blood vessels and the surrounding interstitial cells. This is accomplished through the interplay between hydrostatic and oncotic pressure (also known as osmotic pressure) within the capillary bed. **Hydrostatic pressure** is the "pushing" pressure due to the force of liquid on its container (in this case a blood vessel) and **oncotic pressure** is the "pulling" pressure due to the presence of solutes in a solution (in this case, blood). The key point here is that the hydrostatic pressure drops as you move from the arterial end of the capillary bed to the venous end, but the oncotic pressure remains more or less constant. Therefore, the hydrostatic pressure pushes fluid into the interstitial tissue and the oncotic pressure pulls it back in on the venous end. Dysregulation of this process, either due to excessive hydrostatic pressure or insufficient oncotic pressure, can lead to fluid buildup, known as **edema**.

6. Overview of Gas Transport

Now that we've reviewed the anatomy and physiology of the respiratory and circulatory systems, let's step back and review the ultimate point of both systems: providing tissue with the oxygen necessary for aerobic metabolism and removing carbon dioxide and other waste products. In particular, we'll focus on **gas exchange**, as the next chapter will describe how other forms of waste are removed through the excretory system.

It's not random that the respiratory and the circulatory system were grouped together into the same chapter here. Although they are often studied separately and have distinct anatomical structures, they work together as a single unit from the view of respiration. As you study the physiology of respiration, be sure not to limit it to just the respiratory system. You should also be able to trace the path of gas transport from the first steps of air entering the nostrils to the ways that oxygen is supplied to the tissues that need it. In this section, we'll place a particular focus on the latter question, and review the mechanics of hemoglobin in depth.

The key to gas exchange is **hemoglobin**. Understanding how hemoglobin works is fundamental for the MCAT. You should study hemoglobin with the expectation that you will encounter a couple questions either on hemoglobin specifically or on the principles that explain how it functions.

Hemoglobin is a metalloprotein composed of four subunits. Each subunit is a globular protein that contains a **heme group**, which consists of an Fe^{2+} ion held at the center of a heterocyclic porphyrin ring. The Fe^{2+} ion is what binds oxygen for transport. There are two key facts about hemoglobin-oxygen interactions. First, the affinity between hemoglobin and oxygen varies depending on the chemical composition of the environment, which is what allows it to function as a delivery system. Second, the binding between hemoglobin and oxygen is **cooperative**. When the first heme group on a hemoglobin molecule binds with oxygen, it facilitates subsequent binding.

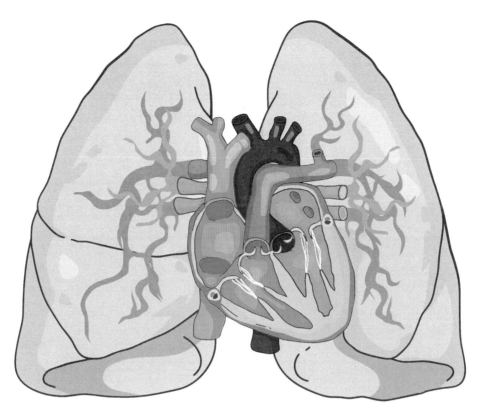

Figure 14. Heart and lungs

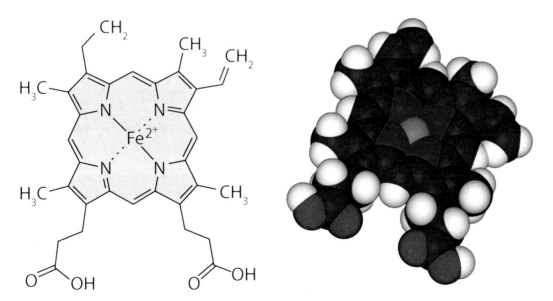

Figure 15. Heme

Let's first review the cooperativity of hemoglobin, because it underlies some terminology that is then used to discuss other factors that affect hemoglobin-oxygen interactions. Hemoglobin has two forms: taut/tense (T) and relaxed (R). The T form has a low affinity for oxygen, and the R form has a high affinity for oxygen. When oxygen binds to the first heme group, it shifts the hemoglobin molecule from the T form to the R form, facilitating further binding. This, technically speaking, is what makes hemoglobin-oxygen binding cooperative. Additionally, hemoglobin-oxygen binding is relatively favored when large amounts of oxygen are present, as indicated by a high partial pressure of oxygen. This results in a sigmoidal shape for the **oxygen-hemoglobin dissociation curve** shown below:

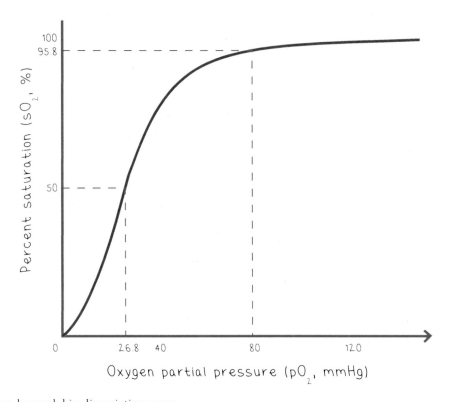

Figure 17. Oxygen-hemoglobin dissociation curve

Be careful to understand what is shown on the dissociation curve. The x-axis indicates the partial pressure of oxygen or the amount of oxygen in the blood. The y-axis indicates the percentage of saturation of heme binding sites on hemoglobin. As you can see, the more oxygen is present in the blood, the more likely hemoglobin is to bind oxygen. The next step is to connect this to the physiological distribution of oxygen versus other gases. Oxygen is plentiful in the alveolar capillaries of the lung, allowing hemoglobin to "load up" with oxygen. Then, hemoglobin is transported to blood vessels in other tissues of the body, where the partial pressure of oxygen is lower. The resulting higher levels of dissociation between hemoglobin and oxygen allow oxygen to be "delivered" to the tissues. The partial pressure of oxygen is even lower in areas where exercise is happening, allowing even more oxygen to be delivered precisely where it is needed.

However, the regulation of hemoglobin is even more complicated due to allosteric regulation by carbon dioxide, H^+, and a byproduct of glycolysis known as 2,3-bisphosphoglyceric acid (2,3-BPG). Let's start with the effects of carbon dioxide and pH. Recall the **bicarbonate equilibrium** reaction, discussed earlier in the chapter but reproduced below:

$$CO_2 + H_2O \rightleftharpoons H_2CO_3 \rightleftharpoons HCO_3^- + H^+$$

The bicarbonate equilibrium reaction means that an increase in carbon dioxide due to increased metabolism in active muscles is manifested as a lower pH due to a higher concentration of H^+ ions. H^+ ions allosterically regulate hemoglobin and in particular they stabilize the T form, which has a lower affinity for oxygen. This means that H^+ causes hemoglobin to have less affinity for oxygen at a given partial pressure of oxygen, which is manifested as a rightward shift of the oxygen-hemoglobin dissociation curve. This is known as the **Bohr effect**. 2,3-BPG also causes a rightward shift of the curve. A leftward shift of the dissociation curve would reflect a greater affinity for oxygen. In fact, this takes place in fetal hemoglobin because fetal hemoglobin is less strongly affected by 2,3-BPG. This allows fetal hemoglobin to "take" oxygen from maternal hemoglobin.

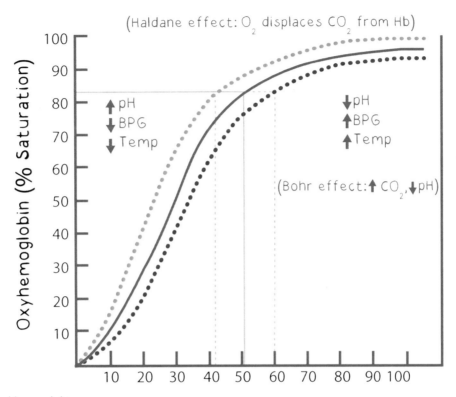

Figure 18. Shifted hemoglobin curves

Carbon dioxide can be carried by hemoglobin, but is not responsible for the majority of carbon dioxide transport. Again, the bicarbonate equilibrium reaction is crucial for understanding how carbon dioxide is excreted. The enzyme **carbonic anhydrase** converts carbon dioxide gas to carbonic acid (H_2CO_3), a process that would otherwise take much longer. Carbonic acid then dissociates into bicarbonate ion and H^+. Since bicarbonate ion is charged, it moves freely through the aqueous blood. Carbon dioxide as a gas is then exhaled in gas exchange in the lungs, where it diffuses down its concentration gradient and out of the body. At the same time, oxygen diffuses down its concentration gradient to bind with hemoglobin in the newly oxygenated blood.

MCAT STRATEGY >>>

As always, the key to MCAT success is going from passive learning in the initial stages of your content review to active mastery. Shifted hemoglobin curves are an excellent place to practice this. Set yourself the goal of explaining to an intelligent but not biochemically sophisticated friend (perhaps a non-premed humanities major?) what a shifted hemoglobin curve means. You will find that to do so, you truly have to master the content. This is the point of studying: actually taking the MCAT is not the time to derive the implications of leftward versus rightward shifts from scratch. You want it to have become a reflex by then.

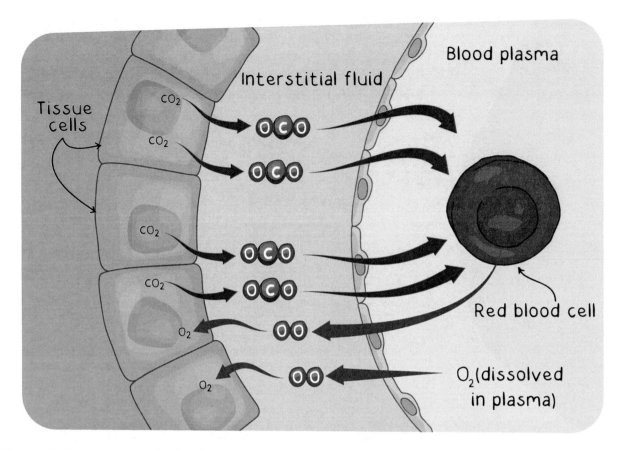

Figure 20. Capillary beds and gas exchange

7. Must-Knows

> Respiratory anatomy: nasal/oral cavity → pharynx → trachea → bronchi → bronchioles → alveoli. Pleura surround lungs in the thoracic cavity. Surfactant covers alveoli to decrease surface tension and prevent them from collapsing.

> Negative-pressure respiration: diaphragm contracts, expanding lungs; greater volume = lower pressure, air comes in from outside.

> Ciliated cells and mucus in trachea and bronchi help trap particulate matter and push it up to be either expelled or swallowed.

> Basic point of respiration: carbon dioxide produced as waste product of metabolism needs to be exhaled, and oxygen for aerobic respiration needs to be inhaled.

> Connection between CO_2 and pH due to bicarbonate equilibrium:

$$CO_2 + H_2O \rightleftharpoons H_2CO_3 \rightleftharpoons HCO_3^- + H^+$$

> Blood contains plasma (non-cellular component), platelets (thrombocytes), white blood cells (leukocytes) and red blood cells (erythrocytes).

> Erythrocytes lack nuclei and membrane-bound organelles; rely on anaerobic metabolism, have biconcave shape, and are packed with hemoglobin (which carries oxygen and some carbon dioxide).

> Basic cardiovascular anatomy: venae cavae → right atrium → tricuspid valve → right ventricle → pulmonary semilunar valve → pulmonary artery → capillaries (gas exchange) → pulmonary veins → left atrium → bicuspid (mitral) valve → left ventricle → aortic semilunar valve → aorta → systemic circulation.

> Arteries take blood *away* from heart, veins take blood *to* heart.

> Aorta > arteries > arterioles > capillaries > venules > veins > venae cavae.

> Pressure decreases as blood moves through the circulatory system, and velocity decreases from arteries to capillary beds.

> Hemoglobin: a protein composed of four units, each with a heme group that contains an iron ion which binds oxygen.

> Hemoglobin-oxygen binding is cooperative. Hemoglobin has T form, which is resistant to binding, and R form, which facilitates easier binding. The first bond stabilizes the R form.

> Rightward shift of oxygen-hemoglobin dissociation curve means a lower affinity. Caused by ↑ CO_2, ↑ H^+, ↓ pH, (Bohr effect), and ↑ 2,3-BPG. Leftward shift means higher affinity. Caused by opposite of above conditions and in fetal hemoglobin.

> Biochemical properties of hemoglobin allow it to pick up oxygen in the lungs and deliver it to where it is needed in tissues undergoing active metabolism.

End of Chapter Practice

The best MCAT practice is **realistic**, with a focus on identifying steps for further improvement. For those reasons, we recommend completing practice questions in an online setting that simulates the real MCAT interface, and taking advantage of advanced analytic features to help you determine how best to move forward in your MCAT study journey.

With that in mind, **online end-of-chapter** questions for Biology, Biochemistry, Chemistry + Organic Chemistry, Physics, and Psychology/Sociology are available through your Blueprint MCAT account.

As a further supplement, given the importance of active learning for effective studying, we also suggest that you consult the Must-Knows at the end of each chapter as a basis for creating a study sheet, in which you list out key terms and test your ability to briefly summarize them.

This page left intentionally blank.

This page left intentionally blank.

Digestive and Excretory Systems

0. Introduction

In this chapter, we'll deal with some of the most basic realities of human existence: obtaining nutrients from food, processing those nutrients, and excreting the resultant waste products. You should approach this chapter with two goals in mind: first, you should study the anatomy carefully, because basic anatomy/structure questions are fair game on Test Day. While any single point of anatomy is relatively unlikely to be tested, the cumulative likelihood of getting one or two questions that require you to draw on an understanding of the anatomy of these systems is high. Second, and more importantly, you must master the underlying physiology, which means understanding how the digestive and excretory systems allow the organism to obtain nutrients and maintain homeostasis. As you have seen, this is a recurring theme for physiology-related topics on the MCAT: you're not generally expected to have a complete command of all of the details, but you are absolutely expected to have a solid understanding of the fundamental principles and how all of the main physiological systems of the body fit together.

1. Digestive System Anatomy

Let's begin this chapter by reviewing the path of a piece of food. In this section, we'll cover the relevant anatomy and the basic functions of the organs of the digestive system, and then in the next section we'll take a closer look at digestion from a physiological standpoint. We should start, though, by clarifying some terminology. First, we need to distinguish digestion from absorption. **Digestion** refers to the breakdown and processing of food, while **absorption** refers to how nutrients actually enter the body. Digestion does not necessarily imply absorption. Unabsorbed but digested food is a major component of feces.

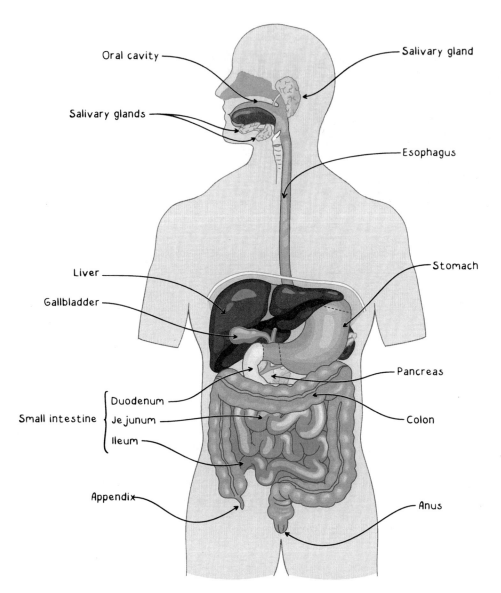

Figure 1. Anatomy of the digestive system

Food is first ingested and chewed in the mouth, where **saliva**, which is produced by the salivary glands, provides lubrication. What enters your mouth as a piece of food exits as a "**bolus**"—a term used in digestive anatomy and physiology to describe a ball-shaped mixture of food and saliva (in fact, "bolus" means "ball" in Latin). Saliva has other functions in addition to lubrication. Most notably, it contains some enzymes, including alpha-amylase (or salivary **amylase**), which begins to break down starch. The activity of salivary amylase explains why starchy foods such as rice or potatoes begin to taste sweet if you chew on them for long enough: amylase breaks down starch to form disaccharides, which are perceived as sweet. Saliva also contains the antimicrobial enzyme lysozyme. Although the antimicrobial properties of saliva are nowhere near strong enough to kill off the extensive microbiota of the oral cavity, they are strong enough for saliva to be considered part of the innate immune system.

>> **CONNECTIONS** <<

Chapter 11 of Biology

Once food is swallowed, it passes down the **esophagus**, a fibromuscular tube that runs behind the trachea and passes through the diaphragm. The esophagus empties into the stomach through a sphincter that goes by various names: the lower esophageal sphincter, gastroesophageal sphincter, or the

230

cardiac sphincter (this name refers to the fact that the esophagus enters into the upper part of the stomach, which is known as the cardia). Dysfunction of the lower esophageal sphincter can lead to gastrointestinal reflux, in which the highly acidic contents of the stomach back up into the esophagus. This leads to a painful condition known as heartburn, and when it persists, it can result in gastroesophageal reflux disease (GERD).

The lumen of the stomach is highly acidic. In the **stomach,** proteases such as pepsin begin to break down proteins, turning the bolus of food into a semi-digested substance known as **chyme**. The stomach stores food, churns it, and continues to digest it, although very little absorption happens in the stomach. Exceptions to this include water, some medications, caffeine, and, to some extent, ethanol (although most ethanol is absorbed later). The gross anatomy of the stomach is shown in Figure 2. Some features of note include the greater curvature and the lesser curvature, the presence of folds known as rugae along the lining of the stomach, and the fact that the top of the stomach is known as the fundus and the bottom area as the pylorus. **Gastric acid** is secreted by **parietal cells**, and contains highly concentrated HCl that is used to keep the stomach at a pH of 1.5-3.5. This low pH is optimal for the functioning of digestive enzymes in the stomach, and also helps to kill off bacteria.

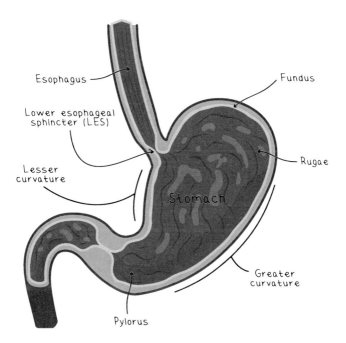

Figure 2. Stomach

A major challenge the body faces with the stomach is how to protect itself from the low pH and digestive enzymes that it contains. On a conceptual level, a similar point can be made regarding acidic lysosomes in cells, but the stomach is much larger and has an even lower pH, making this an especially important task. **Mucous cells** secrete bicarbonate-rich mucus that helps protect the stomach lining from the acidity of its contents. Additionally, protections are built into the sequence of events leading to the activation of digestive proteins. In particular, chief cells do not secrete pepsin directly, because doing so would run the risk of proteolytic activity being initiated immediately. Instead, chief cells release the precursor pepsinogen (an example of a zymogen), which is then cleaved under intensely acidic conditions to create the active form, pepsin.

As mentioned, **pepsin** is a digestive enzyme secreted in the stomach. Pepsin primarily cleaves proteins at the site of aromatic residues. As such, it breaks proteins down into smaller peptides but does not complete their digestion. Additionally, the stomach secretes intrinsic factor, which is necessary for the proper absorption and processing of vitamin B12. The stomach also secretes water to dilute the bolus, as well as signaling molecules to help regulate digestion, as discussed further in Section 2.

The next step in the journey that food takes through the body is to pass through the pyloric sphincter, which connects the stomach with the **small intestine**. The small intestine is where we shift gears from digestion to absorption, although this is not a watertight distinction since, as we've seen, only a little bit of absorption happens in the stomach, while digestion continues in the small intestine in addition to absorption. The small intestine is subdivided into the **duodenum**, which is a fairly short structure, and the longer structures of the **jejunum** (the midsection of the small intestine) and the **ileum**.

MCAT STRATEGY >>>

The acronym "Dow Jones Industrial" can be used to remember the sequence of the duodenum → jejunum → ileum in the small intestine.

A lot happens in the small intestine, so it's worth stepping back and reviewing the main things that need to be accomplished. Having a clear sense of these tasks will help keep track of which organs are responsible for which components.

> The chyme coming from the stomach is highly acidic and needs to be neutralized.
> When the chyme enters the small intestine, little chemical digestion has happened, with the exception of the contribution of salivary amylase and proteases such as pepsin. Digestion needs to continue.
> Nutrients and vitamins need to be absorbed.

Let's first briefly review how digestion continues in the small intestine. Several organs contribute to this process. The small intestine itself releases **brush-border enzymes** through cells contained in structures known as **microvilli** (which are discussed more below). Some brush-border enzymes, known as disaccharidases, break down disaccharides (recall that disaccharides are a common form in which carbohydrates are consumed), while a different group of enzymes, known as peptidases, break down proteins. The **pancreas** also contributes significantly to digestion in the duodenum by directly secreting an alkaline fluid containing several types of digestive enzymes, capable of digesting all major classes of biomolecules. The **liver** also contributes to digestion via the secretion of **bile**, which is an alkaline, dark green to yellowish fluid that contains bile salts, bilirubin, and some fats. Its main function is to emulsify lipids and help convert them into micelles. The reason this is important is because the enzymes that digest lipids are water-soluble, so it is important to break up lipids and expose the greatest amount of surface area possible to the action of those enzymes. An interesting fact about bile is that it is secreted by the liver but stored and concentrated in the gallbladder, from which it is released into the small intestine.

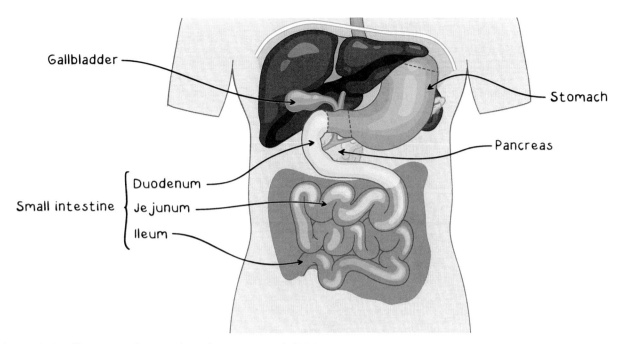

Figure 3. Small intestine: large scale with anatomic subdivisions

The Gallbladder

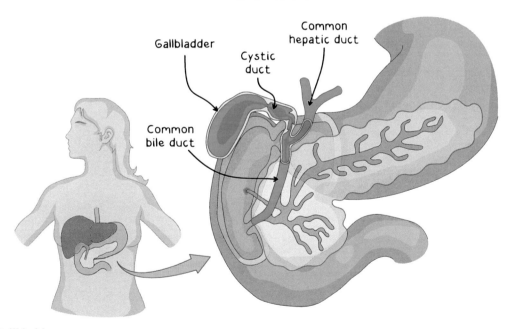

Figure 4. Gallbladder

Next, let's look at how the highly acidic chyme from the stomach is neutralized. An elegant aspect of this process is that it is, to a great extent, combined with the digestive processes reviewed above. As mentioned, the fluid secreted by the pancreas that is rich in digestive enzymes is an alkaline solution rich in bicarbonate. Likewise, bile is also slightly alkaline, with a pH roughly between 7.5 and 8. Additionally, the duodenum itself secretes bicarbonate buffer via the Brunner's glands. The additive effect of these secretions results in the duodenum becoming a slightly alkaline environment, which is optimal for the various digestive enzymes.

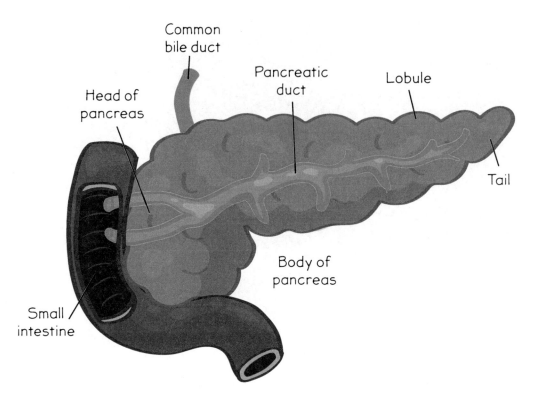

Figure 5. Pancreas

Once food is sufficiently digested, the resulting nutrients need to be absorbed. This is primarily the job of the small intestine: the **jejunum** and the **ileum**. The small intestine is characterized by structures known as **villi**, which are finger-like projections that extend into the lumen of the intestine that dramatically increase the available surface area. The surfaces of villi are lined with enterocytes (the cells of the intestinal lining), and the enterocytes themselves are characterized by microvilli, which are finger-like projections from the cell membranes of enterocytes that greatly increase the surface area available for cellular functions.

Chyme now travels to the **large intestine**. The large intestine is subdivided into the cecum and appendix, followed by the **ascending colon**, **transverse colon**, **descending colon**, **sigmoid colon**, and **rectum**. The **cecum** is a pouch that is connected with the ileum of the small intestine through the ileocecal valve. The **appendix** is attached to the cecum. Traditionally, the appendix has been thought to be a vestigial organ—that is, an organ that has lost the function it had in our evolutionary ancestors—but emerging research has called this into question. The last component of the large intestine is the rectum, which stores feces before it is expelled through the anus.

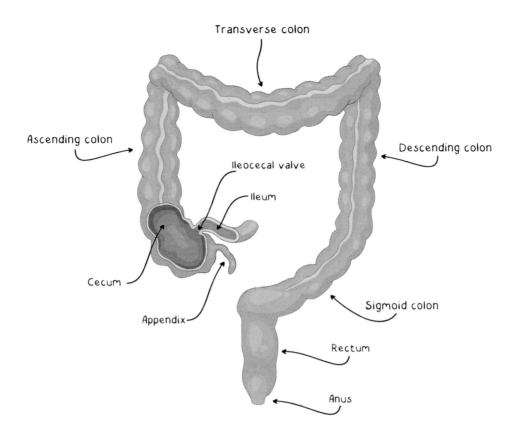

Figure 6. Large intestine

The **large intestine** has several functions. First, it absorbs water from the food undergoing digestion, which is a large component of how watery chyme becomes solid feces. Second, it hosts the largest community of bacteria in the human body, referred to as the **gut microbiota** or the **gut flora**. The relationship of these bacteria to their human host is a symbiotic relationship that ranges from commensal to mutualistic. Bacteria that provide a benefit to the human body by synthesizing necessary vitamins such as vitamin K and vitamin B_7 (biotin) are called mutualistic bacteria, and bacteria that provide neither benefit nor harm to their host are called commensal bacteria. While you do need to be aware of these terms for the MCAT, you should also be aware that they are simplifications, as modern research efforts into the gut flora suggest that the entire gut biome may have complex effects on human health that we are only now aware of. No chemical digestion takes place in the large intestine, but absorption of remaining nutrients (either from food or the metabolic products of bacteria) takes place to some extent. You don't have to be aware of the details for the MCAT, but they may come up in a passage.

After passing through the large intestine and into the rectum, food has now been fully transformed into **feces**. Feces primarily contain indigestible material and water. In healthy individuals, a major example of indigestible material would be plant cellulose, because humans lack the enzymes to break down the carbohydrate polymers contained in cellulose. However, pathological conditions can result in different substances becoming indigestible, with ramifications for the content of feces. For example, liver dysfunction can lead to impaired production of bile, which leads to impaired digestion of lipids because bile plays a major role in emulsifying lipids to allow digestive enzymes to do their work. If lipid digestion is impaired, more fat can be excreted in the feces, a condition known as steatorrhea. Steatorrhea itself is not required content for the MCAT, but this is an example of the kind of chain of logical reasoning that the MCAT often incorporates into passage-based questions.

2. Overview of Digestion

In this section, we'll take a closer look at some of the physiological processes that underpin digestion, and also review digestion from the perspective of how specific nutrients are digested.

First, we may ask ourselves: how, exactly, does the bolus/chyme/feces move through the digestive system? The answer is a combination of **peristalsis** and **sphincters**. Peristalsis refers to an involuntary process of contractions and relaxation of the smooth muscle in various parts of the digestive tract. These contractions proceed in a concerted manner to create a peristaltic wave that pushes material along. As we saw in our review of the anatomy of the digestive tracts, various sphincters connect different digestive organs, such as the lower esophageal sphincter, which connects the esophagus and the stomach, the pyloric sphincter, which connects the stomach and small intestine, the ileocecal valve (also known as the ileocecal sphincter), which connects the small intestine and the large intestine, and finally, the anal sphincter, which regulates the release of feces from the rectum.

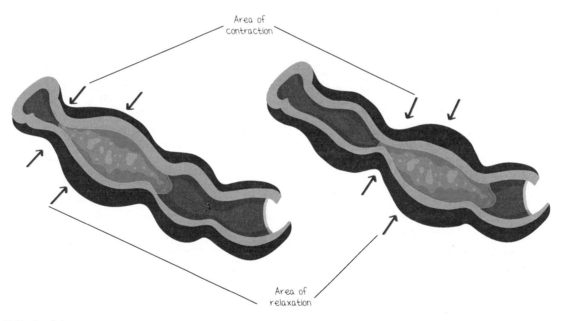

Figure 7. Peristalsis

Additionally, digestion is subject to complex patterns of endocrine and nervous control, which makes sense as it must be regulated closely in order to ensure that the organism responds appropriately to various external and internal stimuli. The hormonal control of digestion incorporates everything from our perceptions of hunger to very fine-tuned control over the release of enzymes from one digestive organ to another.

Hunger is principally regulated by the hormones **ghrelin** and **leptin**. Ghrelin is often known as the hunger hormone (think "grrr," like how your stomach growls when you're hungry). Ghrelin is secreted by specialized cells in the upper part of the stomach and in the pancreas, and is released when the stomach is empty. It promotes appetite. In contrast, leptin is secreted by adipocytes (fat cells) and promotes feelings of satiety, or fullness. Interestingly, emerging research has demonstrated that these hormones have effects on a surprisingly broad range of target organs throughout the body, but this goes well beyond what is necessary for the MCAT.

In the stomach, G cells secrete **gastrin**. Gastrin generally promotes digestion, with the main effect of stimulating parietal cells to secrete gastric acid (HCl). Acidic chyme in the duodenum of the small intestine triggers the release of **secretin** from S cells. As the name suggests, secretin triggers the secretion and release of bicarbonate-rich mucus from the pancreas to neutralize the acidic chyme and promote the optimal functioning of the digestive enzymes that do their work in the small intestine. **Cholecystokinin (CCK)** is also secreted by cells lining the small intestine, and stimulates the secretion and release of digestive enzymes from the pancreas and the release of bile from the gallbladder. You can therefore think of secretin and CCK as being on the same team, in a sense, with secretin having the responsibility for pH levels and CCK being responsible for the actual enzymes and compounds that do the work of digestion. CCK also inhibits appetite, which makes sense because it is only secreted if the body is already working on digesting food and therefore doesn't need any more at the moment.

However, digestion also sometimes needs to be slowed down. This is where **somatostatin** comes in. Somatostatin is released from several areas of the digestive tract and has the effect of inhibiting the release of many hormones involved in digestion, including some that we have already discussed, such as gastrin, CCK, and secretin. It also decreases the rate at which the stomach empties and inhibits the secretion of pancreatic hormones such as insulin and glucagon. Additionally, somatostatin (released from the hypothalamus) inhibits the release of growth hormone, leading to its use as a treatment for gigantism. This gives a sense of its broad-range inhibitory effects, the result of which is that the most effective way to think about somatostatin is a signaling molecule that basically puts the brakes on digestion.

> ## MCAT STRATEGY >>>
>
> Somatostatin is an example of how the name of a compound can provide useful hints about its function. "Somat-" means "body," and you can associate "stat" with "static," indicating that it means slowing something down. So, somatostatin is basically what slows your body down. This is a perfect indication of its very general effects on the body.

In addition to endocrine control, the digestive process is also regulated by nervous system control. In fact, it has an entire subdivision of the nervous system: the **enteric nervous system**, which is sometimes called a "second brain" due to its complexity and autonomy. Although the enteric nervous system is connected to the rest of the nervous system, it can actually function autonomously even if important connections with the rest of the nervous system are severed. The autonomic nervous system also has important effects on the gastrointestinal system. Recall that the sympathetic nervous response (also known as "fight or flight") is triggered in response to acute stresses and generally predisposes the body to urgent responses, while the parasympathetic system ("rest and digest") has the opposite effect. What this means for the digestive system is that the sympathetic nervous system contracts the vessels supplying the digestive tract, reducing blood flow and shunting it towards muscles. In times of danger, digestion can wait while you run away or fight. In contrast, the parasympathetic nervous system kicks in when the acute stress has passed, at which point digestion becomes a good idea again.

Next, let's take a closer look at how nutrients are absorbed. Although it is easy to skim over this point, but this is a complicated question that leads us to important physiological topics such as the hepatic portal system and the functions of the liver.

As discussed above, the main action in terms of absorption takes place in the small intestine, although some absorption of certain compounds happens in the stomach, while water and vitamins can be absorbed in the large intestine. To understand how absorption takes place, we need to take a closer look at the anatomy of **villi** and **microvilli** in the lining of the small intestine. To review, villi are finger-like projections that dramatically increase the surface area available for absorption, and microvilli are similar projections from individual cells located on the villi that increase the available surface area even more. Villi contain capillaries and a lacteal. Capillaries drain into the hepatic portal vein, which takes water-soluble nutrients for the liver for what is often referred to as first-pass metabolism. Meanwhile, lacteals drain lipids into the lymph vessels.

What needs to happen in absorption is for nutrients to get into the epithelial cells lining the small intestine, and then get out of those cells to enter the capillaries or lacteals. This process is different for amino acids and carbohydrates (which are soluble in aqueous solution) than it is for lipids (which are non-soluble in aqueous solution). This is a common recurring theme when it comes to membranes. Note, for instance, how the membrane interactions for steroid hormones (lipids) and peptide hormones are fundamentally different, with functional implications as discussed in Chapter 7.

>> **CONNECTIONS** <<

Chapter 7 of Biology

Carbohydrates must be broken down into monosaccharides to be absorbed. Secondary active transport coupled to Na$^+$ is used to transport glucose and galactose into the epithelial cells, while facilitated diffusion is used for fructose. All three of these monosaccharides then leave the epithelial cells and enter the circulatory system via facilitated diffusion. Similarly, single amino acids and short chains of two to three amino acids enter the epithelial cells through secondary active transport (via specific transporters), and then leave the epithelial cells and enter the bloodstream through facilitated diffusion. Facilitated diffusion can be used to push these molecules into the bloodstream because the constant flow of blood through the capillaries means they will always be moving down their concentration gradient.

Lumen of small intestine

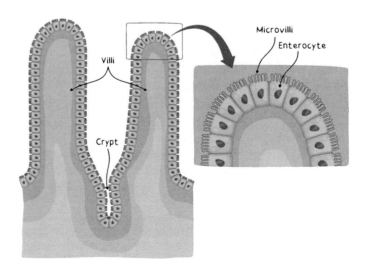

Figure 8A. Small intestine microstructure

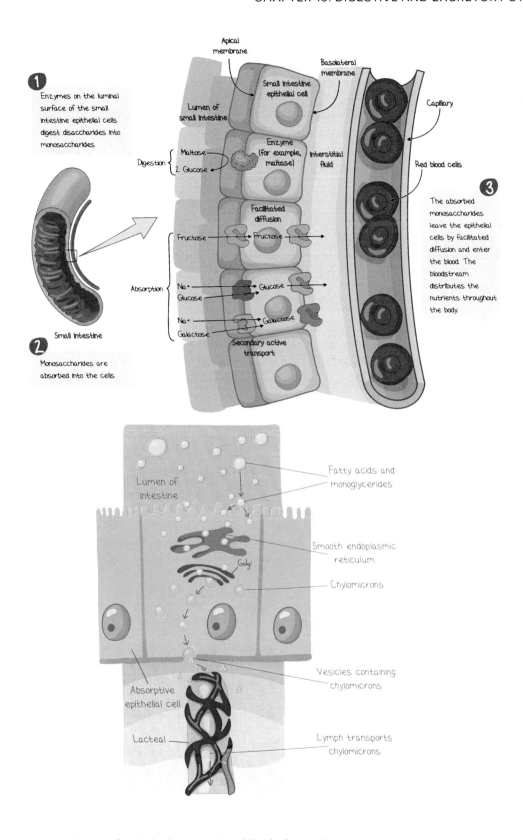

Figure 8B. Absorption pathways of carbohydrates (top) and lipids (bottom)

Lipids, however, are more complicated. Lipids form into **micelles** with the aid of bile salts, and individual lipid molecules break away from those micelles to be absorbed into the epithelial cells. No special transport mechanism is needed as fatty acids and cholesterol can diffuse through the plasma membrane. This creates an interesting challenge. If simple diffusion explains this process, how can the body prevent the concentrations from simply equalizing, at which point the absorption would stop? To prevent this from occurring, the epithelial cells in the small intestine combine fatty acids and monoglycerides to form triglycerides. This reduces the concentration of free fatty acids and monoglycerides so that they can continue to diffuse into the cells. Next, the cell needs to get rid of the lipids. Triglycerides and other lipids (as well as lipid-soluble vitamins) are combined into fat droplets known as **chylomicrons**, which are then released into the interstitial space, from where they move on to the lacteals. Lipids pass through the **lymphatic system** and eventually drain into the venous circulation of the body.

The capillaries of the small intestine eventually drain into the **hepatic portal vein**, which runs to the **liver** and the hepatic portal system. The hepatic portal system is one of several portal systems in the body. Another example is the hypophyseal portal system in the hypothalamus. Portal systems are systems of blood vessels with a capillary bed at each end. Because of the hepatic portal system, blood from the small intestine is processed by the liver before entering the systemic circulation. This gives the liver the chance to perform important metabolic tasks, including the following:

> Detoxifying compounds, either absorbed from the external environment or produced by metabolic processes.
> Metabolizing medications and drugs (this has important implications for routes of drug delivery, because this "first-pass" metabolism can dramatically reduce the efficacy of certain drugs when administered orally).
> Storing excess carbohydrates as glycogen or excess fatty acids as triglycerides.
> Mobilizing lipids into circulation in the form of lipoproteins and breaking down glycogen to release more glucose if necessary.

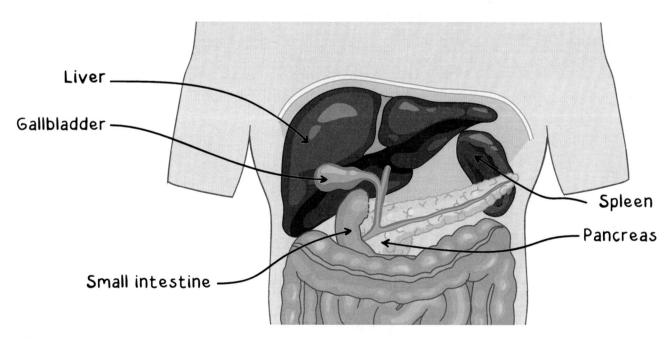

Figure 9. Liver

Finally, let's review the path taken by each major class of nutrient (proteins, carbohydrates, and lipids) as they go from your mouth to a state where they can be used by the cells of the body.

Proteins are broken down in the stomach by pepsin and continue to be broken down in the small intestine by peptidases, the most notable of which are trypsin and aminopeptidase. Trypsin cleaves proteins on the carboxyl end of lysine or arginine (except when followed by proline), and aminopeptidases are a class of enzymes that break down proteins from the amino end. Single amino acid residues then enter the epithelial cells of lining the lumen of the small intestine, from which they pass into the circulatory system.

Carbohydrates begin breaking down in the mouth, where the enzyme amylase breaks down starches into disaccharides, but they are primarily broken down in the small intestine by various enzymes. The enzymes active in the small intestine include pancreatic amylase, which breaks down starch and disaccharidases, such as sucrase, lactase, and maltase. The monosaccharides produced enter the epithelial cells of the small intestine and from there move into the circulatory system. Cellulose and undigested starch then move into the large intestine, where they may be broken down or digested by the gut flora. This results in short-chain fatty acids that are used by the body and may mediate some of the health effects associated with the gut microbiota, and gas, which is expelled as flatulence.

Triglycerides begin to be digested in the mouth by lingual lipase. An interesting fact about lingual lipase is that it functions at slightly acidic pH levels, so it continues to work to some extent as the bolus continues into the stomach. The majority of the digestion of triglycerides, though, occurs through pancreatic lipase. The resulting free fatty acids and monoglycerides are separated by bile salts into micelles that also contain cholesterol and other lipids. Lipids then enter the cells lining the small intestine, are packaged into chylomicrons, and released into lacteals, which drain into the lymphatic system.

3. Vitamins

Vitamins are non-macronutrient compounds that are vital for healthy functioning and most cannot be synthesized in adequate quantities by the body, meaning that they must be obtained from external sources. They are an interesting topic for the MCAT, because they have many different effects on a variety of physiological systems, so they often come up in various biology chapters—even in biochemistry, as the B vitamins function as coenzymes. However, it can be useful to review the functions of vitamins in one place, which is the goal of this section.

An important distinction is between lipid-soluble and water-soluble vitamins. Vitamins A, D, E, and K are **lipid-soluble**, while the other vitamins—vitamin C and the B vitamins (B_1, B_2, B_3, B_5, B_6, B_7, B_9, and B_{12})—are **water-soluble**. Water-soluble vitamins circulate in the blood and are easily excreted, whereas lipid-soluble vitamins accumulate in adipose tissue. This has ramifications vitamin use as dietary supplements: it is almost impossible to take too much of vitamin C or the B vitamins, because the body will simply excrete excess amounts of those substances in the urine (although some B vitamins are stored in the liver). That is to say so-called "megadosing" with vitamin C will just result in very expensive, vitamin-dense urine. Some cases have occurred in which individuals have experienced negative physical effects due to overdoses of water-soluble vitamins, but this is rare. In contrast, it is quite possible to take too much of lipid-soluble vitamins, resulting in conditions known as hypervitaminosis A, hypervitaminosis D, hypervitaminosis E, and hypervitaminosis K.

Table 1 below presents the basic functions of all the vitamins, followed by a further discussion of some vitamins of special note for the MCAT.

VITAMIN	CHEMICAL NAME	MAJOR FUNCTION
Lipid-soluble		
Vitamin A	Retinol, retinal (+ carotenoids)	Vision (low-light and color)
Vitamin D	Cholecalciferol (D_3), ergocalciferol (D_2)	Calcium and phosphate absorption from gut
Vitamin E	Tocopherols, tocotrienols	Antioxidant
Vitamin K	Phylloquinone, menaquinones	Coagulation
Water-soluble		
Vitamin C	Ascorbic acid	Cofactor for reactions in collagen synthesis, antioxidant
Vitamin B_1	Thiamine	Coenzyme in important metabolic reactions
Vitamin B_2	Riboflavin	Coenzyme involved in electron transport chain, precursor of FAD (which is involved in many key reactions)
Vitamin B_3	Niacin, niacinamide	Precursor of NAD and NADP, which are involved in many key reactions
Vitamin B_5	Pantothenic acid	Required for synthesis of CoA, as well in metabolism
Vitamin B_6	Pyridoxine, pyridoxamine, pyridoxal	Used as a coenzyme in many metabolic reactions
Vitamin B_7	Biotin	Cofactor for several carboxylase enzymes in metabolic reactions
Vitamin B_9	Folic acid	Ensures proper neurological development in pregnancy, required for fertility and red blood cell synthesis
Vitamin B_{12}	Cyanocobalamin + derivatives (ending in -balamin)	Coenzyme in metabolic reactions, especially DNA synthesis and lipid/amino acid metabolism

Table 1. Vitamins

A few background points are helpful for understanding vitamins. First, you might wonder why several of the vitamins, especially the lipid-soluble ones, correspond to multiple chemical names. You may also wonder about the naming conventions. In a sense, both of these points can be thought of as a historical legacy from the initial period of research into vitamins, which was conducted before modern techniques for characterizing molecular structures emerged.

Vitamins were discovered as a result of research into nutritional deficiencies. The most famous example is probably **vitamin C deficiency**, which used to be common among sailors who spent extended periods of time away from land without access to fresh food. In fact, scurvy - which is caused by a lack of vitamin C - has caused the deaths of millions of sailors over the centuries. A deficiency of vitamin C leads to symptoms of weakness, gum disease, and excess bleeding, and can eventually be fatal. There are a few takeaway points you should know about vitamins in general for the MCAT:

> Vitamins are compounds essential to our health. They generally cannot be synthesized in adequate quantities by the body and therefore must be obtained externally, generally from the diet, although vitamin D is synthesized in the skin in response to sunlight.
> Some vitamins actually reflect families of related compounds that are interconverted metabolically and/or contribute to the same overall effect.
> Vitamins and vitamin derivatives often serve as coenzymes/cofactors in essential reactions.
> The descriptions of vitamins given in Table 1 only scratches the surface of their range of functions, covering the most important points that are testable on the MCAT. In reality, vitamins play an astonishingly diverse and complex set of roles in the human body, and are still the subject of ongoing research.

For the most part, knowing the difference between fat-soluble and water-soluble vitamins and the short descriptions presented in Table 1 is enough for the purposes of the MCAT. There are a few vitamins, however, that require a bit more attention.

Vitamin A is essential for vision because it binds with opsin to form a protein known as rhodopsin, which is present in the rods of the retina and is used for low-light vision. The way that vitamin A contributes to the function of visual processing is interesting chemically in ways that overlap closely with some high-yield organic chemistry processes. Thus, it is worth having a detailed overview of how vitamin A functions.

CLINICAL CONNECTIONS >>>

A range of studies have shown correlations between vitamin D deficiencies and poor health outcomes. Does this mean that supplementation of vitamin D is a good preventive measure? Interestingly, research into this question remains controversial. It has been surprisingly difficult to document the benefits of vitamin D supplementation in a way that rules out the possibility of vitamin D deficiency and poor health outcomes both stemming from underlying disease processes, meaning that vitamin D supplementation would just be covering up the underlying problem. The utility of supplementation remains a controversial question that primary care physicians (for example) address frequently in their patients.

First, vitamin A occurs in a variety of forms characterized by different terminal functional groups. Although it's not exactly correct to say that any one form is the base form biochemically, it's useful to consider the alcohol form, retinol, to be the base form from which others are derived. In fact, retinol is the form in which we absorb vitamin A in the small intestine. However, retinol, like alcohols, is fairly reactive and is therefore not ideal for long-term storage. To counter this, a fatty acid can be used to create a retinyl ester. **Retinyl esters** are used for long-term storage and are the form in which we consume vitamin A in food (the conversion to retinol happens during digestion). You may see references to retinol as vitamin A's storage form and while this does occur, it is more often the case for shorter-term storage. Retinol itself is not biologically active. It can become biologically active in one of two ways: (1) being converted into retinal, which is used for vision; or (2) oxidation to retinoic acid, which is used in various pathways involving growth. The conversion between retinol and retinal is reversible under physiological conditions, whereas the oxidation of retinol to retinoic acid is an irreversible step. Thus, vitamin A provides an excellent real-life example of the oxidation and reduction of oxygen-containing organic compounds.

The mechanism through which retinal triggers visual input also overlaps with a high-yield organic chemistry concept: the stereochemistry of double bonds. The form of retinal that binds to opsin is 11-*cis*-retinal. Light causes 11-*cis*-retinal to isomerize to all-*trans*-retinal, which triggers the transduction of a signal along the optic nerve and the temporary dissociation of retinal from opsin.

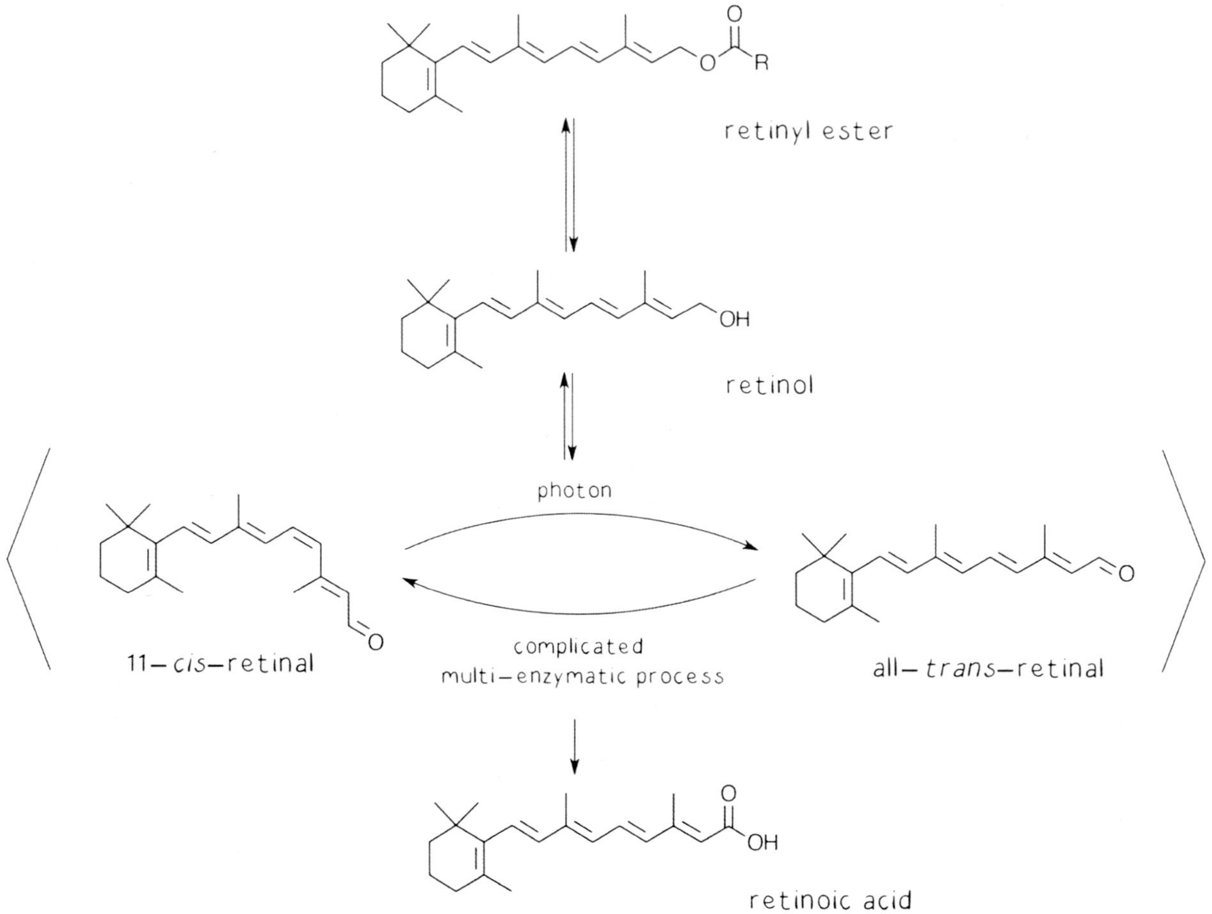

Figure 11. Forms of vitamin A

Vitamin D is also noteworthy because it has multiple forms and acts as a hormone, regulating calcium and phosphate concentrations in the bloodstream and promoting growth, as well as increasing the absorption of calcium, phosphate, and other minerals from the intestine. The major forms of vitamin D are: vitamin D_2 (ergocalciferol) and vitamin D_3 (cholecalciferol), which are metabolized by the liver to form 25-hydroxyvitamin D or 25(OH)D_2. This compound is then converted to calcitriol, which exerts the hormonal effects of vitamin D.

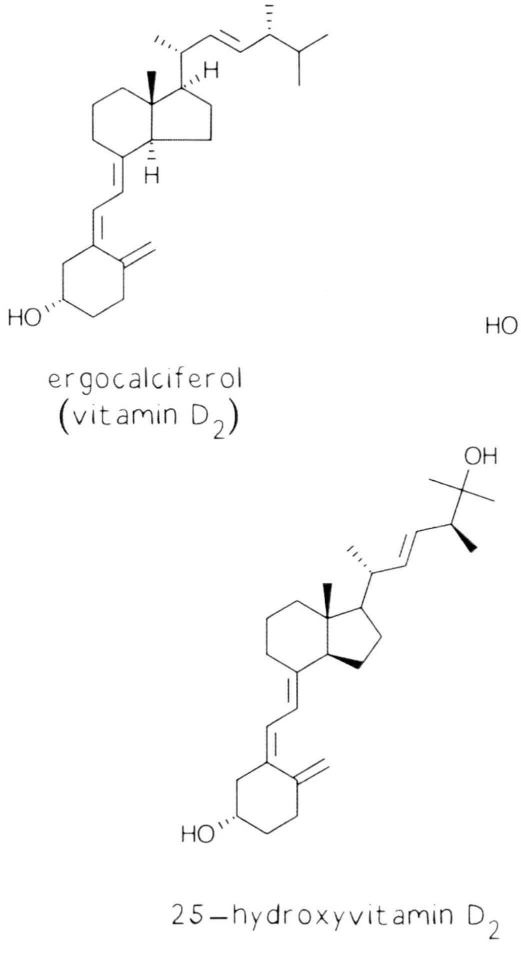

ergocalciferol
(vitamin D$_2$)

cholecalciferol
(vitamin D$_3$)

25-hydroxyvitamin D$_2$

Figure 12. Forms of vitamin D

For the other vitamins, a general knowledge of their function suffices for the MCAT, although there are some isolated points of information that may prove useful. The bacteria in the gut, for instance, play a major role in the synthesis of **vitamin K**. In particular, plants contain ample amounts of vitamin K$_1$, but bacteria in the gut transform it to vitamin K$_2$, which then goes on to be the source of various active derivatives in the body. This is another piece of evidence pointing towards the idea that bacteria play an integral role in human health. **Vitamin B$_{12}$** is similarly of note because it cannot be produced by plants, fungi, or animals. However, humans can obtain vitamin B$_{12}$ from animal sources in their diet. This may seem paradoxical, but some animals (such as cows) can absorb the vitamin B$_{12}$ produced by their gut flora and concentrate it in their tissues, making meat, liver, eggs, and milk sources of B$_{12}$ for humans. A consequence of this is that vegans must be very careful regarding vitamin B$_{12}$, which they can obtain from fortified foods or supplements.

4. Anatomy of the Excretory System

Next, let's turn to the excretory system. **Urination** may at first seem like a simple topic, but in reality it is tremendously important physiologically. Defecation played a relatively small role in our discussion of the digestive tract above, whereas multiple sections of this chapter are dedicated to urination. Why the discrepancy? Essentially, with a few exceptions, such as pancreatic secretions and bile salts, the contents of feces (primarily water, fiber, bacteria, and bile salts) are derived from substances external to our body. In fact, the entire gastrointestinal tract can be thought of as a series of tubes that pass material through our body while minimizing and tightly regulating the transfer of substances between the body and the lumen of the gastrointestinal tract, because it would be disastrous to simply absorb food directly.

In contrast, though, we also have to get rid of waste products generated in the body. This is the role of the excretory system. As such, the excretory system plays a crucial role in maintaining homeostasis in the body, as discussed in more depth in Section 6. First, though, let's review the basic anatomy of the excretory system.

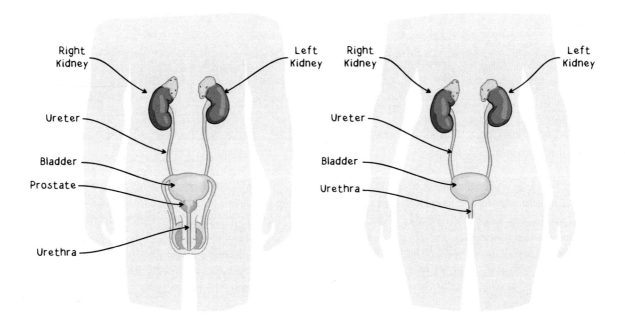

Figure 13. Diagram of excretory system

Blood is filtered to form urine in the **kidneys**, which are located towards the back of the abdominal cavity. Humans have two kidneys, one on each side. They are supplied with blood by the renal arteries, and then drain into the renal veins. The outside of the kidney is surrounded by the protective tissue of the **renal capsule**. The kidney itself is divided into the renal cortex (outer region) and the renal medulla (inner region).

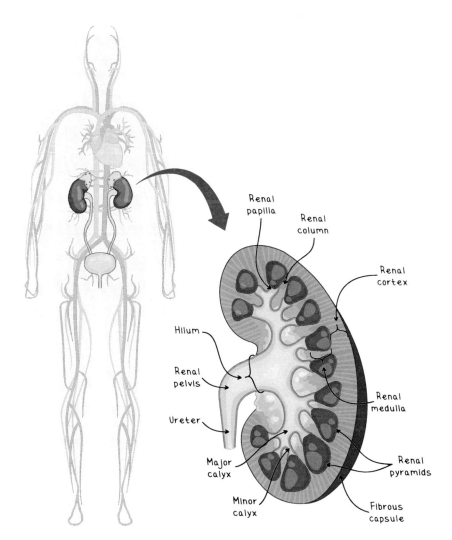

Figure 14. Kidney anatomy

Nephrons are the functional unit of the kidneys that produce urine. They are divided into two major parts. The **renal corpuscle** is the part of the nephron that carries out the initial filtration, and is located in the renal cortex. The **renal tubule** then projects downward into the medulla before returning up to the cortex, at which point urine drains into a **collecting duct**. Collecting ducts empty via structures known as the medullary pyramids into minor calyces (singular = calyx), which drain into major calyces, which drain in turn into the **renal pelvis**. The renal pelvis then becomes the **ureter**.

The ureters drain downwards from the kidneys into the **urinary bladder**, which rests on the pelvic floor. The bladder is a muscular and flexible structure that can generally hold approximately 400 mL of urine. Urine is then released from the bladder into the **urethra**, where it exits the body. The anatomy of the urethra differs between males and females. In females, the urethra exits the body anteriorly to the vagina, while in males the urethra exits the body through the penis, where it is used both for urination and ejaculation.

Release of urine through the urethra is controlled by the **urethral sphincter**, which has two components: the external urethral sphincter (which differs anatomically between males and females but has the same basic function) and the internal urethral sphincter. The internal urethral sphincter is composed of smooth muscle and is controlled by the autonomic nervous system, meaning that it is not subject to voluntary control. The external urethral sphincter, in contrast, is composed of skeletal muscle and is under voluntary control. Both sphincters must be open for urine to flow.

5. Physiology of the Excretory System

In this section, we'll take a closer look at how urine is produced in the nephron and how urination is regulated.

As mentioned above, the nephron can be divided into the **renal corpuscle** and the **renal tubule**. The renal corpuscle contains the **glomerulus** and **Bowman's capsule**. The glomerulus is a bunched-up set of capillaries through which water, ions, and small molecules filter out and are gathered into Bowman's capsule, which wraps around the glomerulus. Blood is supplied to the glomerulus through an afferent arteriole and exits through an efferent arteriole. The fluid collected in Bowman's capsule is known as the **glomerular filtrate**.

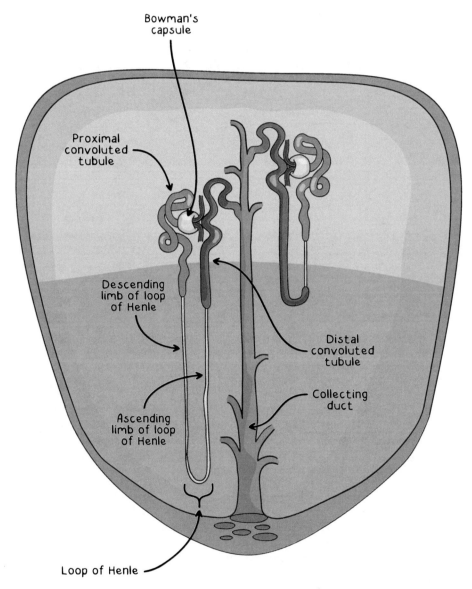

Figure 15. Nephron

The renal tubule is composed of three main parts: the **proximal convoluted tubule**, the **loop of Henle**, and the **distal convoluted tubule**. The body must solve one basic problem in the renal tubule: adjusting the volume and concentration of urine appropriately. A tremendous amount of blood is filtered by the kidneys on a daily basis—in fact, the entire blood volume of the body is filtered many times per day! It would be tremendously wasteful to eliminate even a small fraction of that fluid. Therefore, the body has to figure out how to keep enough water to maintain health while getting rid of the wastes that need to be removed. The activity and structure of the renal tubule are relatively complex because this is a critically important task that must be regulated carefully.

In the **proximal convoluted tubule (PCT)**, two-way exchange happens. From the perspective of sheer volume, absorption predominates in the PCT. In particular, large amounts of sodium ions are reabsorbed, as well as other salts, water-soluble vitamins, free amino acids, glucose and water. However, secretion of waste products into the urine also happens in the PCT. In particular, hydrogen ions, nitrogen-containing compounds such as creatinine and ammonia, and some medications are secreted into the urine via the PCT. This may seem surprising at first, because you might wonder where these waste products are coming from. In fact, a rich vascular plexus supplies the renal cortex, so the wastes in question come from the blood but are mediated via the cells of the PCT.

The **loop of Henle** is the next step in the nephron. It is a U-shaped tube that consists of a descending limb and an ascending limb. The basic goal of the loop of Henle is to create an osmotic gradient in the medulla and to reduce the amount of water and salts in the filtrate. The need for tight regulation is why the structure itself is quite complex. An important point to have in the back of your mind while studying the loop of Henle is that the deeper you go into the medulla, the greater the concentration of solutes is, which facilitates the processes of osmosis throughout the loop of Henle.

MCAT STRATEGY >>>

The loop of Henle is one of the most common points of confusion in terms of MCAT physiology. The secret to understanding it is first to focus on its overall function (reabsorption of water and salt and the creation of an osmotic gradient in the medulla) and then break that down into two subtasks: first, water is reabsorbed in the descending limb, and salt is transported out of the ascending limb. This topic contains a general lesson about studying physiology topics for the MCAT: always focus on the function *first*, and learn the anatomy in the context of that function.

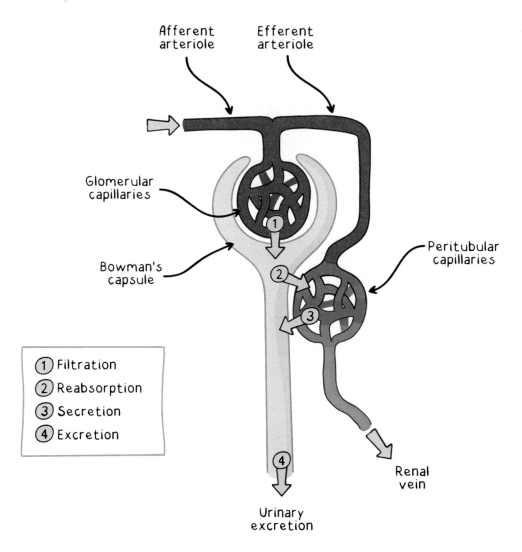

Afferent
arteriole

Efferent
arteriole

Glomerular
capillaries

Peritubular
capillaries

Bowman's
capsule

1 Filtration
2 Reabsorption
3 Secretion
4 Excretion

Renal
vein

Urinary
excretion

Excretion = Filtration − Reabsorption + Secretion

Figure 16. Diagram of excretion through the kidney

The **descending limb** of the loop of Henle is permeable to water but not to ions. This means that, as the descending limb plunges deeper into the increasingly hypertonic medulla, more and more water flows out of the loop of Henle and into the medulla, where it is eventually absorbed by the vasculature in the region (vessels known as the vasa recta) and brought back into circulation. Thus, the filtrate at the bottom of the loop of Henle is quite concentrated. The **ascending limb** of the loop of Henle, in contrast, is impermeable to water. Ions are transported out of the ascending limb, resulting in a much lower osmolarity by the time the filtrate completes its path through the loop. The top part of the ascending limb is known as the thick ascending limb, and this area also allows the active transport of sodium, potassium, and chloride ions. The end product of this is filtrate that is less concentrated in terms of osmolarity than the initial filtrate, and has a significantly decreased volume.

The mechanism through which the loop of Henle operates is known as a **countercurrent multiplier**. This seemingly abstract term describes how the concentration gradients leading to solute and water flow are established and maintained. If the blood vessels responsible for draining the solutes back into the systemic circulation went in the same direction as the flow through the loop of Henle, the concentration gradients would just equalize and transport would grind to a halt. To visualize this better, keep in mind that the blood supply near the loop of Henle is provided by vessels known as the vasa recta (or "straight vessels"), which run parallel to the loop.

The nephron has two more areas where water balance can be adjusted: the **distal convoluted tubule (DCT)** and the **collecting duct**. Aldosterone can act on both sites to promote sodium reabsorption, which in turn promotes water reabsorption (in the presence of ADH) mediated by the osmotic effects of this process. The DCT can also increase calcium reabsorption in response to parathyroid hormone, and can contribute to pH regulation by secreting or absorbing hydrogen ions as needed. The collecting duct, in turn can be affected by antidiuretic hormone (ADH, or vasopressin), which increases water reabsorption directly. Atrial natriuretic peptide (ANP) has the opposite effect of aldosterone in that it promotes excretion of sodium in the urine, which draws water with it, increasing the amount of water expelled in the urine and decreasing blood pressure. Once the urine drains into the renal pelvis, its composition and concentration are established.

6. Homeostasis and the Excretory System

The details of the excretory system can be overwhelming, but the MCAT often expects you to apply your detailed knowledge to evaluate hypotheticals or in the context of new information. To do so, you must understand the principles of how the excretory system regulates homeostasis. In this section, we'll review the four major domains of homeostasis regulation through the excretory system: blood pressure, osmoregulation, acid-base balance, and the removal of soluble nitrogenous waste.

Blood pressure can be influenced by many parameters, such as the elasticity of the blood vessels, and the peripheral resistance. However, this list omits a physiologically fundamental contributor to blood pressure: total fluid volume, which is regulated by the excretory system, which can either eliminate more water in urine or make the urine more concentrated in order to preserve water. As briefly reviewed in the previous section, there are three main hormones that affect fluid balance:

> **Aldosterone** promotes water retention by increasing sodium absorption:
  $\uparrow$ aldosterone = $\uparrow$ Na$^+$ reabsorption = $\uparrow$ H$_2$O reabsorption (in the presence of ADH) = $\uparrow$ plasma volume of blood = $\uparrow$ blood pressure
> **Antidiuretic hormone (ADH; vasopressin)** promotes water retention directly by increasing water reabsorption in the collecting duct: $\uparrow$ ADH = $\uparrow$ H$_2$O retention = $\uparrow$ plasma volume of blood = $\uparrow$ blood pressure. Because it only promotes water retention, ADH acts to reduce the osmolarity of the blood.
> **Atrial natriuretic peptide (ANP)** is the opposite of aldosterone, as it promotes sodium excretion in the urine: $\uparrow$ ANP = $\downarrow$ Na$^+$ reabsorption = $\downarrow$ H$_2$O reabsorption = $\downarrow$ plasma volume of blood = $\downarrow$ blood pressure.

Aldosterone release is regulated by the kidneys via the **renin-angiotensin-aldosterone axis**. Juxtaglomerular cells in the afferent arterioles of the kidneys release a substance known as renin in response to reduced blood pressure (detected by intrarenal baroceptors), reduced sodium levels, or signaling from the sympathetic nervous system (which raises blood pressure as part of the "fight or flight" response). Renin causes angiotensinogen to be cleaved to form angiotensin I, which is then converted to angiotensin II by an enzyme known as angiotensin-converting enzyme (ACE). Angiotensin II increases blood pressure through vasoconstriction and also triggers the release of aldosterone.

>>**CONNECTIONS**<<

Chapter 7 of Biology

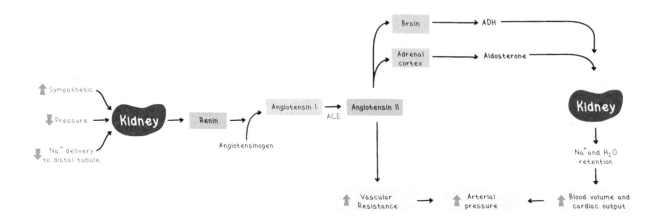

Figure 17. Renin-angiotensin-aldosterone axis

As suggested by the fact that the mechanisms of aldosterone and ANP involve modulating sodium reabsorption, the excretory system is also involved in regulating solutes. The overall **osmolarity** of the blood (as distinct from the specific concentrations of individual solutes) is important to maintain fluid balance within the body. As discussed in Chapter 9 on the respiratory and circulatory systems, an interplay between **hydrostatic pressure** and **oncotic pressure** (the osmotic pressure due to proteins in blood) drives fluid exchange between capillaries and the interstitial space. Blood osmolarity must be maintained within a very tight range, and this is largely accomplished by fluctuations in the relative quantities of water and solute reabsorption or excretion.

The excretory system also regulates **blood pH**, which must be kept within a range of between 7.35 and 7.45. Many factors can impact blood pH, such as active anaerobic metabolism that generates H^+ as a byproduct, or levels of CO_2, which increases the acidity of blood by participating in the bicarbonate buffer equilibrium. However, one easy way to decrease the acidity of blood is to excrete more H^+ in the urine, and one way to increase the acidity of blood is to inhibit the excretion of H^+. As discussed in Chapter 9, the respiratory system also modulates pH. It is useful to think of the respiratory system providing the short-term response to pH changes because the respiratory rate can either increase or decrease very quickly. In contrast, the excretory system helps regulate pH on a medium-term to longer-term scale.

Soluble nitrogenous waste is also removed by the excretory system. In particular, this applies to **urea**. Urea ($CO(NH_2)_2$) can be thought of as a carbonyl-containing carrier of excess amine groups that need to be excreted. Ammonia (NH_3) is a byproduct of the metabolism of nitrogen-containing compounds such as amino acids, but excessive levels become toxic to the body. Therefore, the liver converts ammonia to urea, which is secreted into the nephron for excretion.

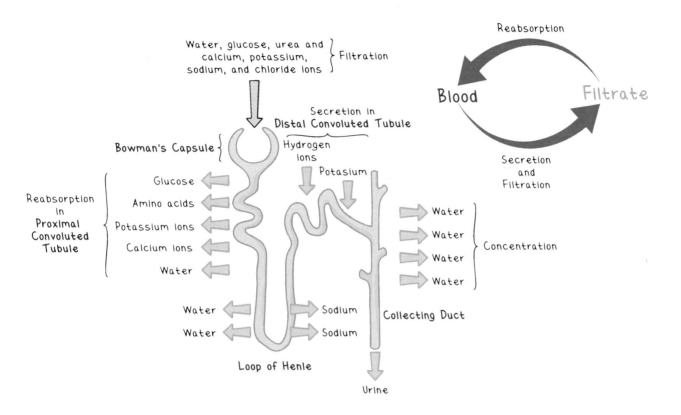

Figure 18. Steps in the formation of urine

7. Must-Knows

> Basic path of food through the digestive system: oral cavity → esophagus → stomach → small intestine (duodenum, jejunum, ileum) → large intestine (cecum, ascending colon, transverse colon, descending colon, sigmoid colon) → rectum.
> Stomach has very low pH due to gastric acid. pH becomes slightly alkaline in small intestine.
> Bile: generated in liver, stored in gallbladder, released to small intestine to emulsify fats.
> Pancreas: secretes digestive enzymes and bicarbonate and releases them to small intestine.
> Small intestine: main site for digestion and absorption of nutrients.
  – Villi multiply surface area of small intestinal lining; microvilli on surface of cell increase surface area available for absorption.
> Large intestine: re-absorption of H_2O, large microbial community, absorption of microbe-generated substances (vitamin K, short-chain fatty acids).
> Carbohydrates: salivary amylase in mouth → digestive enzymes (pancreatic amylase + disaccharidases) in small intestine → monosaccharides absorbed into small intestine cells → hepatic portal vein for liver processing → bloodstream.
> Proteins: pepsin in stomach → various peptidases in small intestines; isolated amino acids primarily absorbed in small intestine, as well as some dipeptides → absorbed into small intestine cells → hepatic portal vein for liver processing → bloodstream.
> Fats: lingual lipase starts digesting triglycerides → pancreatic lipase continues → bile salts in small intestine emulsify → absorbed into small intestinal cells → lacteals in villi → drain into lymphatic system as chylomicrons → bloodstream.
> Vitamins: A, D, E, K = fat-soluble; B vitamins and C = water-soluble.
> Vitamins have range of functions. Notably A helps in function of vision, D in calcium/phosphate metabolism, K in clotting, C in collagen synthesis, and B vitamins are many important coenzymes/factors.
> Basic urination path:
  – Nephron: glomerulus (blood vessels) → capsular space of Bowman's capsule → proximal convoluted tubule → loop of Henle (descending & ascending), distal convoluted tubule → collecting duct.
  – Collecting duct → minor calyx → major calyx → renal pelvis → ureters → urinary bladder → urethra.
> Nephron has two major functions: (1) filtering various substances in blood; (2) appropriately regulating fluid/salt content of urine.
> Loop of Henle has countercurrent multiplier mechanism to greatly reduce liquid volume in urine by first making urine concentrated (descending limb) and then removing solutes (ascending limb).
> Aldosterone: ↑ Na^+ reabsorption = ↑ H_2O reabsorption (in the presence of ADH) = ↑ plasma volume of blood = ↑ blood pressure; ADH: ↑ H_2O retention = ↑ plasma volume of blood = ↑ blood pressure; ANP: ↓ Na^+ reabsorption = ↓ H_2O reabsorption = ↓ plasma volume of blood = ↓ blood pressure.
> Excretory system: regulates blood pressure, pH, excretion of nitrogenous wastes.

End of Chapter Practice

The best MCAT practice is **realistic**, with a focus on identifying steps for further improvement. For those reasons, we recommend completing practice questions in an online setting that simulates the real MCAT interface, and taking advantage of advanced analytic features to help you determine how best to move forward in your MCAT study journey.

With that in mind, **online end-of-chapter** questions for Biology, Biochemistry, Chemistry + Organic Chemistry, Physics, and Psychology/Sociology are available through your Blueprint MCAT account.

As a further supplement, given the importance of active learning for effective studying, we also suggest that you consult the Must-Knows at the end of each chapter as a basis for creating a study sheet, in which you list out key terms and test your ability to briefly summarize them.

This page left intentionally blank.

Immune System

0. Introduction

The immune system refers to the complex set of mechanisms that the body uses to protect itself against foreign invaders and malfunctioning cells originating from the body. The immune system is incredibly complex. The MCAT only expects you to have a relatively basic knowledge of the fundamental components and principles of the immune system, but this is a non-trivial task. For the MCAT, you should break your approach to the immune system into two parts: first, become familiar with the components of the immune system, how they are classified, and how they relate to each other. Second, develop a thorough understanding of the key principles of immunology, such as antigen-antibody interactions and how the body distinguishes between self and non-self.

Special care must be taken when studying the immune system because of the abundance of classifications applied to its components. Especially as such classifications sometimes have been outpaced by modern research. For example, the distinction between "humoral" and "cell-mediated" immune responses (discussed in more detail below in Section 3) dates from the early stages of modern research into immunology, and the term "humoral" itself derives from the ancient Greek system of medical thought. In reality, these two aspects of the immune response interact with each other, and can only fully be understood in relation to one another. Therefore, you have a twofold task as you study the immune system: first, to know the definitions, and second, to understand how the actual immune response is coordinated on a physiological level.

The highest-level distinction in the immune system is between the innate (or non-specific) immune system, (which responds generally to threats but does not learn to recognize specific foreign bodies/molecules) and the adaptive immune system, (which responds to specific foreign pathogens and molecules). In this chapter, we will cover fundamental concepts in immunology, explore the differences between the innate and adaptive immune systems, and then discuss the anatomy of the immune system, the lymphatic system, and allergies and autoimmune disorders.

1. Concepts in Immunology

In order to make sense of the immune system, it's key to have a solid understanding of the basic principles that govern its function. It may be worth reading this chapter twice, as understanding the principles will help you make sense of the tremendous diversity of cells and pathways discussed later in this chapter.

The most basic principle of the immune system is the interaction between **antigens** and **antibodies**. This is also one of the most common sources of confusion among students preparing for the MCAT, so let's review the details carefully. One way of thinking about antigens and antibodies is to visualize it as a system through which information is communicated. The body has ample resources it can mobilize to destroy cells/viruses/debris, but it will do so *if and only if necessary*. Failure in either direction can have major negative consequences: if the body fails to recognize and respond to a real threat, it could potentially die, but if the body responds inappropriately to objects that aren't actual threats (like body cells), serious illness can result. Such illnesses are known as autoimmune disorders and are discussed in Section 6.

Antibodies have to be able to do two things: recognize substances/cells that need to be eliminated, and be recognized by other components of the immune system. The term "antigen" is used to refer to what antibodies recognize. There is no specific structural property that defines an antigen, although they often are macromolecules (especially proteins) expressed on a cell surface or a viral envelope/capsule. However, external substances like pollen can also serve as antigens, causing pollen allergies.

The structure of an antibody provides a bridge between these two functions. As shown in Figure 1, antibodies have a Y-shaped structure consisting of **two heavy chains** and **two light chains** that are linked by **disulfide bonds**. Five classes of antibodies exist, which are classified according to the details of their heavy chains: immunoglobulin (Ig) A, IgD, IgE, IgG, and IgM. The details of these classes go beyond the scope of the MCAT. The "top" ends of the Y-shaped structure have a **variable antigen-recognizing area**, and another region is recognized by other immune system cells. The specific site on an antigen that an antibody recognizes is the **epitope**. Extensive random recombination of the antigen-recognizing area of the antibody (also known as the paratope) allows the generation of antibodies that recognize potentially infinitely many different antigens. How the adaptive immune system uses antibodies are detailed in Section 3 below.

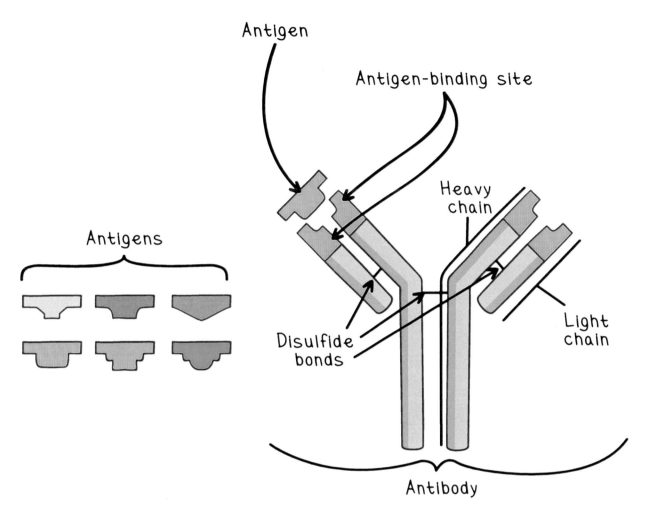

Figure 1. Antibody-antigen interactions

A fundamental issue for the immune system is how to distinguish between self and non-self/damaged-self materials and cells. This is often framed just in terms of self versus non-self, but it is also important for the immune system to be able to recognize cells that have been damaged by viral infections or have malfunctioned in ways likely to turn them into cancer cells. This is primarily the role of T cells. T cells either directly attack compromised/foreign cells or mobilize an immune response based on antigen fragments that are presented by **major histocompatibility complex (MHC) class I and II**.

MHC class I is a protein expressed on the plasma membrane of all nucleated cells that is unique in each individual. It receives protein fragments from inside the cell and then presents them extracelluarly, on the outside of the cell, as antigens that T cells can respond to. If a cell is healthy, T cells will not respond to MHC I-antigen complexes, as the "antigens" are just normal pieces of cellular machinery, and T cells that would inappropriately respond to such stimuli were eliminated during their maturation process. However, cells infected by viruses can present viral antigens on MHC class I, and incipient tumor cells are likely to fail to present appropriate proteins.

MCAT STRATEGY >>>

The best way of thinking of MHC class I is as a spot-check, in which the cell presents a sample of its products to T cells, which play the role of quality control checkers.

MHC class II, on the other hand, is expressed in a smaller range of cell types. Specifically, MHC class II is expressed primarily on macrophages, macrophage-like cells such as dendritic cells, and B cells. Whereas MHC class I serves as an *internal* checkpoint that relays information about the internal health of the body's own cells, MHC class II serves as a source of *external* information. For instance, when macrophages consume a microbe (or any foreign object), some of its fragments will be displayed as a complex formed with MHC class II on the cell membrane. This complex is recognized by helper T cells, initiating a larger immune response.

The process by which cells present antigens on their membranes is known as **antigen presentation**. All nucleated cells can be considered antigen-presenting cells as they express MHC class I, whereas the more specialized cells that express MHC class II are considered professional antigen-presenting cells. Antigen presentation is also a major mechanism in the maturation and activation of B and T cells. This is discussed in more detail below.

>> CONNECTIONS <<

Chapter 5 of Biology

Immunological principles are also commonly used in laboratory techniques. In western blotting and enzyme-linked immunosorbent assays (ELISA), a technique known as **immunohistochemistry** or **immunostaining** is used to visualize specific proteins. Here, the protein of interest serves as an antigen that is visualized after it reacts with an antibody that has been modified so that it can be visualized using fluorescence or staining with an appropriate dye.

2. Innate Immune System

As mentioned above, the **innate** (or **non-specific**) **immune system** is the immune component that coordinates a broad-spectrum defense, but does not involve the recognition of specific foreign bodies and molecules. The innate immune system is split into non-cellular and cellular components. The **non-cellular component** includes anatomical barriers and signaling molecules such as cytokines and complement proteins, while the **cellular component** includes a range of white blood cell types (leukocytes) that play various roles in threat response. The various components of the innate immune system can act independently or be coordinated in the inflammatory process.

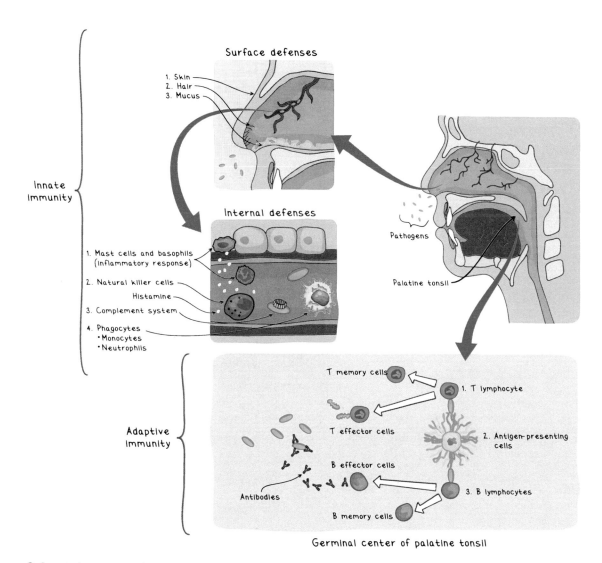

Figure 2. Innate immune system

The most obvious anatomical barrier to external pathogens is the **skin**. The tightly packed cells of the epidermis provide a formidable physical barrier to the entry of pathogens, and mechanisms such as sweat and the shedding/replacement of skin cells also contribute to the ability of the skin to function as a barrier. Additionally, cellular components of the adaptive immune system are "stationed" in and around the skin, allowing a prompt response to any incursions. The gastrointestinal tracts and the respiratory system are other pathways through which external materials enter the body, and therefore it is not surprising that they also provide anatomical barriers against infection.

The protection that the **gastrointestinal tract** provides against infections starts with the **oral cavity**, in which the lysozyme contained in saliva helps to break down bacterial cell walls. Interestingly, lysozyme is also present in other fluids, such as mucus, breast milk, and tears. The extremely low pH of the stomach also constitutes a physical barrier against pathogens, as many microorganisms cannot survive in such acidic conditions. The gastrointestinal tract also contains some less obvious physical features that contribute to immunity. First, **peristalsis** provides a physical way of moving microbes through the digestive tract, so that bacteria/viruses that do not immediately find a way to adhere to the gastrointestinal lining or invade body cells will be rapidly flushed out. Second, the abundant bacterial flora of the large intestine can be thought of as an anatomical barrier, as the **gut flora** are well-balanced and play a role in maintaining intestinal health by preventing pathogenic bacteria from colonizing the intestine by potentially outcompeting them.

The role of microflora in creating a barrier in the innate immune system can be extended to other areas of the body with sizable microbial populations, such as the skin, oral cavity, and female reproductive tract. For instance, recent research has indicated that maintenance of a healthy vaginal microbiome, with abundant lactobacilli, can help prevent bacterial vaginosis and yeast infections.

The **respiratory system** also contains mechanisms for protecting the body from invasion. The mucus secreted throughout the upper respiratory tract contains lysozyme, which has antibacterial properties. Mucus also traps microbes in a viscous fluid that can either be expelled from the body or swallowed into the highly-acidic stomach. The mucociliary escalator in the bronchi and trachea combines mucus with the ability of cilia to push trapped microbes up the pharynx.

Next, let's turn to the cellular component of the innate immune system, which include most of the **white blood cells** (**WBCs**, or **leukocytes**). The white blood cells have a diverse range of functions. In this section, we will review the various types of WBCs, starting from the most common types to the least common types, and then briefly discuss their classification. However, despite their diversity, WBCs have some common features: they all have nuclei (unlike red blood cells) and they are all produced in the bone marrow.

Neutrophils are the most common type of WBC, making up over 60% of WBCs in circulation. Their main role is to phagocytose invading bacteria, and can be thought of as the first responders to infection. As a result of this, an elevated neutrophil level in a complete blood count may be a sign of an acute inflammatory response or an acute infection.

The next most common type of WBC, comprising about 30% of circulating WBCs, are **lymphocytes**. This is a tricky category as lymphocytes span the innate and adaptive components of the immune system. The major categories of lymphocytes are **B cells**, **T cells**, and **natural killer (NK) cells**. B cells and T cells are involved in the adaptive immune system and are therefore discussed in Section 3. NK cells, on the other hand, are considered to be part of the innate immune system. Their role is to respond to cells infected by viruses and tumor cells. NK cells can recognize such cells by alterations in how affected cells present themselves as "self" (see Section 1 for a review). Additionally, NK cells can be thought of as straddling the innate and adaptive immune systems because they respond to cells that have been "tagged" by antibodies and destroy them.

Next come **monocytes**, which make up about 5% of circulating WBCs. The main role of monocytes is to travel to various tissues in the body and then differentiate further into **macrophages** or **dendritic cells**. Dendritic cells tend to be found in parts of the body in contact with the external environment, and bridge the innate and adaptive immune systems by interacting with external substances to present antigens to T cells. Macrophages (Greek for "big eaters"), in contrast, are large cells that can be thought of as the non-specific garbage processors of the body, as they phagocytose cellular debris, tumor cells, non-cellular foreign substances, microbes, and so on. **Eosinophils** make up approximately 3% of circulating WBCs, and primarily target parasitic infections. **Basophils** make up under 1% of the circulating WBCs and are involved in allergic responses, particularly the release of histamine and heparin (an anticoagulant) as part of inflammatory responses. **Mast cells** function similarly to basophils, but tend to be located specifically in mucous membranes and connective tissue.

The term "**phagocyte**" refers to any cell that engages in phagocytosis. The engulfment and destruction of one cell by another. Phagocytes include neutrophils, monocytes, macrophages, dendritic cells, and mast cells. The MCAT expects you to know the difference between macrophages and phagocytes. Don't be fooled by the fact that they both have "phag-" in their name! Macrophages are a specific subset of phagocytes.

However, the innate immune system is not limited to cells. A system known as **complement** is also a major component of the innate immune response. Complement refers to a signaling cascade of 30 proteins (if receptors and regulatory proteins are counted) that tag pathogens for destruction. This process is known as **opsonization**, and is used to recruit phagocytes to destroy the pathogens in question, and/or to initiate an inflammatory process. There are actually three main pathways of complement activation, but the details go beyond the scope of the MCAT. Antibodies play a role in determining which cells are "tagged" by complement proteins, but the complement system is still considered to be part of the innate immune system because its components do not change over time.

The details of the **complement system** can be challenging to study because its constituent proteins were named C1, C2, …, C9 in order of their discovery. While this naming system may have been reasonable at the time, an unfortunate consequence is that there is no logical connection between the name of a complement protein and its function, and very little traction for mnemonics to help. The good news, though, is that the MCAT does not expect you to be aware of the specific steps of the complement system (that's what medical school is for!). Just be aware of its existence and general function.

In addition to the complement system, **cytokines** are a broad and diverse class of signaling proteins (at least dozens) that are involved in coordinating the immune response and inflammation. Many cytokines have been found to exert multiple functions: for example, the interleukin 1 (IL-1) family is involved in body temperature control, innate immunity, and inflammation, just to name a few examples. The details certainly go beyond the MCAT, but you should be aware that cytokines exist and what their general function is.

Interferons are a subset of cytokines that are best known for having antiviral effects. They are released by infected cells when receptors located in the cytoplasm or the plasma membrane recognize certain microbial biomolecules (such as viral glycoproteins). Once released, they have two major effects: they signal nearby cells to prepare themselves to defend against a viral infection and they upregulate the overall immune response.

Inflammation is a response to cellular injury or pathogens that results in the clinically noticeable signs/symptoms of redness, heat, pain, swelling and loss of function. On a mechanistic level, acute inflammation involves cells belonging to the innate immune system, including neutrophils, monocytes, macrophages, dendritic cells, and mast cells. The inflammatory signal cascade ultimately results in vasodilation in the affected area and increased permeability of blood vessels. **Vasodilation** results in increased blood flow, and increased permeability results in plasma being able to migrate from the blood into the

CLINICAL CONNECTIONS >>>

A phenomenon known as the "cytokine storm" may be responsible for abnormal deaths among young healthy adults who were victims of the 1918 influenza pandemic and the SARS epidemic in 2003. In a cytokine storm, a pathological positive feedback emerges between white blood cells and the cytokine system, resulting in a hyperintense immune reaction that can cause organ failure and death. It is also thought that cytokine storms are part of what makes the Ebola virus so deadly.

CLINICAL CONNECTIONS >>>

Until recently, interferon was commonly used, along with an antiviral drug, as part of the treatment of hepatitis C, a chronic liver infection estimated to affect 3.5 million people in the United States. One of the disadvantages of interferon treatment is that it causes side effects like flu-like symptoms, fever, and vomiting, which are ultimately due to the upregulated immune response.

affected tissue. Combined, these two factors result in redness and swelling, but also have the physiologically useful result of allowing a large number of immune cells to move in quickly to address the situation. Similarly to the complement system, the details of the inflammatory signaling cascade are quite complex and go beyond the scope of the MCAT. However, you should also be aware that chronic inflammation—that is, inflammation that persists for a long time—has been increasingly associated with the pathogenesis of a range of major health conditions, including cardiovascular and cerebrovascular disease.

3. Adaptive Immune System

The **adaptive immune system**, in contrast to the innate immune system, is the part of the immune system that "learns" to recognize specific invaders/pathogens. There are two main classes of cells at work in the adaptive immune response: B cells and T cells. Both B cells and T cells are lymphocytes that are produced in the bone marrow and mature in the lymphatic system.

When you hear **B cells**, think **antibodies**, as the role of B cells is to learn to recognize antigens and to differentiate into plasma cells which secrete large amounts of antibodies in response (B cells can also present antigens and secrete cytokines, but the MCAT is unlikely to test you on these points). After being produced in the bone marrow, B cells move to lymphatic tissue, such as the lymph nodes and the spleen. At this point, before they have "seen" an antigen, they are known as "**naïve B cells**." Through random recombination, naïve B cells express receptors for many different antigens, and some may never actually encounter a matching antigen at all. However, once a B cell is presented with a matching antigen, generally by antigen-presenting cells such as dendritic cells, it proliferates in a process known as clonal expansion. Activated B cells have one of two fates: either they become plasma cells, which are short-lived cells that secrete massive amounts of antibodies in an infection, or they become memory cells, which persist for the entire life of the host. Memory cells "remember" the antigen they were activated by, allowing the body to mount a significantly quicker and stronger response the next time it encounters the antigen in question.

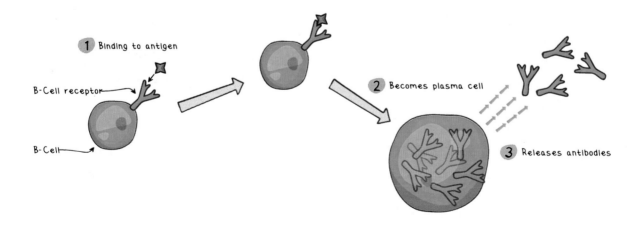

Figure 3. B cells

B cells are involved in **humoral immunity**, which specifically refers to the immune effects of antibodies, whereas T cells, as we'll discuss below, are involved in cell-mediated immunity. You may object that this distinction doesn't make sense because the elements of humoral immunity (antibodies) are secreted by cells and are therefore cell-mediated in a sense. This objection is logical, but many divisions of the immune system reflect scientific progress as it happened. In particular, the division between the humoral and the cell-based systems of immunity arose from the observation that some properties of the immune response can be retained and transferred in the absence of cells. These properties were dubbed "humoral immunity," based on a reference to the ancient Greek medical system of the humors.

T cells correspond to the **cell-mediated branch** of the adaptive immune system. The basic role of T cells is to respond to the major histocompatibility complex (MHC) classes I and II. MHC class I is present in all nucleated cells, and presents proteins from inside the cell as antigens. **Cytotoxic CD8⁺ T cells** recognize and destroy cells that present abnormal **MHC class I proteins**, which are indicative of a viral infection or transformation into a tumor. Unlike macrophages, which engulf target cells, CD8⁺ T cells inject their target cells with substances that induce apoptosis. **MHC class II** is expressed in a smaller range of cells in the immune system, and is used to present antigen fragments from external sources. **CD4⁺ helper T cells** respond to these cells by secreting specialized cytokines that recruit other immune cells to mount a reaction.

MCAT STRATEGY >>>

You can remember which T cells interact with which MHC class proteins by remembering that the numbers involved must multiply to 8. Therefore, CD8⁺ T cells interact with MHC class I ($8 \times 1 = 8$) and CD4⁺ T cells interact with MHC class II ($4 \times 2 = 8$).

CLINICAL CONNECTIONS >>>

Human immunodeficiency virus (HIV) is a retrovirus that attacks CD4⁺ T cells. When the population of CD4⁺ T cells declines beyond a certain point, the body becomes very vulnerable to infections that would otherwise be unlikely to harm a healthy individual. This condition is known as acquired immunodeficiency syndrome (AIDS). HIV is fatal without treatment. It emerged in the late 1970s and 1980s. Its effects in the United States peaked around 1995, when nearly 42,000 Americans died from AIDS. Subsequently, highly effective combination treatments were introduced, allowing individuals with HIV to potentially live full lifetimes. However, AIDS remains a major public health issue worldwide.

In addition to these two main classes of T cells, memory T cells "remember" antigens they have been exposed to, similar to memory B cells, and regulatory (suppressor) T cells function to reduce the immune response once an infection has been adequately dealt with and to help prevent self-reactivity, which can cause autoimmune diseases (see Section 6).

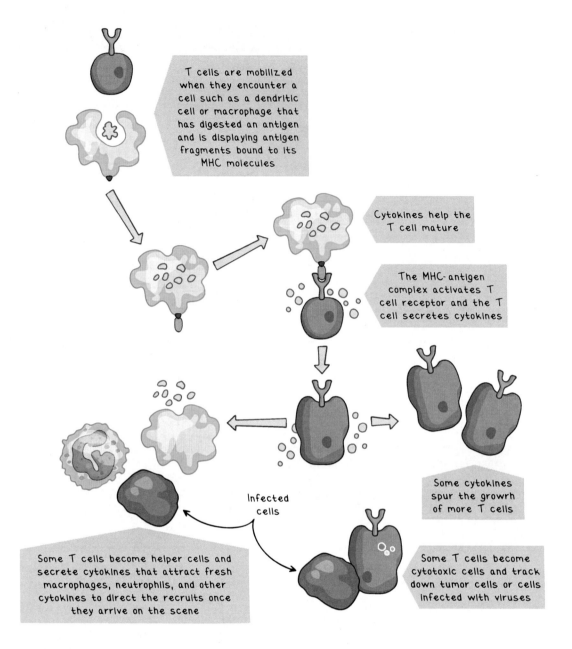

Figure 4. T cells

Although **T cells** are produced in the bone marrow, they mature in the thymus, and the vast majority of immature T cells are discarded. T cells that fail to respond appropriately to MHC class I and II proteins are eliminated in a process known as **positive selection**, while T cells that are over-reactive (in particular, reactive against self cells) are eliminated in a process known as **negative selection**. The combination of positive and negative selection ensures that T cells in the body will reliably respond against only invaders and unhealthy cells.

Figure 5 below presents an overview of the immune response that ties together the contributions of the innate and adaptive immune systems.

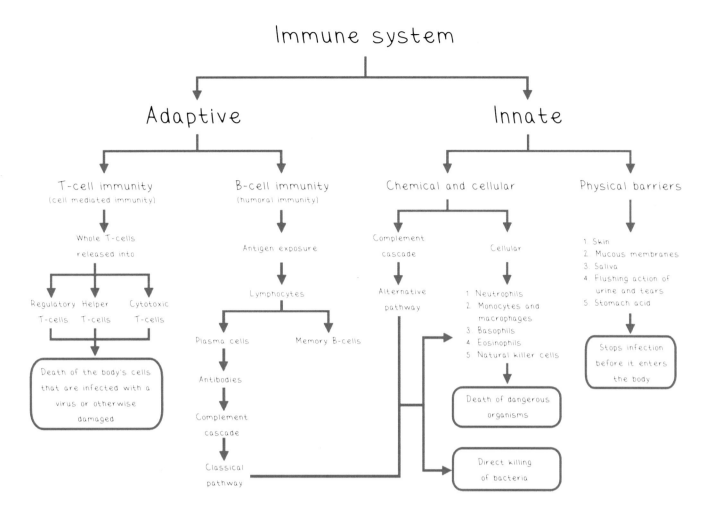

Figure 5. Diagram of immune response

4. Anatomy of the Immune System

The anatomy of the immune system is distributed diversely across the body as shown in Figure 6. However, there are some structures that are particularly important for the immune system.

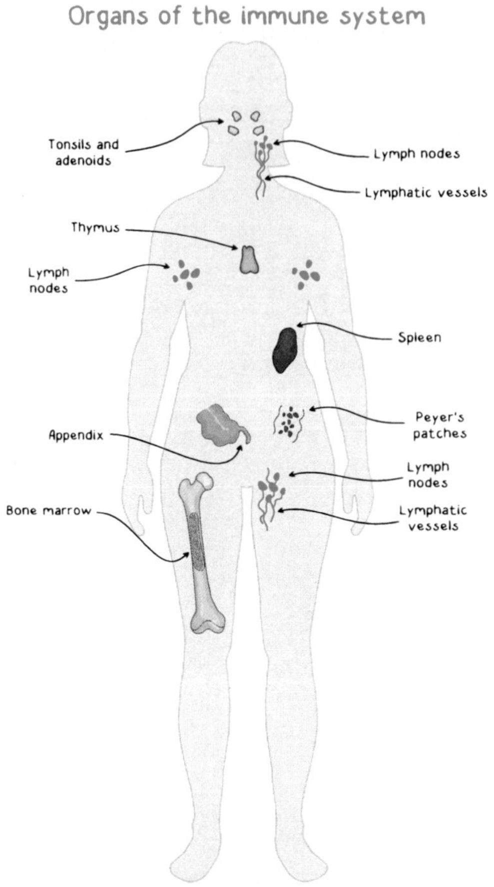

Organs of the immune system

Figure 6. Anatomical view of organs relevant for the immune system

As briefly discussed in Section 2, white blood cells (WBCs) are produced in the **bone marrow**, as are platelets and red blood cells (although red blood cells do not play a role in the immune system). In general, you can think of bone marrow as what is on the inside of bones. Its main role is the production of the formed elements of blood (red blood cells, white blood cells and platelets), known as **hematopoiesis**. In hematopoiesis, hematopoietic stem cells divide into either lymphoid stem cells or myeloid stem cells. Lymphoid stem cells further differentiate into lymphocytes (B cells, T cells, and NK cells), while myeloid stem cells differentiate into all other types of blood cells, including other types of WBCs as well as red blood cells and megakaryocytes (a large cell from which platelets are derived). The structure of the bone marrow is further discussed in Chapter 12.

> > CONNECTIONS < <

Chapter 12 of Biology

The **spleen** is another organ that plays an important role in the immune system. It is located in the left upper quadrant of the abdomen. The spleen contributes to the circulatory system by breaking down senescent red blood cells and holding a reserve of blood, but the areas of the spleen known as the white pulp contributes to the immune system. It is rich in lymphocytes and is a site for the activation of B cells, which will differentiate into plasma cells to produce great quantities of antibodies. Since the spleen does double duty as a blood filtration/processing center and as an organ rich in T and B cells, it is an especially important nexus for coordinating the immune response. Lymph nodes (and the lymphatic system in general) are quite important for the immune system, and are discussed separately in Section 5 below.

A final immune organ to be aware of is the **thymus**, which is located in the central part of the anterior chest. The thymus is where T cells mature, as discussed above in Section 3.

5. Lymphatic System

The **lymphatic system** is a part of both the circulatory and immune systems. Let's review its circulatory function first, and then explore how it operates as part of the immune system.

In a nutshell, the lymphatic system is a parallel circulatory system that drains interstitial fluid from the space surrounding the cells of the tissue. Fluid moves from the capillary beds into the extracellular space in the tissues and most of it is returned to the circulatory system at the venous end of the capillary. However, some of the excess tissue fluid is returned to the circulatory system via the lymphatic system. **Lymph capillaries** collect this fluid, and empty into **lymph vessels**, which converge into the right lymphatic duct and thoracic duct. The right lymphatic duct empties into the circulatory system at the intersection of the right internal jugular vein and the right subclavian vein; the thoracic duct empties into the circulatory system at the intersection of the left internal jugular vein and the left subclavian vein. The lymphatic system also has a connection with the digestive system because it is used to transport lipids, in the form of chylomicrons, to the circulatory system.

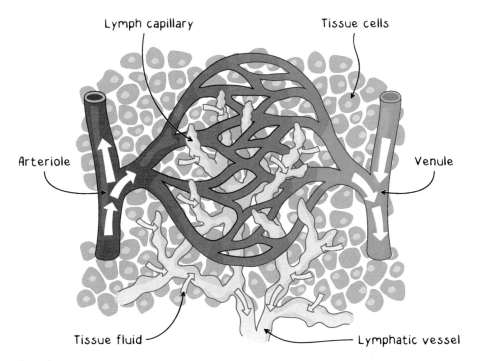

Figure 7.. Lymph node

The lymphatic system is dotted by hundreds of **lymph nodes**, which are organized clusters of lymphatic system that can be thought of as filtration points for the lymphatic fluid where reservoirs of B and T cells are stored. Distinct clusters of lymph nodes are located in the head, neck, chest, underarms, abdomen, and groin. They are often palpated as a part of routine physical examinations because swollen lymph nodes may be a sign of conditions such as infection or cancer.

CLINICAL CONNECTIONS >>>

Lymphedema is peripheral swelling (edema) caused by blocked lymphatic vessels. It can be an aftereffect of the treatment of cancer that has spread to the lymph nodes, and in developing countries, can be caused by parasitic infections.

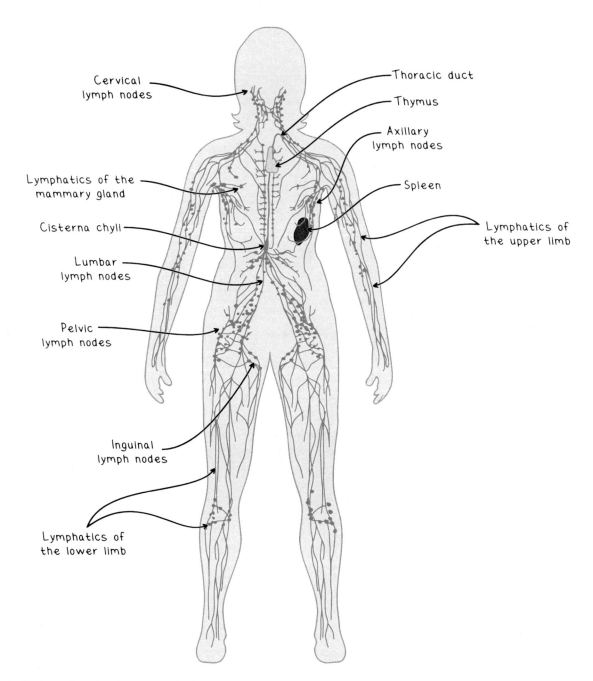

Figure 8.. Lymph nodes throughout body

The **thymus**, where T cells mature, is considered to be part of the lymphatic system, as is the spleen. The **red bone marrow**, which is where blood cells are produced, is also a key organ in the lymphatic system.

Thus, the lymphatic system can be thought of as having the following major functions:

> Maintenance of fluid balance (by draining fluid out from the interstitial space in tissues and returning it to circulation).
> Transport of other materials from the interstitial space back into the bloodstream.
> Lipid transport from the digestive system into the bloodstream.
> Production and maturation of lymphocytes.

6. Allergies and Autoimmune Disorders

In light of how intricate the machinery of the immune system is, and how many checks and balances exist to ensure its proper function, it is unsurprising that the immune system can become dysregulated. Disorders of the immune system, in the form of allergies and autoimmune disorders, are mainstays in the daily clinical practice of medicine.

Allergies occur when the immune system mounts a response against some exogenous stimulus that is actually harmless. Common examples include pollen and food allergies.

Autoimmune disorders, in contrast, occur when the body mistakenly recognizes self cells as being non-self and mounts an immune response against them. Common examples of autoimmune diseases include inflammatory bowel disease, multiple sclerosis, lupus, and rheumatoid arthritis. The MCAT does not expect you to know the details of all of these conditions, but it does expect you to be aware of the general concept of autoimmune disorder and the steps the body takes to minimize the likelihood of such disorders emerging.

Figure 11, on the next page, shows how autoimmunity can be thought of as the result of an 'overactive' immune system, in contrast to an underactive immune system that leaves one vulnerable to infection. Although the actual mechanisms underlying autoimmune attacks are more complicated, this way of visualizing autoimmune disorders helps contextualize them within the overall spectrum of immune function.

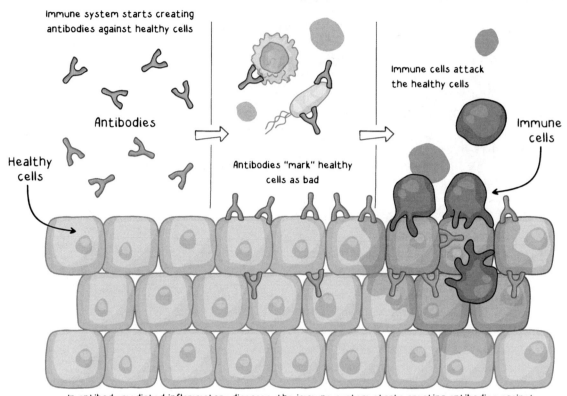

Immune system starts creating antibodies against healthy cells

Antibodies

Healthy cells

Antibodies "mark" healthy cells as bad

Immune cells attack the healthy cells

Immune cells

In antibody-mediated inflammatory diseases, the immune system starts creating antibodies against healthy cells. Once marked "bad", the healthy cells become the target of the immune cells' attack.

Figure 9. Autoimmune disorders

7. Must-Knows

> Antigen: any substance that stimulates an immune response.
> Antibody: Y-shaped molecule that recognizes antigens and allows an immune response to be mobilized. Has two heavy and two light chains linked by disulfide bonds.
> Antigen-antibody interactions: like lock in a key, antibodies are specific for certain antigens.
> Self/non-self: mediated by major histocompatibility complex (MHC) class I and II:
>   − MHC: unique to every person.
>   − MHC class I: expressed in all nucleated cells, shows fragments of proteins from inside cell. Can be thought of as internal quality check. Abnormal in cases of viral infections or tumorigenesis. CD8⁺ T cells destroy.
>   − MHC class II: expressed in some immune cells (macrophages, etc.), shows fragments of antigens from external invaders that have been engulfed; CD4⁺ helper T cells recruit response.
> Innate immune system:
>   − Anatomical barriers: skin, digestive enzymes, lysozyme in saliva/tears/breastmilk, mucociliary elevator in respiratory tract.
>   − White blood cells: neutrophils (phagocytose bacteria), NK cells, monocytes (differentiate into macrophages ("big eaters") and dendritic cells), eosinophils, and basophils.
>   − Complement: proteins involved in signaling cascade to tag pathogens, recruit phagocytes, and initiate inflammatory process.
>   − Cytokines: signaling proteins that coordinate immune response/inflammation. Interferons are cytokines that specialize in response to viruses.
> Adaptive immune system:
>   − B cells differentiate into plasma cells for: *antibody production.* Produced in bone marrow and are activated in lymphatic organs or tissues. When activated, clonal expansion → many copies; short-lived plasma cells produce antibodies in response to current infection, memory cells remain present and react next time a threat appears.
>   − T cells: mature in thymus through positive/negative selection. Most are discarded.
>   − CD4⁺ helper T cells: coordinate response to abnormal MHC class II (bacterial/fungal/other infection).
>   − CD8⁺ cytotoxic T cells: kill cells with abnormal MHC class I (virus/tumor).
>   − Other T cells: suppressor T cells (also called regulatory T cells) moderate immune reaction when response has been sufficient. Memory T cells "remember" previous antigens.
> Anatomy of immune system: bone marrow, lymphatic system, spleen, thymus, and other lymphatic tissues (appendix, tonsils, etc.)
> Lymphatic system: regulates fluid balance, is home for lymphocytes (B and T cells), drains fats from digestive system into bloodstream, returns substances from interstitial space to circulation.

End of Chapter Practice

The best MCAT practice is **realistic**, with a focus on identifying steps for further improvement. For those reasons, we recommend completing practice questions in an online setting that simulates the real MCAT interface, and taking advantage of advanced analytic features to help you determine how best to move forward in your MCAT study journey.

With that in mind, **online end-of-chapter** questions for Biology, Biochemistry, Chemistry + Organic Chemistry, Physics, and Psychology/Sociology are available through your Blueprint MCAT account.

As a further supplement, given the importance of active learning for effective studying, we also suggest that you consult the Must-Knows at the end of each chapter as a basis for creating a study sheet, in which you list out key terms and test your ability to briefly summarize them.

This page left intentionally blank.

This page left intentionally blank.

Musculoskeletal System and Skin

0. Introduction

In the final chapter of the Biology book, we'll focus on the musculoskeletal system and skin. These topics are important for the MCAT in their own right and because they interact with other physiological systems we have already discussed, which means they provide an opportunity for the MCAT to test you on important themes in physiology. In this chapter, we'll first review the broad category of connective tissue, discuss some aspects of skeletal anatomy, and then review bone from a physiological perspective. Next, in Sections 4 and 5, we will discuss muscle tissue and how it contracts, and then finally, in Section 6, we will discuss the skin, the largest organ of the body.

1. Connective Tissue

Connective tissue is an extremely broad category that corresponds to one of the four basic types of tissue (the others being epithelial, nervous, and muscle). The MCAT does not expect you to have a detailed knowledge of the anatomical and histological properties of connective tissue, but you should know that it generally carries out the role of holding the body and its organs together (hence its name). Connective tissue includes bone, blood, and adipose tissue as well as cartilage, ligaments, and tendons (as well as a few other types).

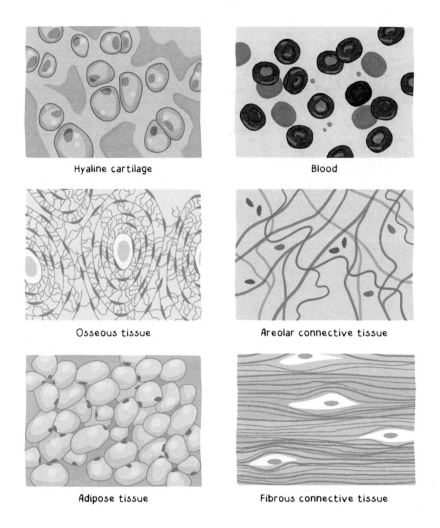

Figure 1. Connective tissue types

Cartilage is a type of connective tissue that does not contain nerves or blood vessels, and is primarily made up of cells known as **chondrocytes**. Chondrocytes produce abundant amounts of **collagen**, which is a structural protein that is prevalent in the human body, and is found in the extracellular matrix of many types of connective tissue. Cartilage is also a very accessible tissue type in that it comprises the tip of the nose and portions of the outer ear, so you can easily reach and feel the texture of cartilage in and around your face. Additionally, cartilage protects the ends of bones at synovial joints, and is part of many other structures in the body, including but not limited to the rib cage.

Ligaments and **tendons** are tough bands of collagenous fibers that connect components of the body. The main difference between ligaments and tendons is simply the kind of connections that they make: ligaments connect bones with other bones, whereas tendons connect muscles with bones.

2. Anatomy of the Skeletal System

The **skeletal system** has multiple important functions. It provides the body with structural support, and some specific skeletal structures provide important protection for organs. For example, the bones of the skull protect the brain, and the rib cage protects the heart and lungs within the thoracic cavity.

It is not necessary to know all of the 200+ bones of the human body for the MCAT, but it is worth investing some time to obtain a general sense of the major bones and skeletal structures of the body, because they may be mentioned in passages.

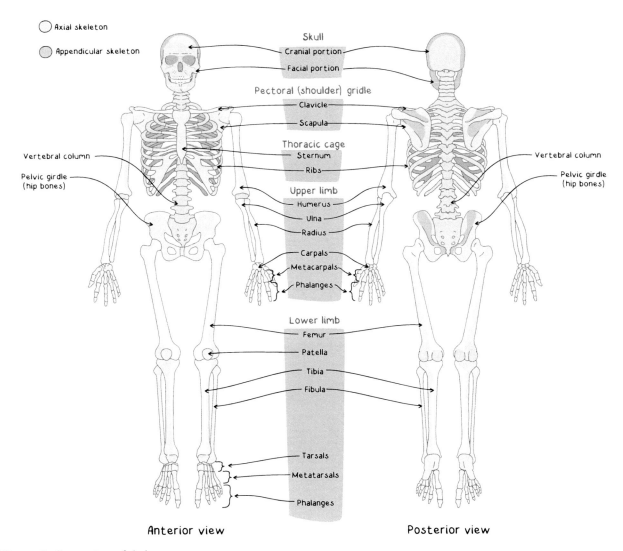

Figure 2. Gross view of skeleton

The skeleton is subdivided into the **axial skeleton** and the **appendicular skeleton**. The axial skeleton starts with the skull and runs downward to the bottom of the vertebral column, while the appendicular skeleton accounts for the upper and lower extremities (medical speak for the arms/hands and the legs/feet, respectively), the shoulder girdle, and the pelvic girdle. On a basic level, the axial skeleton can be thought of forming the core of the organism, including protecting the central nervous system and protecting the lungs and heart. The appendicular skeleton, on the other hand, can be thought of as comprising the structures needed for mobility. Some of the most important skeletal structures are listed below:

> Skull. The skull contains 22 bones (eight cranial bones and 14 facial bones). The frontal, parietal, occipital, and temporal bones of the skull correspond to important brain regions that are discussed in Chapter 6. The facial bones form intricate structures that go beyond what you are required to know for the MCAT, although it may come in handy to remember that the mandible is the lower jaw bone, while the maxilla is the upper jaw bone.

> Vertebral column. The vertebral column includes 24 distinct vertebrae, the sacrum, and the coccyx. The sacrum and the coccyx are each single bony structures that form from vertebrae that fuse during development. Moving from top to bottom, the vertebral column is divided into the cervical spine (seven vertebrae, C1-C7), the thoracic spine (12 vertebrae, T1-T12), the lumbar spine (five vertebrae, L1-L5), the sacrum, and the coccyx.

> Rib cage. A total of 12 pairs of ribs curve out from the spine and meet at the sternum in the front of the chest. The rib cage protects critical organs such as the heart and the lungs.

> Upper extremities. The bones of the wrist are quite complicated and go beyond the scope of the MCAT, but you should know the basic structure of the arm. The humerus is the upper bone of the arm, stretching from the elbow up to the shoulder. The forearm is composed of two bones: the ulna and the radius. If you place your arms to your side with your palms facing forward (in what is known as anatomical position), the ulna is closest to the body.

> Lower extremities. The uppermost bone in the leg is the femur, which is the largest bone in the body. The patella is the kneecap, and is an interesting example of a sesamoid bone (or a bone that is encased in tendon or muscle). The lower leg includes two bones: the tibia and the fibula. The tibia is the larger and more anteriorly located of the pair, while the fibula is more slender and ultimately runs down to become part of the ankle joint.

Bones can be classified into five major types:

1. Long bones are probably the most familiar type of bone, and are exemplified by bones in the upper and lower extremities such as the humerus, ulna, radius, femur, tibia, and fibula. Long bones have a long shaft, known as a **diaphysis**, and a rounded head, known as an **epiphysis**, at each end.

2. Flat bones are exemplified by the bones of the skull: they are relatively thin and flat.

3. Short bones include those present in the wrist and ankle. As the name implies, they are about as wide as they are long.

4. Sesamoid bones are embedded in tendons. The most well-known example is the patella, or kneecap.

5. Irregular bones, such as the ethmoid in the face, do not fit into any of the above categories.

Joints are where bones meet, and they can be classified in several different ways. The basic idea, though, is that different degrees of flexibility are required in various joints, and the anatomical structure of joints therefore varies accordingly to meet those functional requirements.

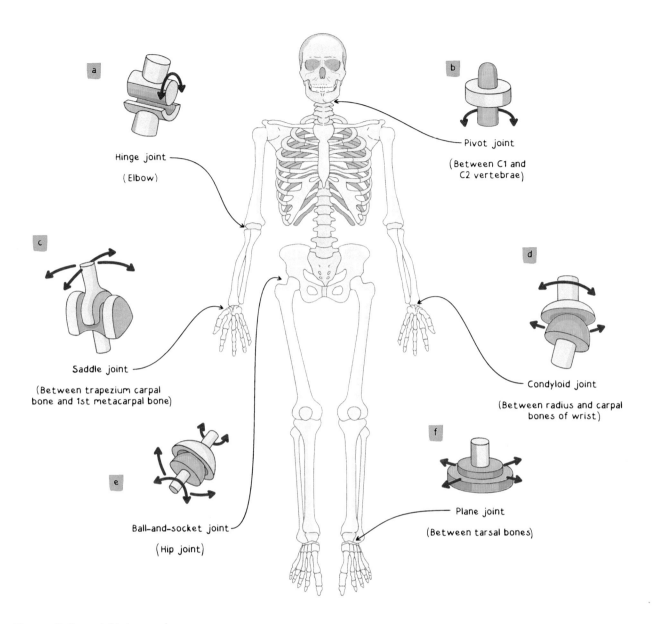

a

Hinge joint

(Elbow)

b

Pivot joint

(Between C1 and
C2 vertebrae)

c

Saddle joint

(Between trapezium carpal
bone and 1st metacarpal bone)

d

Condyloid joint

(Between radius and carpal
bones of wrist)

e

Ball-and-socket joint

(Hip joint)

f

Plane joint

(Between tarsal bones)

Figure 3. Synovial joints and movements

When you think of joints, **synovial joints** are probably what come to mind. These are freely movable joints in which the bones are not actually directly joined together. Instead, the bones meet in an area known as the **synovial cavity**, which allows the bones to have a wide range of motion without scraping onto each other. The term diarthrosis, which refers to free movement, is applied to synovial joints.

On the opposite side of the spectrum, some bones are joined together in a way that allows little to no motion. For example, it is very important that the bones of the cranium stay in place. These joints are known as **fibrous joints** from a structural point of view, because they are held in place by fibrous connective tissue. The term synarthrosis, on the other hand (referring to little or no movement) is applied from a functional point of view. The fibrous joints connecting the skull bones are specifically known as sutures, and are somewhat flexible in fetuses to allow the head to be compressed while passing through the birth canal.

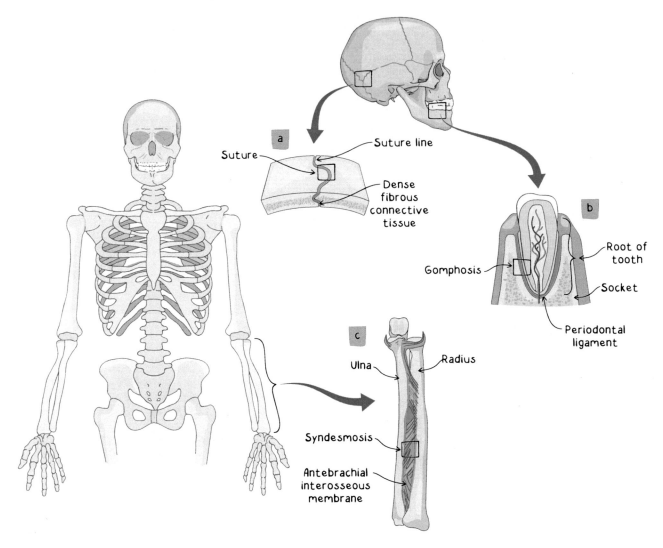

Figure 4. Examples of joints

Another type of joint is the cartilaginous joint. Depending on the specific type of cartilaginous joint, they can either be classified as slightly movable (**amphiarthrosis**) or immovable (**synarthrosis**). A classic example of these joints are the intervertebral discs. In such joints, the bones are connected by a layer of cartilage that allows some movement, while stopping short of the freedom offered by synovial joints.

An additional distinction you should be aware of is the difference between an **exoskeleton** and an **endoskeleton**. Humans, as members of the broad class of vertebrates, contain an endoskeleton: that is, a skeletal system that provides structural support from within the body. Many other organisms have an exoskeleton, which is a tough "shell" that provides structural support on the outside of the body. Exoskeletons in insects, arachnids, and crustaceans are formed of chitin, which is a fibrous polymer of N-acetylglucosamine that is also found in the cell walls of fungi.

3. Bone Structure and Physiology

The structural role of the skeleton, as well as the fact that we generally see skeletons either in the form of artificially constructed display models or as bone samples from no-longer-living organisms, makes it easy to think of bones as static structures that passively provide support. This viewpoint is actually quite misleading: in living organisms, bone is a physiologically active structure that actively participates in the regulation of calcium and phosphate levels in the body, and new blood cells are produced in the bone marrow.

On the most basic level, you can think of bone structure as involving an interplay between non-cellular structural components of the bone and cellular structures. The **non-cellular structural components** of bone are referred to as the matrix of the bone, which consists of water, collagen fibers, and crystallized minerals (primarily hydroxyapatite, which has a chemical formula of $Ca_{10}(PO_4)_6(OH)_2$ and can be thought of as a storage depot of sorts for calcium and phosphate). The **cellular components** of bone tissue are quite diverse, and include epithelial, adipose, and nervous tissue as well as cells and structures unique to the bones.

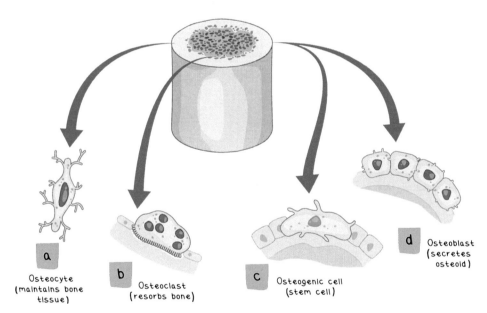

Figure 5. Structural view of bone

An important concept regarding bone cells is the distinction between **osteoblasts** and **osteoclasts**. Osteoblasts are cells that produce osteoid and deposit it into the bone matrix, while osteoclasts break down the bone matrix, mobilizing calcium and phosphate if serum levels of those minerals are too low. Osteocytes are the most common type of bone cell, and can be thought of as osteoblasts that become somewhat inactivated. Osteocytes have a range of roles in regulating bone mass, but for the purposes of the MCAT you can think of them as being relatively inert components of the bone mass.

The balance of activity between osteoblasts and osteoclasts is maintained by hormones. **Parathyroid hormone (PTH)** and **calcitriol**, the active form of vitamin D, work to increase blood calcium and levels through various mechanisms, including the promotion of osteoclast activity. In contrast, calcitonin comes into play when serum levels of calcium are too high. Calcitonin is released by the thyroid and reduces osteoclast activity. This allows the balance to tip in favor of the osteoblasts, reducing serum calcium levels and promoting bone growth

In addition to having various cellular components, different types of bone tissue are distinguished based on how their small-scale structures are arranged. **Compact bone**, also known as **cortical bone** because it forms the exterior shell (cortex) of most bones, is a hard and dense form of bone. As mentioned, it forms the outer layer of bones, providing protection and contributing to the mechanical functions of bone, such as structural support, protection, and leverage for movement. **Cancellous**, or **spongy/trabecular bone**, can be thought of as the spongy interior of bone. It is less dense, and correspondingly has a greater ratio of surface area to mass. Different types of bone have specific distributions of compact and cancellous bone.

There are two types of bone marrow: red and yellow. Red bone marrow is where hematopoiesis takes place, whereas yellow bone marrow is predominantly made up of adipocytes (fat cells). **Red bone marrow** is primarily contained in the flat bones and the proximal ends of some long bones. It is the location of hematopoiesis, or the creation of blood cells. This process includes the constant generation of both red blood cells and white blood cells. As discussed in Chapter 11 on the immune system, the bone marrow can also be classified as part of the immune system due to its role in creating white blood cells that mediate important immune processes. The bone marrow is highly vascularized tissue, as newly synthesized red blood cells must enter the circulatory system.

4. Muscle Tissue

If bones provide the basic structure for our bodies, **muscles** can be thought of as what put our bodies into motion. This motion includes voluntary activities like walking or moving and involuntary but physiologically essential activities like pumping blood through the body and moving food through the digestive tract. In addition to the intuitively obvious function of providing support and mobility, muscles help ensure that circulation takes place (the pumping action of the heart and the smooth muscle in blood vessels), and also play a role in thermoregulation via the shivering reflex. Figure 6 presents a high-level view of some of the major muscles in the body. The MCAT does not expect you to memorize muscle names and anatomy (again, there will be plenty of time for that in medical school), but it's a reasonably good idea to be aware of the location of major muscles like the biceps and to have a general sense of the distribution of muscle tissue throughout the body.

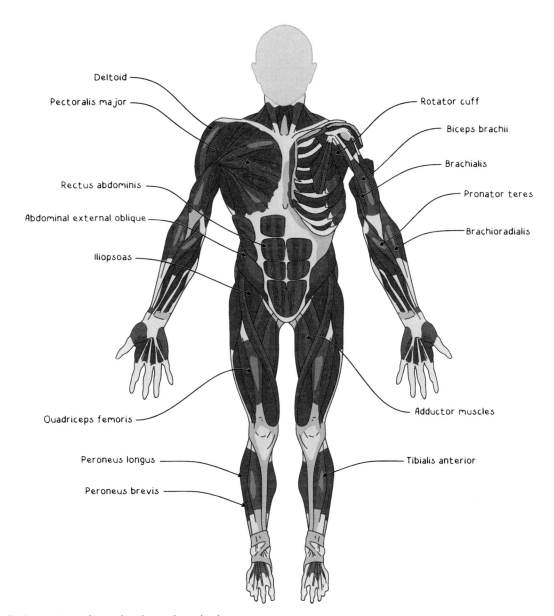

Figure 6. Gross view of muscles throughout body

There are three basic types of muscle: skeletal, smooth, and cardiac. **Skeletal muscle** is under voluntary control, while **smooth muscle** and **cardiac muscle** are involuntary. However, in order for the distinctions among these types of muscle to make sense, we have to step back and consider the structure of a muscle cell. Historically, the study of muscle structure was somewhat of a different specialty from cell biology, which led to the emergence of different terms for muscle cell structures than are used for the corresponding eukaryotic cell structures in general.

First, let's address one common point of confusion: **muscle cells (myocytes)** and **muscle fibers** are different terms that refer to the same thing. This is because muscle cells have structures that are profoundly different from what you may think of as "normal" eukaryotic cells (that is, the standard diagram of a more or less circular cell with organelles that is included in most texts on cell biology). Recall, though, that eukaryotic cells can specialize considerably within organisms, to the point of developing very distinct structures. Common examples of structurally anomalous cell types include neurons, spermatozoa, and myocytes.

Skeletal muscle is the primary focus of the MCAT in terms of cellular structure, so the discussion below will focus on the structure of myocytes in skeletal muscle, and then the ways in which this discussion does not apply to smooth and skeletal muscle will be explored.

Myocytes are long, tubular cells that principally contain **myofibrils**. Myofibrils are long, rod-like bundles of actin, myosin, and other proteins. Actin and myosin form thin and thick filaments, respectively, which are organized into repeating units called **sarcomeres**. The contraction of sarcomeres produces muscle contractions, as discussed in more detail in the next section. Specialized names, generally starting with the prefix "sarco-," exist for the other structures of myocytes. The sarcoplasmic reticulum corresponds to the smooth endoplasmic reticulum, and the sarcoplasm corresponds to the cytoplasm. The cell membrane of myocytes is known as the sarcolemma.

Myofibrils are the essential structures of myocytes from a functional point of view, but myocytes also contain additional structures that allow myofibrils to do their job. Mitochondria are present to various extents in different types of muscle fibers, and the sarcoplasm also contains myoglobin and glycogen. **Myoglobin** is a red-colored protein that stores oxygen. Its general structure and function are similar to hemoglobin, but it only contains one globin chain and one heme group, and bonds to oxygen with a greater affinity than hemoglobin. This allows it to "pull" oxygen from the bloodstream, similarly to how fetal hemoglobin can obtain oxygen from maternal hemoglobin by having a higher affinity. The glycogen stores in the sarcoplasm allow for quick mobilization of glucose for anaerobic metabolism.

The **sarcoplasmic reticulum** wraps around the myofibrils, and has the basic function of storing Ca^{2+} ions. As such, it plays a role in mediating the transmission of nerve impulses and the resulting contractions. In turn, in non-smooth muscle, the sarcoplasmic reticulum is in contact with structures known as T-tubules. T-tubules can be thought of as projections of the sarcolemma (the cell membrane) that reach toward the center of the cell. They contain abundant ion channels that facilitate the rapid transmission of action potentials throughout the muscle fiber, resulting in initiation of muscle contraction.

> **>> CONNECTIONS <<**
>
> Chapter 9 of Biology

> **MCAT STRATEGY >>>**
>
> Take this opportunity to review your knowledge of the physiology and biochemistry of hemoglobin. What would the dissociation curve of myoglobin look like compared to that of hemoglobin? The dissociation curve of myoglobin is left-shifted, because it has a higher affinity for oxygen than does hemoglobin. Its shape is also different. Hemoglobin has a sigmoidal curve due to the cooperative binding among its four subunits, whereas myoglobin has a hyperbolic curve that is more similar to what you see in discussions of enzyme kinetics.

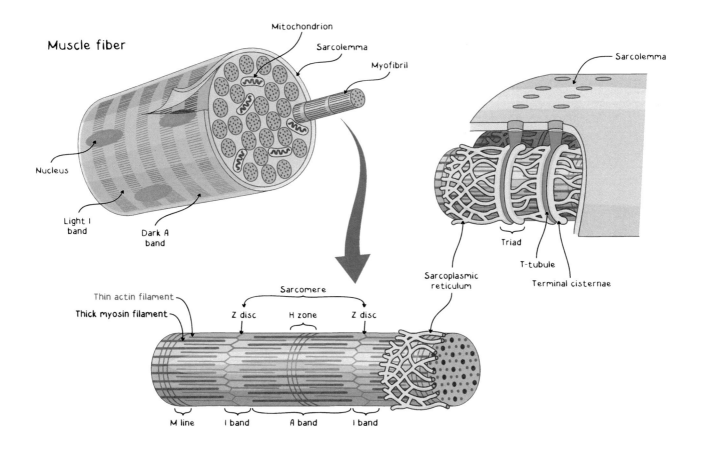

Figure 7. Muscle structure: T-tubule system, contractile apparatus, sarcoplasmic reticulum

With these preliminary considerations in mind, we can now make more sense of the different types of muscles.

Skeletal muscle is innervated by the **somatic nervous system**, meaning that it is under conscious control. It is striated, which means it has extensive linear myofibrils that form striations when viewed with a microscope. Myocytes in skeletal muscles also have multiple nuclei on the periphery of the cell, as they are formed via the fusion of multiple precursor cells. There are two different types of fibers within skeletal muscles: red fibers (slow-twitch fibers) and white fibers (fast-twitch fibers). **Red fibers** obtain their color from the presence of abundant reserves of myoglobin, and are also rich in mitochondria. This means that they prefer oxidative metabolism, and therefore are present in large quantities in muscles that specialize in performing less intense actions over a longer period of time. **White fibers**, in contrast, lack those elements, and tend to mobilize glycogen for quick bursts of intense action followed by fatigue. It has been argued that individuals with a relative predominance of white fibers are natural sprinters, whereas individuals with proportionally more red fibers are natural endurance athletes.

Smooth muscle is innervated by the autonomic nervous system, meaning that it is not under voluntary control. Smooth muscle is found throughout the body, but a particularly common and intuitive example is the digestive tract, where it is responsible for peristalsis. However, it is also found in blood vessel walls, the bladder, the uterus, and other locations. It is non-striated because it does not contain well-organized, linear myofibrils (although it does contain actin and myosin filaments that engage in contraction). Smooth muscle cells contain only one nucleus, and it is found towards the center of the cell.

Cardiac muscle shares some features of skeletal muscle and some features of smooth muscle, but it also has some unique features of its own. Like smooth muscle, it is not under voluntary control. Similarly to smooth muscle, cardiac muscle cells tend to only have one nucleus, although some cells may have two. However, like skeletal muscle, cardiac muscle is striated. A unique feature of cardiac muscle is that its cells are connected by structures known as intercalated discs, which connect the cytoplasm of adjacent cardiac muscle cells, allowing ions to pass from cell to cell. These connections are known as **gap junctions**, and they allow action potentials to pass rapidly from one cardiac muscle cell to another, facilitating the rapid propagation of action potentials.

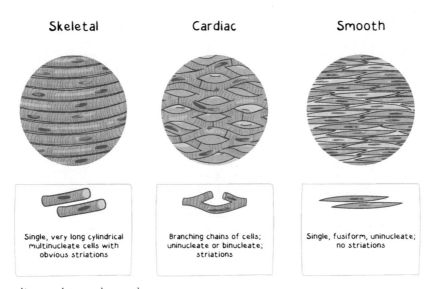

Figure 8. Skeletal, cardiac, and smooth muscle

Myogenic activity, or the ability to contract even without external neural signaling, is an important characteristic of cardiac muscle (although it is also a property of smooth muscle). Cells in the **sinoatrial (SA) node** periodically send out action potentials, which propagate through the gap junctions, causing contraction. The action potential flows from the SA node into the atria, but not into the ventricles because of a layer of insulating tissue. The action potential goes to the **atrioventricular (AV) node**, then travels through the bundle of His, the right and left bundle branches, and then the Purkinje fibers to all the muscle cells of the ventricles.

>> **CONNECTIONS** <<

Chapter 9 of Biology

While the SA node can fire on its own, it is also connected to the autonomic nervous system, which is subdivided into the sympathetic and parasympathetic nervous systems. The parasympathetic nervous system, which is responsible for the "rest and digest" response, slows the heart rate. In contrast, the sympathetic nervous system response ("fight or flight") raises the heart rate. The heart rate is also increased by the hormones epinephrine and norepinephrine, which are released by the adrenal medulla.

5. Muscle Contraction

Next, let's take a closer look at the mechanism of **muscle contraction**. There are a few levels on which muscle contraction can be analyzed: how the sarcomere changes structurally during contraction, the actual molecular mechanism of contraction, and how contraction happens in response to signals from the nervous system.

To review from the previous section, striated muscle fibers contain long rod-like **myofibrils** that are composed of alternating units of thick (myosin) and thin (actin) fibers that overlap with each other. The basic mechanism of contraction is for the interwoven myosin and actin fibers to slip past each other, in what is sometimes known as the **sliding filament model**.

The fundamental unit of contraction is the **sarcomere**, which consists of a band of thick myosin fibers and half of each of the two adjacent bands of thin fibers, as seen in Figure 9. Sarcomeres are divided into the I-band, A-band, H-zone, Z-line, and M-line. This may seem like pointless alphabet soup, but there is some logic to this system. The lines are just definitional: the **M-line** defines the middle of the sarcomere, running through the middle of the thick filaments, while the **Z-lines** define the edges, running through the middle of the thin filaments. The two bands are a way to subdivide the sarcomere. The **I-band** refers to the region where only thin actin filaments are present, and the **A-band** is everything else. That is, the A band is the entire region where thick filaments are present, including areas of overlap with the thin filaments. The H-zone refers to the area in the the A band where only thick filaments are present.

To envision what happens to the sarcomere during contraction, imagine holding a myofibril fragment composed of two or three sarcomeres between your hands and pushing your hands together. Recall that in the sliding filament model of the sarcomere, contraction happens because the actin and myosin fibers slide past each other, not because they are themselves compressed. Therefore, the thin fibers would be pushed towards the center, or the M-line. Let's work through the changes step by step, because this is often a point of confusion.

> M-line: If we place a single M-line at the center of our sarcomere fragment as a point of reference, it would not change, but since the whole system is being compressed, the distance *between* M-lines is decreased.
> Z-line: As the system is compressed, the Z-lines move closer together.
> A-band: Recall that the A-band is defined as the zone where thick filaments are present, *regardless* of whether they overlap with thin filaments. Since the filaments themselves are not compressed during contraction, the A-band stays the same.
> I-band and H-zone: These two areas are defined by the lack of overlap. Recall that the I-band is where *only* thin filaments are present and the H-zone is where *only* thick filaments are present. Since contraction operates by filaments sliding past each other, the overall effect of contraction is to increase areas of overlap between actin and myosin filaments, thereby shrinking areas defined by the lack of overlap.

The shortest way to summarize this would be to say that during contraction, only the A-band does not shrink, because it is the only interval not defined relative to other structures.

MCAT STRATEGY >>>

If you are rushing to memorize the structures of the sarcomere, slow down and make sure you really understand what the different terms refer to. Consider interlocking your fingers and using that as a model for sarcomere contraction, perhaps with lines drawn on your skin to correspond to various structures. Alternately, consider using differently colored slips of paper to correspond to actin and myosin filaments and visualize the structures. Quickly memorizing the features of a structure like this is the path to quickly forgetting them as soon as you turn your energy elsewhere. Your goal should be to connect the terminology to an internalized sense of how the system works, and that takes time.

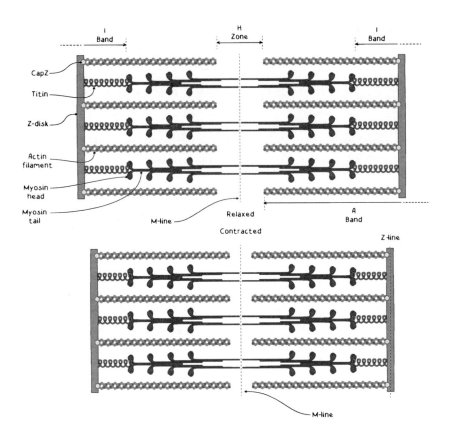

Figure 9. Sarcomeres

Next, let's look at how the actual mechanism of contraction works. The actin and myosin filaments slide past each other through what is known as a **cross-bridge cycle**, in which a cross-bridge is formed between myosin and actin, and a power stroke provides the force of contraction. This is a topic where it pays to slow down and even draw out the structures involved—merely learning the names of the structures involved without a real understanding of the principles may allow you to answer a low-level multiple-choice question right, but it will not be of much help if you encounter a passage that presents this information in a new light or asks you to apply it to solve a novel problem.

Both the actin and myosin filaments have structures in place that permit them to bind to each other when the conditions are right, and then disassociate as needed. This interplay between binding and disassociation is what drives this process, along with conformational changes that take place in response to other factors. Myosin filaments have so-called **heads** that project from the filament. Each head has one site that can bind to ATP and another to actin. Actin filaments have a myosin-binding site that is blocked by the regulatory protein **tropomyosin** in the absence of Ca^{2+}.

As with any cycle, there is no absolute starting point, but a relatively straightforward place to start is immediately after a **power stroke** has happened and a cycle of **contraction** has ended. At this point, myosin and actin are bound together, and the cycle needs to begin again. The first step is for ATP to bind to the myosin head, causing a conformational change that releases it from actin. At this point, **tropomyosin** is free to move back into place to block strong interactions between actin and myosin. The ATP molecule is then hydrolyzed to form ADP + P_i (recall that P_i is inorganic phosphate). This is a strongly exergonic reaction and is used to move the myosin head into the "cocked position." In this position, it can interact weakly with actin, but tropomyosin prevents stronger interactions. Tropomyosin is ultimately removed by Ca^{2+} through a somewhat complex mechanism: Ca^{2+} binds to a protein known as **troponin** that is also located on actin, and the complex formed by Ca^{2+} and troponin causes tropomyosin to dissociate from the actin-myosin binding site. At this point, the myosin head can bind tightly to actin. The final step is for the power stroke to happen. This occurs via a conformational change that happens when P_i is released.

After the **power stroke** happens, ADP is released and actin and myosin are essentially stuck together until another ATP binds to myosin so that the process can start again.

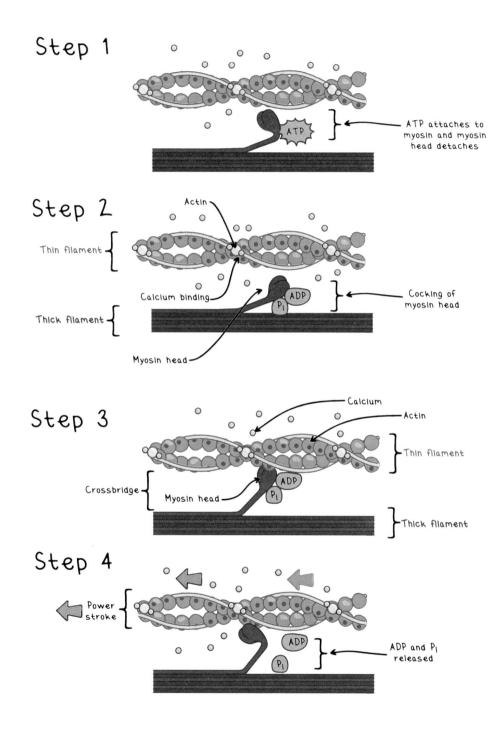

Figure 10. Actin-myosin interactions

Next, let's turn to how muscles receive the signal to contract. An **action potential** propagates down a motor (efferent) neuron, until it reaches the nerve terminal at the neuromuscular junction. The neurotransmitter **acetylcholine** is then released into the neuromuscular junction. As a point of background terminology, the muscle cells innervated by a single neuron are known as a **motor unit**.

Acetylcholine binds to receptors on the cell membrane, which is known as the sarcolemma in muscle cells, and the sarcolemma then depolarizes in response. This results in an action potential, and when the action potential reaches the sarcoplasmic reticulum, Ca^{2+} is released into the sarcoplasm (the cytoplasm). Once in the sarcoplasm, Ca^{2+} can bind to troponin. Troponin causes tropomyosin to move, which exposes the myosin binding site on actin. This allows **contraction** to take place.

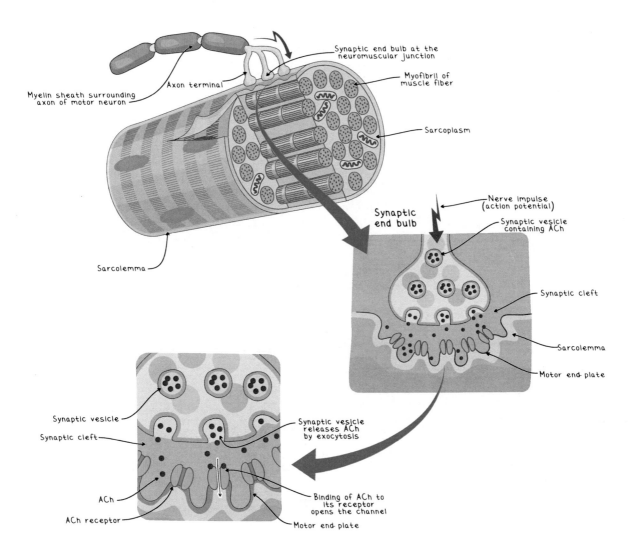

Figure 11. Motor neurons and neuromuscular junction (including how signals happen)

To summarize, contraction has two basic ingredients: ATP and Ca^{2+}, and the job of acetylcholine is to regulate the availability of Ca^{2+} in response to neural signaling.

An isolated contraction is known as a **twitch**, and more coordinated contractions occur in a process known as **summation**. In summation, frequent action potentials mean that muscle fibers do not relax completely between stimuli, and the overall contraction becomes stronger. Hyperstimulation can continue, resulting in a condition known as tetanus that should be differentiated from the disease known by the same name. Tetanus occurs when muscles have been maximally stimulated for some period of time, and to some degree it can occur during normal life, such as if you carry a heavy load for a sustained period of time. It can also be the result of pathological processes (as in the infectious disease tetanus, in which *Clostridium tetani* produces a toxin that causes spasmodic contractions).

All the time that we've spent focusing on contraction should not cause us to overlook the fact that we also must account for **relaxation**. An enzyme known as acetylcholinesterase breaks down the acetylcholine that is released into the neuromuscular junction. In the absence of further stimulation, this allows the sarcolemma to repolarize and for Ca^{2+} to be taken back up into the sarcoplasmic reticulum.

As we've seen, ATP is essential for muscle contractions to happen. The abundant mitochondria and myoglobin in muscle cells help to ensure the constant production of ATP via oxidative respiration, but it is possible for the muscle to run out of oxygen, even though the body does have a range of adaptations to help mobilize oxygen to active muscle tissue. If insufficient oxygen is present, muscles switch to glycolysis. Extensive glycolysis results in a buildup of **lactic acid**, and lactic acid buildup is associated with fatigue. Ultimately, the lactic acid is mostly converted to pyruvate. After exercise, the increase in oxygen consumption is called oxygen debt or excess postexercise oxgyen consumption.

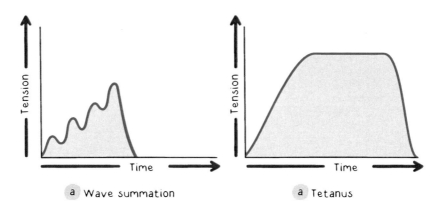

Figure 12. Summation and tetanus

6. Skin

The **skin** is the largest organ of the body by weight, and plays a crucial role in physiology both by serving as a physical barrier dividing the body from the external environment and by making significant contributions to homeostatic regulation.

The skin is divided into three major layers. The **epidermis** is the most external layer, and the basement membrane divides it from the **dermis**, which lies underneath. Below the dermis is the **hypodermis** (which technically is not part of the skin, but is often studied with the skin). We'll review the anatomical features of these structures in some detail, and then review the physiological contributions made by the skin to the overall function of the organism.

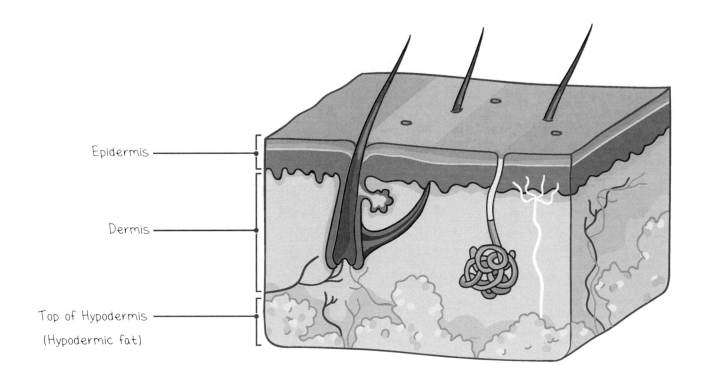

Epidermis

Dermis

Top of Hypodermis
(Hypodermic fat)

Figure 13. Layers of skin.

The **epidermis** is itself divided into five layers: the stratum corneum (most external), the stratum lucidum (only present in skin on the palm and the soles of the feet), the stratum granulosum, the stratum spinosum, and the stratum basale (most internal).

The **stratum corneum** is the layer that most directly provides a physical barrier against the outside world. It is made up of approximately 15 layers of dead keratinous cells known as corneocytes, which are gradually shed as part of the process through which the stratum corneum is regenerated. A lipid matrix surrounds the corneocytes, contributing to the fact that the skin forms a barrier that is largely impermeable to water. The **stratum lucidum** is a clear layer of dead cells only present in the palms of the hands and the soles of the feet. The **stratum granulosum** is where skin cells die and lose their nuclei after forming keratohyalin granules that link keratin filaments together into larger structures capable of serving as a hydrophobic barrier. The **stratum spinosum** and the **stratum basale** are responsible for the formation and development of **keratinocytes** (skin cells that produce keratin). Keratinocytes are produced from stem cells in the stratum basale, and then move upwards into the stratum spinosum where they begin to undergo keratinization. The stratum spinosum also contains **Langerhans cells**, which are antigen-presenting dendritic cells that help alert the immune system to pathogens invading the body via the skin.

The stratum basale contains some additional cell types. **Melanocytes** produce the pigment melanin, which protects against damage induced by ultraviolet light. The expression of melanin is upregulated in response to ultraviolet damage, which is the mechanism behind tanning. Interestingly, differences in the skin color of individuals are not due to the *number* of melanocytes but due to their activity level, which is responsive to a range of stimuli. Merkel cells present in the stratum basale are mechanoreceptors that allow us to perceive the stimulus of touch. They are densely present in highly sensitive parts of the skin, such as the fingertips.

The **dermis** is a much more physiologically active place. It is largely composed of dense connective tissue consisting of collagen and elastic fibers, but has a diverse range of cell types. One particularly notable difference between the dermis and the epidermis is that the dermis is vascular tissue, meaning that it contains capillaries and small lymphatic vessels that supply and drain blood and other fluids. It also contains hair follicles and sweat glands, as well as a broader range of sensory cells. The sensory cells present in the dermis include **Ruffini endings**, which sense stretching, **Pacinian corpuscles**, which sense deep vibration and pressure, and **Meissner corpuscles**, which sense light touch.

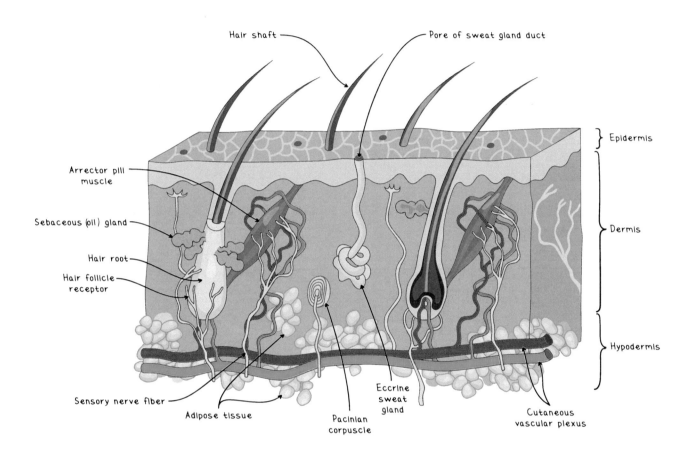

Figure 14. Sweat glands, hair, and erectile musculature in skin

The **hypodermis** lies beneath the dermis, and its main job is to provide structural and immune support. It provides structural support by containing abundant adipocytes (fat cells) that provide padding and insulation, and it provides immune support by containing macrophages that respond to invaders.

With all of the above in mind, we can review the major physiological functions of the skin.

The **epidermis** provides a physical barrier, and this functionality is enhanced in certain parts of the body by the presence of fingernails/toenails and hair (which are both made of keratin) and calluses, which are thicker and tougher areas of skin that emerge in response to friction. In addition to being a physical barrier, the skin protects against invasive microorganisms by hosting abundant populations of immune cells in the dermis.

The skin additionally plays a major role in **thermoregulation**, starting with the fat layer of the hypodermis that provides insulation. Additionally, sweat glands, which are located in the dermis, are a major way in which the organism can avoid overheating. Sweat consists of water combined with very small amounts of minerals. The evaporation of sweat on the skin absorbs heat energy from the body, thereby cooling the blood close to the skin. The arterioles that supply the skin can also be dilated to deal with excess heat (bringing more blood close to the skin to be cooled) or constricted to deal with excessively cold temperatures (minimizing blood flow to the skin to conserve heat). These processes are referred to as **vasodilation** and **vasoconstriction**, respectively. Body hair also plays a role in conserving heat in cold conditions. The arrector pili muscles that surround hair follicles contract, causing the body hairs to become vertical, trapping warm air close to the skin. This manifests as goose bumps, and is technically known as **piloerection**. Since body temperature must be maintained within a very close range, it is tightly controlled by the hypothalamus in response to various stimuli.

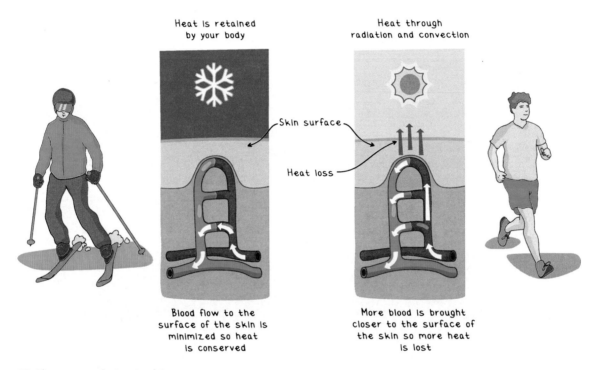

Heat is retained
by your body

Heat through
radiation and convection

Skin surface

Heat loss

Blood flow to the
surface of the skin is
minimized so heat
is conserved

More blood is brought
closer to the surface of
the skin so more heat
is lost

Figure 15. Thermoregulation in skin

7. Must-Knows

> Connective tissue: includes bone, blood, adipose tissue as well as cartilage, ligaments, tendons (as well as a few other types).
>> — Cartilage: avascular, connective tissue.
>> — Ligaments: tough tissue connecting bones to bones.
>> — Tendons: tough tissue connecting muscles and bones.
> Bone types: long (example: humerus, femur), flat (example: skull), short (example: wrist/ankle bones), sesamoid (example: patella [kneecap]), irregular (example: ethmoid).
> Joints:
>> — Synovial: bones connected by lubricated synovial cavity. Example: elbow.
>> — Cartilaginous: bones connected by cartilage. Example: vertebral discs.
>> — Fibrous: bones connected by fibrous connective tissue. Example: skull bones.
>> — Joint mobility: diarthrosis (freely movable); amphiarthrosis (slightly movable); synarthrosis (immovable).
> Bone structure:
>> — Matrix: minerals (hydroxyapatite), collagen, water. Calcium/phosphate reservoir.
>> — Osteoblasts: build up bone; osteoclasts: break down bone.
>> — PTH: $\uparrow Ca^{2+}$ from bone; vitamin D: $\uparrow Ca^{2+}$ from intestine; calcitonin: $\downarrow Ca^{2+}$ in blood by inhibiting osteoclast activity.
>> — Bone marrow: hematopoiesis.
> Muscle types:
>> — Skeletal: voluntary (somatic nervous system), striated, multinucleated. Red (slow-twitch) fibers contain abundant myoglobin, specialize in long-lasting actions requiring oxidative metabolism. White (fast-twitch) fibers contain less myoglobin and specialize in short bursts of action primarily using glycolysis.
>> — Smooth: involuntary (autonomic nervous system), non-striated, uninucleated. Can undergo myogenic activity (contraction in absence of nervous stimulation).
>> — Cardiac: involuntary (autonomic nervous system), striated. Usually uninucleated. Sinoatrial node sets pace of contractions that can be modified by other signaling. Intercalated discs/gap junctions allow signals to spread.
> Muscle contraction: sliding actin/myosin filaments. ATP required to dissociate actin and myosin. ATP → ADP to "cock" myosin head; Ca^{2+} binds to troponin which moves tropomyosin to allow actin & myosin to bind; P_i is released to generate power stroke.
> Sarcomere: I-band (thin filaments only), H-zone (thick filaments only), distances between M-lines (center of H-zone) and Z-lines (center of I-band) contract; A-band (entire area where thick filaments are present) stays the same during contraction.
> Skin:
>> — Layers of the skin, from most superficial to deepest: Epidermis > dermis > hypodermis (although not technically part of the skin).
>> — Epidermis contains layers of dead keratinocytes that provide physical protection, as well as melanocytes (pigment) and Merkel cells (touch).
>> — Dermis: capillaries, lymph vessels, hair follicles, sweat glands, sensory cells.
>> — Skin → thermoregulation via sweating, vasodilation/vasocontraction, piloerection.

End of Chapter Practice

The best MCAT practice is **realistic**, with a focus on identifying steps for further improvement. For those reasons, we recommend completing practice questions in an online setting that simulates the real MCAT interface, and taking advantage of advanced analytic features to help you determine how best to move forward in your MCAT study journey.

With that in mind, **online end-of-chapter** questions for Biology, Biochemistry, Chemistry + Organic Chemistry, Physics, and Psychology/Sociology are available through your Blueprint MCAT account.

As a further supplement, given the importance of active learning for effective studying, we also suggest that you consult the Must-Knows at the end of each chapter as a basis for creating a study sheet, in which you list out key terms and test your ability to briefly summarize them.

This page left intentionally blank.

This page left intentionally blank.

INDEX

This page left intentionally blank.

This page left intentionally blank.

This page left intentionally blank.